Praise for Listen To Your Gut

"No one can be less satisfied with conventional medical treatment for these complaints than the medical profession itself. Patel Thompson gives excellent dietary advice and the clearest message from *Listen To Your Gut* is that one should cease to be a victim of illness and make a determined effort to take charge of one's fate and welfare."
Dr. David Bamford, MD
Gloucestershire, UK

"Conventional medical therapies aren't for everyone, *Listen To Your Gut* is an excellent tool and resource guide for people looking for viable alternatives."
Dr. David Wang Bsc, ND
President, British Columbia Naturopathic Assoc.
Vancouver, Canada

"I have personally witnessed the effectiveness of the diets and methods in this program. It's a well-written manual of holistic treatments that work."
Vivian Szabo MN, Registered Nurse
Calgary, Canada

"The initial diet was quite strict however, I now have quite a regular, normal diet and consume small portions of alcohol. Obviously this is a fantastic situation from the prospect of being told I would need to take pills for the rest of my life to where I take none. Many thanks for the advice in your program."
M.R., Dublin, Ireland

"Your program is the primary reason my UC is in remission and I am also feeling the best I have ever felt! That is due to following many of your tips on diet. One significant change I made as per your program was to eliminate vinegar from my diet. Unbelievable! Everyone who has Crohn's or UC will have a food that is a flash point – mine I believe was vinegar. I also followed many of the other steps. Great book/program – I refer to it often. I also recently

finished 5 months of acupuncture. 3 days a week, 40 minute sessions. Never felt better!"
T.C., Ontario, Canada

"My doctor had never seen anyone getting better from Crohn's and he was very surprised! I followed many of your diets, and after just a few months I began feeling better. A year later I went for another Colonoscopy, and the doctor could not find anything wrong with my small intestine. My illness really took away my energy, and I could not do the activities I loved. But now I am my old self and enjoy running, skiing etc. I don't get tired, I don't start to hyperventilate, and I do not have the "plug" in my ear when I get tired anymore. I hope you are feeling well too, and once again thank you!"
K.W., Oslo, Norway

"I did just one thing suggested in *Listen To Your Gut* and my diarrhea of ten years stopped within three weeks. I would recommend this program to anyone with these diseases."
C.G., Burnaby, Canada

"I have found the book/program (*Listen to Your Gut*) VERY helpful. By following some of the advice, and listening to MY gut, I have greatly reduced the medication I had been taking and feeling better. I recommended the book to my doctor, but … he recommended more drugs."
M.N., Texas, USA

"I need to thank you for saving my life! My "Crohns" attacked my eyes & several of my joints. I was at the point with my eyes that I was running out of time with my prednisone eye-drops (if you take them for too long they cause serious damage) and my collection of Doctors (I had seven all together – from an Internal Medicine Doc to an Ophthalmologist – one specialist for each "hot spot") all wanted me to start taking the "new" immune suppressants – they were really exited about them. This is where you saved my life – your books gave me the tools I needed to start healing. I'm on 6 weeks no eye-drops, my joint inflammation has decreased to the point I am able to start doing Belly Dance & Tai Chi again (no Kung Fu yet-but I'll get there). And I'm totally off the Asacol – and my gut's feeling better all the time!! I don't know if I would have literally died if I had followed the standard medical model, but I do know that my quality of life was so terrible when I was so sick – I was dead.

"Thank you so much Jini- not only has your hard work healed me, it also let me be the wife, sister, daughter, friend, and most importantly mom (I'm lucky enough to have four sweet children) I want to be. Thank you, Thank you, Thank you!"
C.A., California, USA

"I've gave my copy to my friend and ordered another one! I first ordered *Listen To Your Gut* and loved it – particularly the range of subjects covered and the common situations the author and I had experienced. I loaned it to a friend who has a nephew with Crohn's – hoping it would help him, too. But I am ordering it again because I'd like to have my own copy here for review and reference. Thanks for a very helpful program."
D.G., Ohio, USA

"I looked up at the I.V. stand containing the steroid and antibiotic bags and down at the food cart at my pork and jello dinner and determined that the medical establishment doesn't know a whole lot about preventative care. So when I got home I got on the internet and found your book/program. I read it and immediately eliminated many foods from my diet and started on the recommended supplements. A recent trip to the G.I. doctor showed no signs of the disease. So far so good. Thank you for writing *Listen To Your Gut*. It has been an inspiration to me throughout my healing from Crohn's."
T.J., Georgia, USA

"Just wanted to pass on to you my thank you's for your program and the help I received from it. It is by far the best book I have read for my symptoms of IBS, Diverticulitis, and Lactose Intolerance. I followed many of your suggestions and within 3 weeks the pain is gone, the burning has eased, the nausea has subsided and the dreadful diarrhea has stopped!! Keep up the good work!"
D.F., Arizona, USA

"Your program was extremely helpful and supportive when others (including my doctor) could not be. The more I talk about IBD the more I realize that so many folks have to deal with it. At this point I am doing well. I am off Entocort and am up to 123lbs. My cramping has just about completely subsided and my stools are formed and occur about 2 to 3 times/day. Thanks again!"
E.B., Vermont, USA

Other Books, DVDs, & CDs by Jini Patel Thompson

The IBD Remission Diet: Achieving Long-Term Health with an Elemental Diet & Natural Supplementation Plan
Hardcover book

Baby Fart Aerobics: And Other Natural Treatments for Colicky Babies
80 minute DVD with Information Booklet

Stuck in The Seaweed
Murray the Shark Series (Vol. I) 47 minute audio CD

Murray Meets Allie Anglerfish
Murray the Shark Series (Vol. II) 47 minute audio CD

Murray & Friends Build a Bicycle
Murray the Shark Series (Vol. III) 47 minute audio CD

*All are available at Listen To Your Gut Enterprises Inc.
www.ListenToYourGut.com
Toll free: 1.888.866.7745

Listen to Your Gut

THE COMPLETE
Natural Healing Program
FOR IBS & IBD

Revised, Expanded Edition

Jini Patel Thompson

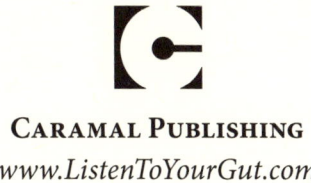

CARAMAL PUBLISHING
www.ListenToYourGut.com

Listen To Your Gut Enterprises Inc.
Caramal Publishing
P.O. Box 29022
Vancouver BC, V6J 5C2
Canada

Copyright © 2000 - 2016 by Jini Patel Thompson

All rights reserved. No part of this book or CD may be reproduced or transmitted in any form or by any means, electronic or mechanical, including photocopying, recording, or by any information storage and retrieval system, without permission in writing from the publisher.

Library and Archives Canada Cataloguing in Publication

Thompson, Jini Patel, 1968-
Listen to your gut: the complete natural healing program for IBS & IBD: Crohn's, ulcerative colitis, diverticulitis, IBS / Jini Patel Thompson. – Rev. ed.
Includes bibliographical references and index.
ISBN 0-9736332-4-7
1. Inflammatory bowel diseases – Alternative treatment.
2. Irritable colon – Alternative treatment. I. Title.
RC862.I53T56 2005   616.3'406   C2005-903626-5

Printed in the United States of America
2000 First Edition
2006 Revised Edition

Cover & Book Design by Mariana Prins – ZWé STUDiOS
www.BaobabCreative.com

Cover Photo by Tamara Roberts
www.tamararoberts.com

CARAMAL PUBLISHING

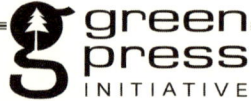

Caramal Publishing is committed to preserving ancient forests and natural resources. We elected to print this title on 30% post consumer recycled paper, processed chlorine free. As a result, for this printing, we have saved:

12 Trees (40' tall and 6-8" diameter)
6 Million BTUs of Total Energy
1,060 Pounds of Greenhouse Gases
5,749 Gallons of Wastewater
384 Pounds of Solid Waste

Caramal Publishing made this paper choice because our printer, Thomson-Shore, Inc., is a member of Green Press Initiative, a nonprofit program dedicated to supporting authors, publishers, and suppliers in their efforts to reduce their use of fiber obtained from endangered forests.

For more information, visit www.greenpressinitiative.org

Environmental impact estimates were made using the Environmental Defense Paper Calculator. For more information visit: www.papercalculator.org.

Disclaimer

This book is designed to provide information in regard to the subject matter covered. It is sold with the understanding that the publisher and author are not engaged in rendering medical, naturopathic, homeopathic or other professional services. If medical or other expert assistance is required, the services of a competent professional should be sought. Every effort has been made to make this book as complete and as accurate as possible. However, there may be mistakes both typographical and in content. Therefore this book should be used only as a general guide and not as the ultimate source of information on intestinal health. Furthermore, this book contains information on IBD/IBS only up to the printing date. The purpose of this book is to educate and entertain. The author and Caramal Publishing shall have neither liability nor responsibility to any person or entity with respect to any loss or damage caused, or alleged to be caused, directly or indirectly by the information contained in this book. If you do not wish to be bound by this disclaimer, you may return this book to the publisher for a full refund.

Listen To Your Gut Enterprises Inc.
Caramal Publishing
PO Box 29022
Vancouver, BC, V6J 5C2
Canada

Acknowledgements

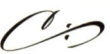

My utmost thanks to Mary and Tony Macer for their tireless and timely editing efforts. Also thanks to Ian Thompson, Dr. Sharad Patel, Anita Patel, Dr. John W. Travis and Stephanie Chimilar for proofreading and feedback. Thank you to Mariana Prins for working so hard to meet a succession of 'impossible' deadlines and for being so good at what you do. Big thanks to Oscar and Zara for letting mummy work all hours to get this out on time!

This book is dedicated to fellow travelers along this pathway to wellness. May you have peace and fulfillment and live a life of unbridled joy and vibrancy.

Please note: Although the anecdotes or 'client stories' told throughout this program are true – names have been changed to protect the identity of the people involved.

Table of Contents

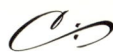

CHAPTER ONE – Take Your Life Back 13
My Healing Journey 15
Cured vs. Healed 21
Etiology And Pathogenesis Of IBD And IBS 24
How Do You See Yourself? 29
The Holistic Healing Journey 34
Children With IBD Or IBS 37
Program Resources 39
The Listen To Your Gut CD 40
Program Implementation 44

CHAPTER TWO – Supplements & Treatment Protocols 47
Using The Supplements In This Program 48
How To Introduce Supplements 55
Symptoms & Recommended Treatments 57
    Anemia 58
    Constipation 65
    Cramping/Spasming Intestines 67
    Diarrhea 68
    Fistulas 77
    Gas & Bloating 84
    Heartburn (Acid Reflux) 87
    Hemorrhoids 91
    Immune System Strengtheners 94
    Intestinal Inflammation, Ulceration & Bleeding 98
        Jini's Healing Implant Enema 108
    Joint Pain & Swelling 117

  Malnutrition... 120

  Mouth Ulcers.. 128

  Rectal Fissures.. 132

  Strictures... 134

Natural Antibiotics / Antimicrobials 140

Wild Oregano Oil... 145

 Jini's Wild Oregano Oil Protocol......................152

Probiotic (Good Bacteria) Supplementation........155

 Jini's Probiotic Retention Enema 181

Vitamin And Mineral Supplementation............. 186

Supplement Introduction Order 191

Chapter Three – Food As Medicine 195

Organic Food And Beverages........................... 196

Restrictions And Guidelines............................ 200

The Healing Diets... 209

 Maintenance Diet................................... 218

 Minimize Gas & Bloating Diet 220

 Reduce Diarrhea Diet 225

 Stop Intestinal Bleeding Diet................... 230

 Bowel Rest Elemental Diet 235

Quick Reference Guides 247

 Maintenance Diet................................... 247

 Minimize Gas & Bloating Diet 248

 Reduce Diarrhea Diet 249

 Stop Intestinal Bleeding.......................... 250

Food Reintroduction Chart 251

Chapter Four – Lifestyle & Environmental Factors 253

Eliminating Toxins 259

Absorption Through The Skin 268

The Toxins In Your Kitchen 270

The Dangers Of Vaccination............................ 276

Implementing Change.................................... 288

TABLE OF CONTENTS

CHAPTER FIVE – Allopathic Medicine..........................291
Drugs...294
Surgery...311
Gastrointestinal Exploratory Procedures.................317
Your Doctor And You.....................................324
Naturopathic Medicine...................................326

CHAPTER SIX – Mind/Body Therapies........................329
Acupuncture...331
Bio-Kinesiology...332
Massage Therapy...334
Craniosacral Therapy....................................335
Emotional Freedom Technique (EFT).......................341
Hypnotherapy..346
Meditation..348
Dialoguing With Your Body...............................350
Colonic Massage...352
   Blockages & Constipation..........................353
   Gas & Bloating....................................354
   Cramping & Diarrhea...............................356
Exercise..357

CHAPTER SEVEN – Use Your Mind To Help Your Body..........361
Affirmations..362
Healing Visualizations..................................364
Controlling Your Bowels.................................368
Transforming Pain.......................................372

CHAPTER EIGHT – Treatments I'm Often Asked About.........377
Ayurvedic Medicine......................................378
Traditional Chinese Medicine............................379
The Blood Type Diet.....................................380
Specific Carbohydrate Diet..............................381
Detoxification Protocols................................383
Colon Cleansing...385
Bacterial Soil Organisms................................386

xi

Plant Sterols/Sterolins 389
Kombucha Tea 390
MSM. 391
Molocure A.M.P. Aloe Vera 391
Ashwaganda 392
Seacure. 392
BC-9 Homeopathic Remedy 393
Trying New Products. 393

CHAPTER NINE – Pregnancy & Breastfeeding 395
Birth Control 399
Natural Menstrual Products. 401
Prior To Conception 402
Supplementation. 404
Breastfeeding 411
Formula Feeding 416
Jini's Formula Supplement Protocol 417
Coping With A Flare-Up Whilst Pregnant 418
The Physical & Emotional Stress of Parenting 420

CHAPTER TEN – How To Use The Listen To Your Gut CD 429
Listen To Your Gut CD Menu 430
Healing Journey Workbook 431
Treatment Summaries 431
Health Assessment & Tracking Tools 432

FOOTNOTES 435

APPENDIX A – Recommended Reading 445

APPENDIX B – Practitioner Resources 449

APPENDIX C – Products & Suppliers 455

APPENDIX D – Research & References 463

INDEX 471

1

Take Your Life Back

"If we listen to our insides, we will also find that inner therapist who says, 'Pay attention! I'm going to make you hurt a bit now so you will wake up.'

For this reason I sometimes call pain and suffering 'God's reset button'.

It is sometimes the only thing that will make people change."

Dr. Bernie Siegel, MD

Since the first edition of *Listen To Your Gut* was published (in 2000) it has gone through three printings and I've received literally thousands of letters, questions and feedback from readers. Therefore, based on your feedback and questions, and due to the continual stream of new information and improved healthcare protocols available, I decided it was time to write a revised, expanded version of *Listen To Your Gut*. This expanded edition is not just a singular book anymore, but rather a complete healing program with detailed implementation tools (on the accompanying CD) to guide you every step of the way and to help you put together the most efficient, effective program for healing your unique body.

This textbook is now your manual of knowledge and treatments, and the CD is your portfolio of treatment assessment and implementation tools. The tools on the CD (*Healing Journey Workbook*, Treatment Summaries and Health Assessment & Tracking Tools) walk you through the information in this manual, step-by-step, and help you to actually implement the treatments and apply the healing protocols to your own life. The tools on the CD are a *very* important part of the program. There is so much information here in the manual that it can be very exciting, but also overwhelming and perhaps confusing. The implementation tools on the CD are what guide you to sift through all the information and decide which treatments to apply to yourself, and in what order.

Although it's possible to just randomly take a few of the recommended supplements here and there and you probably will see positive results from that, for the greatest chance of success (or complete healing), you really do need to implement the complete healing program. Holistic healing does not work like drug therapy; to heal effectively you need to heal *all* the varied aspects of your self. The implementation tools on the CD help you to organize your unique treatment protocol (because we're all different), to action it step-by-step, and to evaluate your progress and make adjustments as needed.

MY HEALING JOURNEY

It is my hope that the contents of this program can be for you, as they were for me, the pathway to autonomy and peace. I initially began work on *Listen To Your Gut* at the suggestion of various healthcare professionals (medical doctors, massage therapists, physiotherapists, etc.) who compared me to all of their other clients diagnosed with Crohn's Disease or ulcerative colitis and couldn't believe how healthy I was. I kept hearing again and again, 'You should write a book about your methods'.

During my initial diagnosis in 1986, the exploratory tests revealed a fairly severe or widespread case of Crohn's with ulceration present throughout the small and large intestine. Coming from a family of physicians and pharmacists, I had complete faith in the sophistication and efficacy of medical science. At the time of my diagnosis, I knew absolutely nothing about alternative medicine. I merely assumed it was a substandard system of healthcare used by people in third world countries who were uneducated and did not have access to modern medicine, or couldn't afford it. Therefore, in complete faith, I did everything the medical establishment told me to do (and not do) for the first three years after being diagnosed with Crohn's Disease. I finally reached my breaking point when I was ingesting thirteen pills per day, terribly weakened from all the diagnostic and exploratory tests and basically had a life that consisted of thinking or dealing with pain and discomfort on a daily basis. Or I would engage in the flip-side of that, which was desperately trying to ignore my physical body in the hope that it would all just go away. Practically everything I ate made me ill (intestinal bleeding, pain, cramping, etc.). By this point my doctors suspected I had Crohn's in my stomach as well, and were pretty much insisting I have surgery. After three years, I finally decided that living like this was no longer acceptable; there had to be something else I could do, something that would give me my life back.

So I went to my gastroenterologist, who headed up a national research team on Crohn's Disease and ulcerative colitis, and I asked him for all the books and papers he had on the subject (this was before the Internet). He

> After three years, I finally decided that living like this was no longer acceptable; there had to be something else I could do, something that would give me my life back.

loaded me up with a stack of textbooks and some of his latest research and I took it home and read everything. That's when I realized that the medical profession had very limited information/knowledge about inflammatory bowel disease. I didn't find anything that could even possibly help me, in my present condition, that I hadn't already tried. That realization, coupled with a horrible course of steroids (Prednisone) and the alarming statistics of recurrence rates following surgery, prompted my departure from the medical establishment. The medical treatment protocols did not work for me and I knew I had to find something that did.

I spent the next seven years researching and experimenting with alternative and indigenous healing therapies as I lived and worked in Japan, England, and Canada. I developed my own methods of dealing with each phase of symptoms. I learned to listen to my body and take responsibility for it. Constantly seeking new knowledge and techniques, I used myself as my guinea pig and conducted multiple, controlled trials to ascertain what worked and what didn't.

However, I didn't want to write and sell a book about healing methods that worked for me, without finding out first whether they worked for others as well. So, in 1995 I drew up a brief sixty-page booklet of my methods and circulated about 200 copies via friends, family and the Internet for the next three years. My main concern was that my diets, techniques, and methods would actually work and help people other than just myself. I wanted to know that the therapies and process that worked for me would also work for others. Based on the positive, affirming feedback I received (along with emails from people exclaiming, 'please publish this!'), I then decided it was time to gather all my information together into a comprehensive book format. That book was the first edition of *Listen To Your Gut*, published in 2000. This current program is the result of that initial research, plus subsequent feedback from thousands of readers and consultation clients, evolving scientific research, improved nutritional information and improved healthcare products and protocols.

The Importance Of Emotional Healing

In detailing my healing process and techniques, I soon realized that I had not one book, but two, and that to relay all the information together in a single volume would simply be too overwhelming for the reader. My healing process is based upon a mind/body/spirit paradigm; in order to heal, we must heal *all* aspects of the Self, not just the physical body. Therefore, I decided to have this program deal primarily with healing the physical body – although I do address the importance of emotional healing throughout the program as well. There are many excellent books already on the market that deal specifically with emotional/mental/spiritual healing (see Appendix A for my suggestions) and I strongly encourage you to look at these aspects of your healing simultaneously. Disease is not just a physical phenomenon. By using the diets, therapies and protocols in this program in conjunction with increasing awareness of the emotional/mental contributors to your dis-ease, you should experience fairly direct results in your physical body. You may be able to reach the stage where you're off all drugs and managing the cycle of your disease, along with flare-ups, by yourself and without (or rarely) having to resort to drugs and hospitalization.

The Brain-Gut Axis

However, for full and complete healing to take place, I cannot emphasize enough that you must also address the emotional and psychological components of your dis-ease. Many people refer to the gut as 'the second brain' and indeed there is even a book by that title that details exactly how the gut biochemistry parallels and interacts closely with the brain. For example, 60% of the neurotransmitters in your body are not found in your brain, but in your gut! Medical journalist Chris Woolston presents this concept well in his article, *Gut Feelings: The Surprising Link Between Mood and Digestion*. Here are some pertinent extracts from his article:

> "If you've ever felt your insides twist in knots before a big speech, you know the stomach listens carefully to the brain. In fact, the entire digestive system is closely tuned to a person's emotions and state of mind, says William E. Whitehead, PhD, a professor of medicine

> "Doctors now see intricate links between the nervous system and the digestive system. The two realms constantly exchange streams of chemical and electrical messages, and anything that affects one is likely to affect the other."
>
> Chris Woolston, Medical Journalist

and an adjunct professor of psychology at the University of North Carolina...Doctors now see intricate links between the nervous system and the digestive system. The two realms constantly exchange streams of chemical and electrical messages, and anything that affects one is likely to affect the other. The connections between the two systems are so tight that scientists often refer to them as one entity: the brain-gut axis. (The brain-gut axis is a hot topic in medicine. In the summer of 2001, more than 100 researchers from around the world gathered in Los Angeles for a convention called "2001: A Brain-Gut Odyssey.")...

It may surprise many people to learn that the gut actually contains as many neurons (nerve cells) as the spinal cord...With all these messages, the connection between the brain and the digestive system is a busy two-way street. The central nervous system releases chemicals (acetylcholine and adrenaline) that tell the stomach when to produce acid, when to churn, and when to rest. Similar signals help guide the movements of the intestines. The digestive system responds by sending electrical messages to the brain, creating such sensations as hunger, fullness, pain, nausea, discomfort, and possibly sadness and joy...

The influence of the mind on the gut goes beyond functional diseases. For instance, people with Crohn's disease or ulcerative colitis – two conditions with clearly physical origins – often suffer flareups during times of emotional stress. And in a recent survey, 68 percent of people with basically healthy digestive systems said stress gives them stomachaches." [1]

In fact, the brain-gut axis (that Woolston refers to in this article) and the undeniable interplay between the mind/emotions and the gut have become so important that a new field of medicine has emerged to specifically study and research this interplay, called Neurogastroenterology.

Before I have my first phone consultation with a client, I ask them to email me their history, if they wish. Most of the time, people send me just the physical information and data about their bodies. Occasionally, a client will mention that a flare was likely triggered by the stress of a particular situation. But I have yet to have anyone write with full awareness of how much and how crucially their mind and emotions affect their physical body. And no one has told me about any therapies or techniques they're implementing to effect healing of their emotional body. When I bring up this important aspect of healing during sessions, some clients get it right away and immediately begin implementing Emotional Freedom Technique (EFT), or craniosacral therapy, or hypnotherapy – and they are the ones that get the quickest results in their healing path. Some clients have the belief that emotional healing is something they might look at *after* their physical symptoms are resolved. And these clients often have very frustrating healing journeys, where for long periods of time it doesn't seem like they're making any progress at all, even though they're doing everything physically possible to heal themselves. You 'll hear me say this often throughout this program: Until you heal your emotional/spiritual body, you will not see the desired results in your physical body, or even if you do, they will not last long-term. You must heal *all* the roots of your illness – physical, mental, emotional and spiritual – to effect long-term healing.

Please try to understand this concept that emotional events, trauma or feelings (past or present) produce clear, measurable results in the gut. When you fully accept and 'get' this concept, your healing will move to a whole new level. Dr Emeran Mayer at the UCLA School of Medicine outlines some of these very real physical consequences of emotions and stress in the digestive system in his article *The Neurobiology of Stress and Emotions*:

> "…the emotion of fear is associated with inhibition of upper GI (stomach and duodenum) contractions and secretions, and with stimulation of lower GI (sigmoid colon and rectum) motility and secretions. The former may contribute to a sensation of fullness and lack of appetite, the latter to diarrhea and lower abdominal pain. Interestingly, when the emotion shifts to anger, the pattern of upper GI activity is reversed, with stimulation of gastric contractions and acid secretion…in humans living in modern societies we are increasingly beginning to realize a phenomenon that has been referred to as the wear and tear, or the allostatic load, of stress. This detrimental

☼ Some clients have the belief that emotional healing is something they might look at after their physical symptoms are resolved. And these clients often have very frustrating healing journeys.

effect of stress may manifest following a one time severe stressor (life threatening situation), following repeated smaller stressors, or following a major sustained stressor over a period of time...while acute stimulation of the immune system has a beneficial effect, chronic stress can be associated with suppression of cellular immunity, and detrimental effects on health. [2]

We were on holiday in Mexico one year with my parents and my Dad was in a grouchy mood one evening. Then he had some wine with dinner (alcohol makes him more aggressive) and at some point vented some of his bad energy on my two year old son by shouting at him. I didn't think much of it as it was a very mild expression compared to what I'd grown up with. But when we were back in our room my son told me that, "Grandad made my tummy feel bad." I was stunned and enlightened at the same time. At that point, I hadn't talked to my son about mind/body connections or feeling via the gut, or anything of that nature. But there it was, the plain truth, in his own words. He was able to recognize immediately the emotional effect of that hurtful experience in his gut. And what would years and years of living with someone who 'makes your tummy feel bad' do to your digestive health? If you want to achieve full healing, you'll also need to look at, connect with, and heal the emotional woundings, fear, anger, etc. that have lodged themselves in your gut.

I once had a series of sessions with an advanced rolfing practitioner (a type of bodywork therapy), named Jeffrey Maitland, who lives in Scottsdale, Arizona. Jeffrey treats professional athletes, dancers, and NBA stars like Charles Barkley, and he is also a Buddhist monk who holds a doctorate in Philosophy. He explained a bit of his view on the mind/body interplay (based on twenty years of treating people's bodies): "All thought/emotion originates in the gut and travels upward through the torso and then through the neck for expression through the mouth. People tend to experience problems in their body dependent on where their blocks or wounds are along this pathway." If you take the time or utilize a therapy that allows you to connect with your gut, I guarantee you'll find past traumas or woundings that are still held in your gut.

You will have the best results from this program if you simultaneously pursue emotional/mental healing along with physical healing. Talk therapy (most forms of counseling and psychoanalysis) are of limited use and not very effective. You need to pursue forms of healing that *integrate* your mind and body. You need to release the trauma or wounding from the cells and tissues of your body, as well as your mind. Therefore, the types of healing therapies that I've found work best are: Emotional Freedom Technique (EFT), hypnotherapy, spiritual or energy healing, craniosacral therapy and acupuncture/acupressure that is combined with emotional release (the craniosacral therapist and acupuncturist needs additional, special training in somato-emotional release). These therapies will be explained in detail in Chapter Six.

> If you want to achieve full healing, you'll also need to look at, connect with, and heal the emotional woundings, fear, anger, etc. that have lodged themselves in your gut.

CURED VS. HEALED

In developing and following the methods and therapies outlined in this program, I have improved my own health to the point where I have been drug and surgery-free for over 16 years. For the most part (although I have my down spells too, which I'll talk about in other chapters), I live a full and active life; I have two children, own my own business, travel every month or two, exercise regularly, etc. As far as I'm concerned, I no longer have Crohn's Disease. However, I eat mostly organic, unprocessed food, live in a toxin-free home, take supplements when needed, utilize EFT when needed, and attend an advanced yoga class where we work with the prana (lifeforce energy) for two hours a week. My digestive system is the most sensitive part of my body and I will always take special care of it. I still experience intestinal disturbances from time to time and still use some of the therapies in this program when required. But, the spectre of "disease" and all its accoutrements (drugs, surgery, hospital visits, exploratory tests, etc.) is no longer a part of my life. Actively seeking better health by hiring a part-time housekeeper, visiting my naturopathic doctor, being careful to eat mostly unprocessed, organic food and seeking ongoing emotional healing is still very much a part of my life.

LISTEN TO YOUR GUT

People ask me, 'are you cured?' The word 'cure' to me means that your body is so healthy that you never even have to *think* about your body again, let alone treat it specially or support it with healing herbs and treatments. If I were to say I was 'cured' then I would be able to eat processed, crap food, drink copious amounts of alcohol and stay up all night for a week – and feel no ill effects. So, I don't use the word 'cured', I prefer the word 'healed'. I can go out and eat a hamburger and fries whenever I want to and feel no ill effects. But, if I ate fast food for a week non-stop I'd feel pretty bad! I can also travel anywhere in the world (except India) and eat the local food with no trouble. But, by the end of two weeks, I'll be feeling the need for better quality food. Actually, the United States is one of the most difficult countries to travel in, since the average restaurant uses a lot of chemical, artificial and processed foods in its cooking. Whereas the average restaurant in Thailand, for example, uses fresh vegetables, seafood, noodles and the only irritants are the hydrogenated oil used for frying and sometimes some MSG in the sauces. I once spent three weeks in Thailand and felt great.

Taking special care of my digestive and immune system will always be a part of my life. I don't have the tolerance levels for toxins that other people have. I can't be stressed or sleep-deprived for months without the effects showing up in my body in the form of colonic or rectal bleeding or low hemoglobin, or flatulence, etc. However, I can heal all those things, very quickly, by addressing the corresponding emotional/lifestyle issue and then following the applicable healing therapies in this program. No matter how bad my condition has been over the years I have never resorted to drugs or surgery, but have always healed myself using the natural methods in this program. I wish for each of you this same freedom and control over your life, body and health.

Instead of viewing your health and healing as an end-point, it will help you immeasurably to view it as a journey. You will be much happier along this holistic healing path if you can view it as a process and celebrate each improvement along the journey – rather than anxiously rushing, pushing and waiting for your body to be cured/healed so you can get back to your

---

☼ No matter how bad my condition has been over the years I have never resorted to drugs or surgery, but have always healed myself using the natural methods in this program.

'regular' life. Instead of looking at how far you still have to go, if you can focus on how far you've come and all the improvements you have made, you will have a lot more peace and happiness along your Healing Journey. Holistic healing is a long, winding path and there are no quick-fixes or silver bullets here (like in drug therapy).

The initial phase of your healing may take the longest and produce the least 'visible' results because you have to build your foundation first. You have to start at the roots of your dis-ease and just like building a house, laying the groundwork and pouring the foundation don't look like much, but they are of crucial importance. For example, let's say you have a mycobacterial (fungal-bacterial hybrid microorganism) infection as one of your 'causative roots'. Treating and resolving such an infection can take anywhere from six months to two years (see Chapter Two), but once you get that infection under control, you'll see improvement. And by the time you completely eradicate that infection, you'll probably have automatically eliminated your diarrhea and colonic bleeding. You will also have restored the integrity of your intestinal walls, mucosal lining, and bacterial flora throughout your gut. Therefore, your digestive and absorptive abilities will now be up to normal. Because you have treated your whole body holistically, you will most likely have cleared up other health issues as well. And by healing your past and present emotional woundings, you will now be creating a job and relationships that support you as a healthy, vibrant person – not as a sick, wounded person.

Initially, it may seem very scary to you to be completely in charge of your own health and to have all the tools and responsibility to heal yourself, no matter what arises. Some people find it easiest to quit the drugs and surgery cold turkey (although strong drugs must always be weaned off gradually) and completely remove it as a treatment option, while others find it easier to go off and on their drugs while incorporating more and more natural healing methods. The first way is definitely a much quicker way of healing, but it has to suit your personality. Remember that stress is a huge component of these dis-eases and anything that causes you stress is not

> ☼ You will be much happier along this holistic healing path if you can view it as a process and celebrate each improvement along the journey – rather than anxiously rushing, pushing and waiting for your body to be cured/healed so you can get back to your 'regular' life.

going to help you heal. Therefore, first and foremost, you must always follow your own gut and introduce change at a pace that feels right for you.

ETIOLOGY AND PATHOGENESIS OF IBD AND IBS

Many people spend a lot of time and energy searching and hoping for the etiology (cause) of inflammatory bowel disease (IBD) and irritable bowel syndrome (IBS) to be revealed. I suppose that most people believe that if we knew what caused IBD or IBS, we would know how to cure it. This is because we are still looking to fulfill the equation of one pathogen (disease-causing agent) equals one disease, which can be cured with one drug. This is the mindset bestowed on us by the commercial medical and pharmaceutical industries that we have accepted easily (even though the scientist knows the truth to be far more complex).

However, ascribing to this model leaves many questions unanswered. For example, autopsies reveal that most people have an average of 16 viruses in their brain. So why is it that most of us experience no abnormal symptoms or diseases as a result of these viruses? In addition, let's say for example, that it is discovered that Virus X causes ulcerative colitis. Okay fine, but that still doesn't explain why you contracted that virus and your twin sister didn't – similar genetic makeup, similar environment, why the difference in susceptibility? If you look at some of the most contagious diseases on our planet, there are always some people who, although exposed, do not contract these diseases. Even when they're living and working in the midst of an entire community of people manifesting a particular illness, some people will not contract that illness. Why not?

The current medical/pharmaceutical model of illness cannot answer any of these questions. Perhaps this is because their construct of disease is flawed. Personally, I think the popular medical model is far too simplistic to adequately portray and understand all the factors involved in the disease/healing/balancing process. I hope this program will stimulate your own thought process and encourage you to open up to unconventional possibilities and ideas, to pursue the many layers of truth and the many

> ☼ I hope this program will stimulate your own thought process and encourage you to open up to unconventional possibilities and ideas, to pursue the many layers of truth and the many facets of reality, rather than latching onto the flat, easy, one-dimensional answer.

facets of reality, rather than latching onto the flat, easy, one-dimensional answer.

Our bodies are not machines, where one plus one equals two. We are complex, many-layered entities capable of containing any number of apparent contradictions simultaneously. We can be both hot to the touch on the outside with sweat pouring off our skin, whilst being freezing cold on the inside – so cold our bones ache and it hurts to breathe. We can feel a well of deep love and attachment to a dysfunctional parent whilst simultaneously hating them for what they have done to us. A father loses his child and his hair turns completely white overnight. A mother lifts a truck single-handedly to save her child trapped beneath it. How are these things possible? As you begin to open to the expansiveness of humanity, you begin to understand. You also begin to glimpse the possibilities that are present within yourself.

What does all this have to do with healing your dis-ease? Quite simply, it opens you to the possibility of delving into and collaborating with your body. Merging with all aspects of your body/self and treading the pathway of healing together – as a multi-dimensional but unified being, with all parts relating to and supporting each other. It releases you from viewing and treating your body or your intestines as something functioning independently of you and your desires. Subscribing to the medical model will cause you to view the malfunctioning parts of your body with impatience and annoyance, even anger. If you see your body in this manner, you'll just want to feed it the right pill and have it perform properly, damnit! But your body is not a machine, you can't separate the parts from the whole. And what place has healing in the midst of anger and resentment?

Opening yourself up to the possibilities of humanity and your unique reality will also create a space for you to integrate the different levels of yourself and begin taking some responsibility for your present state. Taking responsibility for the state of your body and your health may be as simple as saying, "Okay, well, since I got this particular disease and not some other,

> This is your Healing Journey and no one else can walk it for you.

there must be a reason for that. I'm going to start looking at the lesson(s) here for me."

If there was no point in your developing IBS or IBD, no lessons for you to learn, no journey for you to take, then why did you develop this illness? A scientist identifying Virus X as the pathogen (agent of disease) is not going to answer this question. If all the members of your family, or your class, or your community were exposed to the same environment, then why did you contract IBS or IBD when they didn't? Looking for the missing pathogen is not going to give you the answer. Only you can answer these questions. Only you can unite and integrate all the levels of yourself to identify all the contributing and influencing factors in your particular pathogenesis. This is your Healing Journey and no one else can walk it for you.

My Opinion On IBS/IBD Etiology

I have had many readers ask me, 'what do you think caused my colitis/Crohn's/IBS etc.?' Well, I see each of these conditions as points along a continuum, from mild to severe. With IBS at the far left side and Crohn's at the far right. So it would look like this:

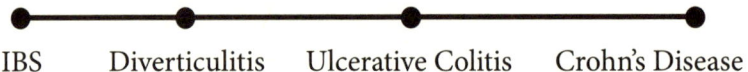

IBS　　Diverticulitis　　Ulcerative Colitis　　Crohn's Disease

Medical doctors maintain that each of these diseases are separate and distinct from each other. But I've heard from far too many people whose IBS has turned into colitis, or whose diagnosis of colitis has metamorphosed into Crohn's. When this happens, doctors tend to say 'oh, well you were misdiagnosed in the first place'. In my opinion each point along this continuum – with it's accompanying symptom profile – is merely an indication of how much your health has been compromised to date and which areas of your body need healing. As you progress along the continuum (from left to right), the symptoms indicate that the damage is not just localized but increasingly more systemic.

> There is seldom just one factor (pathogen) in isolation that causes IBS or IBD.

I believe the causative factors of these conditions are varied. If you go back over your own personal health history, I think you'll find a mix of the following damaging events, that singly or in combination have degraded the health of your gut and immune system:

- **Vaccination** – childhood, adult, flu vaccines, etc. Causes direct damage to bacterial flora of the gut and long-term, immune system damage. See Chapter Four for more details.

- **Antibiotic Use** – any antibiotic therapy that is not followed by full-spectrum probiotic therapy causes lasting, pervasive damage to the bacterial flora of your gastrointestinal tract (from mouth to anus), which in turn leads to increased infestation of yeast, parasites, viruses, bad bacteria and other pathogens. These pathogens degrade the mucosal lining and damage the intestinal wall (symptoms include bloating, gas, inflammation, bleeding, etc.) which leads to Leaky Gut Syndrome, which then triggers allergic and auto-immune response. Certain antibiotic drugs can cause ulcerative colitis all by themselves (like Novo Clindamycin), and the pharmaceutical information that comes with these products even explicitly warns of this. Yet medical doctors continue to prescribe them and also don't follow usage with probiotics.

- **Environmental and Food-borne Toxins** – processed foods with preservatives, Monosodium Glutamate (MSG), artificial sweeteners and flavors, nitrites and other proven toxins and carcinogens, microwaved foods, toxins contained in skin care products, shampoos, cosmetics, furniture, carpets, and the air (to name a few sources) all cause cellular and systemic damage. Lots more on this in Chapter Four.

- **Emotional Trauma or Abuse** – don't underestimate the damaging effects of abusive or traumatic emotional experiences on the body, and the gut in particular. For some of you, this may be damage from your past that was never resolved/healed, and/or ongoing emotional patterns or experiences that continue to degrade your health daily.

> Each of us is capable of identifying our own particular pathology, or the causative factors of our own ill health and then taking the steps that will be particularly healing to each of us.

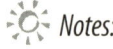 Notes:

- **Parasites & Pathogenic Microorganisms** – if your gut ecology is already weakened or imbalanced, travel to a foreign country or ingestion of tainted food/water can be the 'straw that breaks the camel's back'. If your bacterial flora is already imbalanced with a deficit of beneficial bacteria, then it's very easy for parasites, yeast, molds, bad bacteria, or fungus to flourish. These pathogens then degrade the health of your intestinal mucosal lining, which can result in ulceration, inflammation, bleeding and subsequent damage to your systemic health.

Each of these causative factors – including lesser factors like whether or not you were breastfed, your mother's health while you were in utero, hereditary/genetic weaknesses, heavy metal levels in your body, mercury amalgam fillings in your teeth, pesticide exposure, etc. – will contribute in varying degrees and combinations to your particular pathology. Different people are susceptible to different factors and something that strongly affects your friend adversely, may only mildly affect you adversely. There is seldom just one factor (pathogen) in isolation that causes IBS or IBD. However, I believe each of us is capable of identifying our own particular pathology, or the causative factors of our own ill health and then taking the steps that will be particularly healing to each of us.

This program is designed to assist you in identifying the physical contributors to your dis-ease (or unease) and to provide you with some tools and ideas to correct and balance your physical environment. There are many books available to help you identify the mental, emotional and spiritual elements of your dis-ease and I've listed a few really good ones in the Recommended Reading list (Appendix A) at the back of this book. Maybe you've become very wrapped up in searching for the cause of your illness, thinking that if science could only identify the pathogen, you could then take a drug that would cure you. If this has been causing you stress, for the sake of your own healing, I encourage you to put aside the quest for the etiology of these diseases. Don't worry about it, don't let it frustrate you, don't devote any more time and energy to it. Turn your focus instead to healing yourself, getting in touch with your body and allowing it to heal itself no matter what the cause. The great thing about this program is that the process and therapies will work irrespective of the cause of IBS and IBD. In fact, since all treatment is based on easily identified symptoms, you don't even need an official medical diagnosis to use and benefit from the healing tools provided in this program. All you need is the willingness to connect with your own body and to open yourself to your own wisdom and intuition.

HOW DO YOU SEE YOURSELF?

Please be aware that you also have a choice as to which label or diagnosis you accept for yourself and your condition. How do you define yourself and your health? Do you see your intestinal malfunction as you simply experiencing intestinal problems, or do you see your intestines as diseased, do you see or define yourself as a diseased person? Then think of the implications your mindset has on your healing process. Does your definition or label of yourself and your condition place you in a position of positivity, does it foster a healing environment for your mind/body? Or does it carry an inherent negativity and place you in a defeatist disease environment?

Most of us have accepted the label given to us by the medical community, that of irritable bowel syndrome, or ulcerative colitis, or Crohn's Disease or some other variation. If these labels were used simply as a classification system, as a symbol representing a collection of symptoms, that would be fine and it would be truthful. But there is an insidious aspect to these labels or diagnoses; each one of them also comes with the qualifier of "chronic" or "incurable". This is ridiculous, because it means that no matter how healthy I am, or how long I've been healthy for, doctors will still say to me, "Oh no, you still have Crohn's Disease, you're simply in remission."

I ask you, does any part of this approach or mentality help you? Does any part of this labeling process, this insistence that you are permanently diseased, lead you to positivity? Does it encourage health and a healing environment? Or does it promote despair, negativity and an ongoing disease-environment for your mind and body? I have always felt

☼ Does your definition or label of yourself place you in a position of positivity, does it foster a healing environment for your mind/body? Or does it carry an inherent negativity, and place you in a defeatist disease environment?

that words are very powerful. By accepting the medical profession's label of you as being a permanently diseased person, you are also accepting all the negativity and limiting parameters inherent in a profession that has tended to focus on the disease-process as opposed to the healing process.

In Dr. Andrew Weil's book, *Spontaneous Healing*, he relates a story told by a patient of his with HIV who experienced a similar frustration with medical diagnostics and doctors trying to define his reality for him:

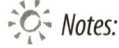 Notes:

> "The medical professionals gave me six to eighteen months to live when I was first diagnosed,' Mark told me when I met him. 'Since 1985 I can't tell you how many doctors have shown me the Curve – that is, the graph showing the percentage of people per year who develop AIDS after infection. They all try to tell me I'm somewhere along it, headed for destruction. This is really Western medicine's fascination with illness. Here I am with normal T cells, in great health, and they have the audacity to tell me I'm on this curve heading for death. When I see doctors now, I tell them right at the start: Look, I don't even want to hear about your curve. Just check me out, answer my questions, and keep your opinions to yourself! They have also all tried to get me to take AZT [the antiviral drug that is conventional medicine's current treatment of choice for HIV], but all of the people I've known who have used it are dead, so I've refused. And none of them have been interested to hear what I'm doing to stay healthy. They pat me on the head and say, "Whatever you're doing, just keep it up!" I have developed an ability not to buy into the medical system..." [3]

New Label – New Framework

My hope for each one of you following this program, is that you get to the point in your healing process where you don't feel you need to accept these medical labels anymore (and maybe you're already there!) and you throw them away. What a wonderful, liberating move to a healing environment for your mind/body/spirit that will be. Keep in mind that this does not involve denying your existing state and physical health, or deluding yourself with positive talk or thinking. It involves full recognition of your existing physical symptoms, but within a framework of healing and positivity. It's the difference between saying, "I'm suffering from an incurable disease" and "I'm having some gastrointestinal problems". Or how about a Chinese Medicine diagnosis: "I have excess wind and fire in my bowels"? Sure you can use the medical label for your condition when dealing with health professionals or people who want the quick answer to, "What's the problem?" But for dealing with and relating to yourself, you may want to use different terminology. When I use the medical labels of Crohn's, ulcerative colitis, IBS and diverticulitis throughout this program, I am using them in reference to a previously defined set of symptoms. However, please keep in mind how I really view and treat intestinal malfunctions and that I do not label any bodily imbalance as "incurable".

You can label and define your own reality using words of positivity within a healing framework that gives you access to positive action. Instead of talking about your disease, you can talk about your healing pathway or your healing journey. This will also help you to start viewing your body as a whole, instead of as separate compartments where the parts and systems of your body function separately and independently. Your digestive tract is not the isolated "bad" part of your body, it is merely the area where your whole-body imbalance is evidenced, or displayed first. I was once talking to Karen Stewart, the owner of NutritionWorks health store in Scottsdale, Arizona, and she said, "All illness is simply an opportunity for growth. It's the body pointing out what you need to work on next. And the body uses the strongest parts of itself to deliver the message." I stared at her, fascinated, as the realization of what she was saying gradually grew in me. "Well think about it," she said, "the body wouldn't use its weakest part to give you the message, it wouldn't risk its life like that, it's going to use the *strongest* part." I found her words very empowering. Instead of viewing your gut as the weak part of your body, where illness shows up first, you can view it as the strongest part of your body, willing to sacrifice itself for your growth and understanding. Regarding your gastrointestinal tract in this manner will also foster a spirit of teamwork within you and gratitude towards your

> Keep in mind that this does not involve denying your existing state and physical health, or deluding yourself with positive talk or thinking. It involves full recognition of your existing physical symptoms, but within a framework of healing and positivity.

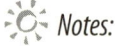 Notes:

gut for offering itself up for your growth and development. In her fantastic book, *Mutant Message Down Under*, Marlo Morgan relates that:

> "The Real People tribe believes that we are not random victims of ill health, that the physical body is the only means our higher level of eternal consciousness has to communicate with our personality consciousness. Slowing down the body allows us to look around and analyze the really important wounds we need to mend: wounded relationships, gaping holes in our belief system, walled-up tumors of fear, eroding faith in our Creator, hardened emotions of unforgiveness, and so on." [4]

When I first began healing myself, I found my healing required equal attention and resolution of both physical and emotional/spiritual/mental issues. However, I'm now at the point in my Healing Journey where symptoms I experience are rarely related to my physical body at all, but rather they are just messages, or indicators of something I need to resolve emotionally or spiritually. As soon as I address the emotional component – for example, resolve a conflict, forgive someone, connect with and share my deepest feelings with a loved one, speak my truth, say 'no' where I need to, etc. – the physical symptom instantly disappears, with no physical intervention necessary. I've also noticed that my body will first give me a feeling, or intuition. If I explore that and connect with my deeper self (or higher/spiritual self), and take appropriate action, the issue is resolved there. However, if I don't, my body will then give me a mild symptom. If I ignore this, a stronger symptom, or escalation of that same symptom will occur, and so on with increasing ramifications in my physical body until I finally stop, connect with my body and my higher self (or subconscious) and receive the message or follow the pathway of emotional/spiritual healing that needs to take place. As soon as I do this, the symptom begins to heal/resolve and in many cases disappears instantly – unless I've allowed things to escalate to the point where physical healing is also necessary.

Give Your Body Time & Space To Heal

I once had a series of consultations with a reader who was following the exclusively elemental diet and supplementation plan outlined in my second book, *The IBD Remission Diet*, but he was finding progress depressingly slow with lots of ups and downs and he was becoming quite discouraged. I was really mystified as to why he was seeing so little improvement until about the third session when he said, "I'm finding it very hard to concentrate at work…" *At work??* It never even occurred to me that he would be working full-time whilst suffering from malnutrition and colonic bleeding! What did this poor man's body have to do to get his attention enough to make him lie down and rest and relax? In addition, it then came out that his family was paying for him to be on the IBD Remission Diet so that he would be perfectly strong and healthy for his wedding in about two months time. Since he was of a certain ethnicity, he had only met his bride once, the wedding would last for three days solid, and there were 350 people invited. Talk about pressure! A normal, *healthy* person would probably get ill under that kind of stress. How could he possibly expect his body to heal under that tremendous workload, emotional stress and pressure?

> We really need to put aside the western concept of 'healthcare': That of using drugs to suppress symptoms so we can go about our business as usual.

We really need to put aside the western concept of 'healthcare': That of using drugs to suppress symptoms so we can go about our business as usual. If your body is ill, it is crying out for you to pay attention, slow down and listen to it, and give it the time and space to heal. Another reader said to me, "I can't take any time off, I can't afford it." Nonsense! If you were in the hospital you wouldn't be going to work, would you? The longer you let things escalate, the longer it will take you to heal. Natural healing cannot take place without giving your body adequate rest. True, root-level healing requires a lot of energy. If you use up your available energy by going to work or looking after your kids and household full-time, or being completely stressed out, how will your body get the energy it needs to heal itself? Try to remember that your physical body (although responding to physical factors) is also being directed by your higher/spiritual self – which is not trying to punish you or make your life hard, it is simply trying to communicate a very important message to you and really has only your best interest at heart. The sooner you slow down, take some time out, connect with your higher/subconscious self (see Chapters Six and Seven for details on how to do this), and resolve your emotional distress, the sooner your physical body will begin to heal.

THE HOLISTIC HEALING JOURNEY

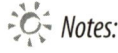 *Notes:*

As you tread this path of holistic healing, keep in mind that healing of any sort is rarely a linear, progressive process. Usually it occurs in cycles or spirals, but it's important to keep in mind that the spirals do spiral upward, so there is continuous improvement overall. Alternatively, you could view the healing process as one where you're doing well, moving in a straight line upwards, then you have a rough spot (often referred to as a healing crisis), so the line dips down for a bit, but then the line climbs upwards again as your healing continues. Symptoms experienced during a healing crisis can include skin eruptions, nausea, headache, sleepiness, unusual fatigue, constipation, diarrhea, head or chest cold, ear infections, boils, or any other method the body uses to loosen and eliminate toxins. A healing crisis will usually last around three to seven days – and occasionally longer if you're very run down and weakened.

There are numerous different theories as to why the body doesn't just heal in a straight, uninterrupted manner. Personally, I think it's because the body heals in layers, starting with the easiest imbalances and then moving progressively deeper into the more difficult, serious imbalances or malfunctions. As well, part of the healing and balancing process involves the periodic release of toxins, which may make you feel sicker and temporarily worsen your symptoms. As unpleasant and scary as this may be, toxin release and elimination is still an integral part of the healing process. When this happens, even though it feels like you're getting sicker, you've got to try to remember that it's actually part of you getting better. At times like this, you can get really scared and it's very tempting to feel that the natural healing methods just aren't working for you and to get back on your drugs again. But whilst the drugs will suppress the symptoms (in the short term) and relieve your immediate fear and worry, they will continue to damage your body and degrade your health overall. Drugs do not heal. They merely suppress symptoms whilst damaging the body further.

True, root-level healing (healing the cause, not just masking symptoms) is a winding pathway with ups and downs along the way, but always improving overall. I know this is a very confusing process. Discerning between whether you just need to give your body time, or whether the treatment you're pursuing isn't working for you, is a very difficult decision to make. Unfortunately, there's no simple formula I can give you in these instances, since everyone's body is unique and there are so many factors involved in the healing process. You're just going to have to really tune in to your body and your intuition during these times (see *Dialoguing With Your Body* in Chapter Six) and trust your body and higher/spiritual self to lead you step by step along your healing pathway. I cannot emphasize enough how much it helps to have a support network of family, or friends, or like-minded healthcare practitioners around you at these times. When you get really scared or frustrated, nothing is as valuable as someone who can pray with you, or give you a bodywork treatment that helps you connect with yourself and your strength, or just be there to listen, or hold you while you cry or vent. Having a caring support network will greatly increase your chances of success with natural healing.

> Keep in mind that healing of any sort is rarely a linear, progressive process. Usually it occurs in cycles or spirals, but it's important to keep in mind that the spirals do spiral upward, so there is continuous improvement overall.

I think there's also another more nebulous phenomenon at work in the healing process, and the best way I can describe it is to give you an analogy. Let's look at a middle-aged man (for example) who's got a good career, a nice house, a wife and kids. This man appears to be leading a pretty good life. What the outsider can't know is that this man was sexually abused as a child, but he's never discussed it with anyone or dealt with the memories. He was bullied terribly at school and had few friends in college. All his life, he's held himself tightly wrapped and under control and so appears fairly stable and 'together'.

However, severe interpersonal problems with his wife lead this man into counseling. It's only when he begins to acknowledge his trauma, when he

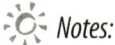 Notes:

begins the process of healing his wounds, that the tight, rigid bonds that have held him together begin to unravel. All of a sudden, this apparently healthy, successful man can't sleep at night and begins to perform poorly at his job. He doesn't get his yearly bonus so he and his wife have to sell one of their cars. You see, this man seems to be degenerating, he seems to be falling apart and getting worse, but what is really going on is that he is healing himself. He is actually getting better. For the first time in his life he is actually dealing with and healing all the deep-seated, tightly controlled wounds he's been carrying around.

I believe a similar process occurs when we start to access and heal the deeper layers of our physical body. Regardless of the depth and severity of your dis-ease, the balancing homeostatic mechanism will have caused your body to hold on tightly for as long as possible, to assume some form of control or pseudo-balance in order to keep your body functioning. Although there may be *very* serious long-term imbalances present in your system, they may not be apparent initially. However, as you start to heal your body and nurture and support it in its natural healing process, your body will gradually release its hold over these imbalances and offers them up for healing. When your body unmasks a long-term, systemic imbalance, you can become very ill quite suddenly. It may *appear* that your condition is suddenly and drastically worsening, and you may panic thinking the holistic healing methods aren't working at all. I know it's hard (especially the first time it happens) but try to remember that it's probably only temporary and your body needs your support and positivity the most at this time. I really encourage you to try not to panic when this happens. It helps to have someone close to you who can act as your sounding board, to help you stay rational and determine whether you actually do need additional help, or whether you just need to give it a few more days to settle down again. It's helpful if you can find a very skilled and empathetic naturopathic doctor to help you assess whether you're in danger, or whether you're just going through a healing crisis. Someone who can pray with you or offer some kind of spiritual healing is also invaluable at this time and will *really* help you to get through the fear that may overwhelm you, without resorting to drugs (which will only set your healing back). As you implement more and more of the therapies and diets in this program, you'll come to have a lot more confidence in the methods listed and in your own healing ability. But again, only do or don't do what you feel is right and safe for you. Don't give your power and authority over your own body away to anyone, especially not to me or the guidelines in this program!

CHILDREN WITH IBD OR IBS

As the parent of a child with IBD or IBS, you're going to have to walk a fine line between ministering to your sick child, and not letting their dis-ease take over your family or obliterate your other children's needs. Please try to spend quality time with your other children and remember that just because they're physically healthy, it doesn't mean they don't have needs that are just as crucial to their mental, emotional and spiritual health. Devoting all your time and energy to your sick child doesn't serve them or their siblings (or your spouse/partner) in the long run. Strive to maintain a balance of interaction and attention within your family and it will only impact positively on your child with IBS/IBD. Dr. John Harrison, MD, who wrote one of my favorite books, *Love Your Disease – It's Keeping You Healthy*, has a wonderful approach to maintaining a healthy family dynamic:

> "Children respond very quickly to a change in the reward system and are very aware of its ramifications, as demonstrated by the five-year-old client of mine overheard by his parents as he pointed out to his three-year-old sister: 'If you want Mummy to look after you, just get sick, that's what I do.' When children come into my office and one member of the family is ill, I am careful to pay equal attention to the healthy. Since some of them like coming to see me, I arrange times for them to visit when they are well. They begin replacing illness with wellness." [5]

There are entire books written on the family dynamics surrounding and often supporting illness, but for now, the main factor to be aware of is to spend quality time with and give attention to your healthy children as

☼ Remember that children are mirrors and our greatest teachers. If your child is ill, also look to yourself and your own actions. What message, or gift of teaching is your child trying to give you? What do you need to change or heal within yourself?

well. Your ill child can also be a caring, contributing member of the family too. Look for and point out ways (no matter how small) that they can demonstrate caring and concern for other family members. This will help your child to feel like a more equal, capable member of the family, whilst balancing the family dynamic. Also, waiting on your sick child night and day and catering to their victim status is not going to help them be well. It's just going to help them be weaker.

Try to come up with words and actions that make your child feel strong. Give them as much autonomy and decision-making responsibility as you can. Help your child to feel that he/she is in control, that she has options, that he has the strength to make decisions and reclaim his body. A child that's been subjected to the damaging, invasive, traumatic exploratory tests, drugs, or surgery involved with an IBD diagnosis is going to feel very violated and probably victimized and helpless. It's up to you to restore your child's feelings of control, safety, and empowerment with his/her body.

I once read a letter in *Mothering* magazine (www.mothering.com) from a mother whose two year old son began having violent epileptic seizures along with various other symptoms. They gave their child, at the age of two, complete control over his health and healing. He made the decisions regarding which doctors he wanted to see (they took him to medical, naturopathic and homeopathic physicians) and also which drugs, herbs, or homeopathic remedies he wanted to take and when. They basically gave him complete and total control, trusting that he was able to connect with and know his body better than anyone. At the end of a year they discovered that he had some very rare but severe allergies and if they had made him take the prescription drugs (which would have suppressed the frightening seizures, but not addressed the root cause), he would have suffered permanent brain damage as a result. It took a winding journey, or healing pathway, of a year to pinpoint the exact problem, but then the child was then completely healed and symptom free. I was awed by their story, and to this mother (and father) I give the utmost respect and admiration. So if you think your child is too young to make his/her own decisions about their health and body, keep this testimonial in mind.

> Help your child to feel that he/she is in control, that she has options, that he has the strength to make decisions and reclaim his body.

Remember that children are mirrors and our greatest teachers. If your child is ill, also look to yourself and your own actions. What message, or gift of teaching is your child trying to give you? What do you need to change or heal within yourself? If your child is hyper and stressed, look to your own energy – are you stressed, or tense, or controlling, or worried, etc? How's your relationship with your spouse or partner? When my husband and I are in conflict, our kids go nuts. As soon as we resolve the issue between us and restore an energy of peace and joy to the home, our children instantly, automatically, follow suit. Healing your child will also involve healing yourself in some manner. Pursuing a pathway of natural healing together will also involve lessons and gifts of wisdom for you as well as your child.

PROGRAM RESOURCES

The contents of this program comprise the results of my personal research and experimentation into alternative, natural healing methods.
Their results and effectiveness have now been confirmed by thousands of readers worldwide. But like any endeavour in life – whether it's a weight-loss program or an innovative business plan – people often feel the need for additional support and resources along the way. Therefore, I've set up a website: *www.ListenToYourGut.com* with many useful resources and services available – be sure to check it out.

I've also set up a blog (linked to from *www.ListenToYourGut.com*) where people specifically post their experience or results with certain experimental treatment protocols (you'll learn more about this in Chapter Two). So you can check here for ideas and feedback, and also to post your own experience so others can benefit.

Telephone Consultations

A private telephone consultation can be helpful if you get stuck, or need some additional ideas, or the benefit of my experience. I often consult to people who have a good healthcare team in place, but they want to discuss their particular situation with me and also reap the benefits of information

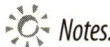 *Notes:*

I can provide on other clients (all confidential, of course) and what they did in a similar situation. Alternatively, I often have clients who are in smaller towns who simply cannot find supportive healthcare professionals, so they use me as their support and feedback person. Information and booking for private phone consultations is available at: www.LTYGShoppe.com.

THE *LISTEN TO YOUR GUT* CD

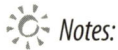 Notes:

Affixed to the cover of this manual, you will find a computer disc containing all the companion workbook and implementation materials that are an integral part of the *Listen To Your Gut* program. This manual gives you all the knowledge and information you need to heal yourself using natural methods, but the CD gives you all the tools to actually put that information into action and apply it to your life, body, and self. These tools are presented on a computer disc that you can insert into your computer and print out the various tools as often and repeatedly as you need to. Following are descriptions of exactly what's on the CD:

Healing Journey Workbook

The *Healing Journey Workbook* consists of a list of questions or activities to help you explore for yourself the contents of each chapter of *Listen To Your Gut*. This Workbook is where you take the techniques and concepts presented as a result of my experience, and other readers' experience, and turn them into the techniques and concepts that will work for you, as a result of your experience, who you are, and where you're at in your life. In short, the *Healing Journey Workbook* is where you take all the information presented here and make it your own. This is where you will organize and integrate all this new information, and map out a detailed, clear treatment program for your unique body. The Workbook is perhaps the most important part of this program. Don't let this be just one more book that you read and say, "Oh yeah, great ideas, I'm really excited, this sounds as if it will actually work!" and then put the program aside and never do anything with it. The knowledge and techniques in this program can only help you if you put them into practice.

Begin while the feeling and motivation is still fresh within you. You can do the Workbook sections in order as you read through *Listen To Your Gut*, chapter by chapter, or you can read the whole manual first and then go back and do the Workbook sections. If you read the entire manual first, you may want to re-read each chapter of *Listen To Your Gut* again right before beginning the corresponding Workbook section in order to stimulate your thoughts and feelings.

The Workbook is formatted so that you can print it out and write your answers directly on the pages. I suggest you get a binder for your *Healing Journey Workbook*, and if you need extra room to write certain answers, then just insert a blank page where needed. Alternatively, if you prefer, you can get yourself a spiral-bound notebook, or an esthetically pleasing diary notebook of some sort (something that feels special), and write down your Workbook answers, thoughts and ideas in your special notebook. You could title the notebook "My Healing Journey" (or something similar) and keep it for any future exercises or writings you might have.

The important thing is to actually *write down* your answers to the questions in the *Healing Journey Workbook*. Just answering them in your head will *not* result in the same enlightenment and integration as that of committing your thoughts to physical form. Also, you'll need to have your answers written down, as you'll be using them to compile your summary for *Jini's Optimum Treatment Plan* – outlined below.

Yes, it will be difficult. Yes, you'll probably be tempted to put off actually doing it. Wading through the jungle of our Self is a difficult and time-consuming process. But if you want to restore yourself to wholeness, then you must take the time and you must discipline yourself to face your tangled jungle, one step at a time. Don't be discouraged, you don't need to sit down and go through every page at once. You could choose the easiest chapter for you to start with and simply begin there. Take as much time as you need to thoroughly work through your issues and practices involved with that section of the Workbook and make the necessary changes. Then you may need to take a break and just 'be' for a while. Excellent!

> The *Healing Journey Workbook* is perhaps the most important part of this program. The knowledge and techniques in this program can only help you if you put them into practice.

Then, when you feel ready to handle the next step, go back and choose another chapter to work on. Get ready to see your weaknesses transformed into strengths and your limitations into opportunities as you reclaim your natural state of wholeness and completeness.

Treatment Summaries

By the time you finish reading *Listen To Your Gut* your head will probably be swimming with the mass of information contained here. The Treatment Summaries folder provides you with a bullet-point outline, or broad-strokes map, of how to pull all the relevant information together for your particular condition. There are three separate action plans in the Treatment Summaries folder that give you a step-by-step summarized treatment plan for what you need to do to heal yourself. Some plans are more thorough and comprehensive than others. For example, for the first plan, you'll need to have completed the *Healing Journey Workbook*. The other two plans are for you to use if you haven't yet completed the Workbook. Therefore, you can choose which plan to follow depending on your current motivation, energy, and time available:

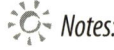
Notes:

- ▶ ***Jini's Optimum Treatment Plan*** – This is the best plan to ensure whole body healing. It guides you through creating your unique, customized, Optimum Treatment Plan based on your answers in the *Healing Journey Workbook*. This is the best treatment plan of the three offered, since it is the most thorough plan, and completely customized to your specific needs. *Jini's Optimum Treatment Plan* presents you with the highest chance of success in implementing the healing protocols in this program. However, you need to have completed the *Healing Journey Workbook* in order to fill out this plan.

- ▶ ***Jini's General Treatment Plan*** – If you haven't had time yet, or don't want to complete the *Healing Journey Workbook*, then this plan contains a summary of generalized treatments for each illness (IBS, diverticulosis, colitis, Crohn's). Using a General Treatment Plan is not as good as compiling your own, individualized Optimum Treatment Plan, but it is the next best thing.

▶ *Jini's Quick & Easy Treatment Plan* – This plan is a list of quick-action points, for those of you who don't have the time or energy to follow either the Optimum Treatment, or General Treatment plans. Even if you just implement the first item on this list, you'll see an improvement in your health. Once you see an improvement, maybe you'll then have the energy or motivation to implement one of the more comprehensive treatment plans.

Health Assessment & Tracking Tools

These are a collection of charts and questionnaires that give you a self-assessment method of mapping out your current symptoms and understanding what your symptoms are telling you about your state of health or dis-ease in the various systems of your body (e.g., nervous, endocrine, digestive, etc.). I have also included some tests to evaluate whether you have a *Candida albicans* (yeast) infection underlying your IBS or IBD. The Symptom Tracking Charts then provide you with a concise way of tracking and monitoring your symptoms at a glance.

You will be directed in the *Healing Journey Workbook*, and in the Treatment Summaries, to fill out these tests and charts at various points throughout the program. Since the tools are on CD, you can print them out and fill them in as often as you need to, and then keep them in a file for reference and comparison. This will help you to track your progress and also to pinpoint areas that need addressing. Again, remember what I wrote earlier in this chapter about the holistic healing process: As your body heals, it can suddenly unmask a deeply-seated imbalance that you were not previously aware of, and offer it up for healing. When your digestive system is so ill (for example) you may not be aware that your endocrine/hormonal system is in serious trouble – because your digestive system is more urgent, and healing that takes all your attention and energy. However, as you heal your digestive system, your body may feel it's time to draw your attention to your endocrine system, so you can focus on healing that. The Health Assessment & Tracking Tools will provide you with methods of assessing and tracking this process, and guiding you on what to address next.

☼ Get ready to see your weaknesses transformed into strengths and your limitations into opportunities as you reclaim your natural state of wholeness and completeness.

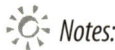 Notes:

PROGRAM IMPLEMENTATION

Choose the area from this program that is easiest for you to work on and begin with that first. As anyone with intestinal problems knows, stress is the number one trigger and inflamer of these disorders, so don't increase your stress (or your child's stress, if your child is the one who's ill) in your efforts to heal yourself or your child! Just take it slowly and easily, realize and accept that you're on a long, winding path and there are no miracle cures or quick-fix remedies. Your dis-ease (unease) encompasses your environment, upbringing, past issues/occurrences, financial state, career satisfaction or lack thereof, diet, family, intimate relationships, lifestyle, stress, stability, security, peace, self-love, exercise, genetic make-up, your doctor-patient relationship and drugs ingested, to name a few.

The diets, therapies, and techniques in this program demand that you take full responsibility for your health and healing, and appoint only yourself as your final, ultimate authority. Do not give this authority away to anyone, not to me, not to your physician, your naturopathic or homeopathic doctor, your spouse or parent. You have everything you need to heal yourself – it is your responsibility, and you are the only trustworthy repository of final authority for your body/mind/spirit. There are many pathways to healing. This program may comprise part, or all, of your pathway. Only you know what's best for you, only you possess the map of your Healing Journey.

All the information included in this program is of my own personal opinion and experience. My only intent is that you examine it from your point of view, take what you need, adapt whatever you want, and feel free to discard whatever you don't need. Some of the information and ideas presented in this program may be difficult for you to accept. Some of my approach (e.g., no pharmaceutical drugs) may be too radical and you may feel it's not safe for you – no problem! Just listen to yourself and only do what you feel comfortable with. You know yourself better than I do and you should certainly stick to what you feel is true and works best for you. I often got emails from readers saying, "I'm going to follow your program because I feel I can trust you, so I'm going to do what you say." And I would write back saying, "No, do NOT give your power and authority away! Use my programs as a resource or guidebook, but always trust yourself first and foremost. You are the only one who knows the best/right path for your body."

It will probably take you quite a while to work through and incorporate the diets, protocols and therapies outlined in this program, but it will also be well worth it. Imagine what it would be like to be 100% drug free. Imagine what it would be like to go for years without seeing your gastroenterologist (intestinal specialist), or having to go through any more torturous scans and scopes. Imagine what it would feel like to go to yourself first whenever you have a flare or attack (or healing crisis) and be able to deal with and heal the fear and pain without having to rush to the emergency room or resort to damaging drugs or surgery. Yes, the path is difficult, and time-consuming, and at times nothing can be more frustrating than having to face your own self. However, as you begin to achieve this freedom, you'll also come to realize, beyond a shadow of a doubt, that nothing is more worthwhile.

Turn now to the *Healing Journey Workbook* – on the *Listen To Your Gut CD* – and complete the section for Chapter One.

> As anyone with intestinal problems knows, stress is the number one trigger and inflamer of these disorders, so don't turn 'healing yourself' into one more stressor!

2

Supplements & Treatment Protocols

"The most commonly accepted fallacy is that using herbs is really a primitive form of medicine. But what would you say if I told you that in 1965, over 130 million prescription drugs were written which came from plants? Or if I told you that over 75% of the hormones used in medicine today are derived completely from plants?

It hardly does justice to herbs to call them primitive and backward, and at the same time, to label drugs as advanced and modern, when so many drugs are in fact derived from herbs. But there's more. All drugs which are extracted out of plants are not in a whole natural state. This is the reason there are so many side effects, which is a medical problem in itself.

For example, everyone has heard of quinine. Quinine is very efficient in reducing fever, especially malarial fever. This drug comes from the Peruvian bark in South America. You can take all the Peruvian bark tea you want and you won't have any problems. But take a little too much of the quinine extracted from the Peruvian bark and you will grow deaf. Take a still larger dose and you will die."

Dr. John R. Christopher, ND, MH

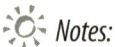 Notes:

The herbal remedies in this chapter have been organized according to which symptom they relieve or heal. Therefore, certain multi-functional remedies are listed more than once, as they're useful for relieving more than one symptom. In this way, you can pick and choose the healing remedies that are appropriate for your specific set of symptoms. Or, if you have a new symptom appear, you can quickly look up what you need to do to heal that particular condition. Supplementing with these herbs is a relatively easy endeavor that you can get started on right away and see a significant improvement in your health and well-being fairly quickly.

USING THE SUPPLEMENTS IN THIS PROGRAM

Make a list of your current symptoms now, and as you read through the chapter you can note down which herbs and supplements will address your particular condition. Of course, many symptoms are often interrelated and/or share a common root cause, and I've tried to point this out where applicable. A cornerstone treatment for healing the root cause of many IBD symptoms is eradicating pathogenic (disease-causing) microorganisms (like yeast, fungus, bad bacteria, viruses, parasites, etc.) from the gut environment, and then re-populating the gut with beneficial bacteria. Also key is healing the mucosal lining and restoring/repairing the intestinal wall. This is accomplished by eliminating pathogenic or infectious microorganisms (see *Natural Antibiotics / Antimicrobials* section) followed by probiotic supplementation (see *Probiotic Supplementation* section), and supplementing with substances that specifically heal the mucosal lining and repair gastrointestinal tissue. As this process takes several weeks (or months) to complete, along with this foundational treatment I also provide other remedies that provide quick relief from the symptom. Therefore, you can obtain immediate relief from your diarrhea (for example) whilst simultaneously addressing the root cause, which will provide long-term resolution of the problem.

Use Herbal Medicines Holistically

Many people in the Western world who have embraced herbal/plant-based medicine are still automatically using it within the parameters of Western (modern) medicine. People are using herbal supplements in the same manner as they use drugs – once they find a supplement that helps them, they take it every day, indefinitely. This does not fit the paradigm of holistic healing. Proper use of herbal medicine involves using the supplement(s) to address/heal the root cause of the imbalances in your body. Once your body is balanced (i.e. healed) then you don't need to keep using those supplements. If you continue to use an herbal medicine your body no longer has a need for, you'll just unbalance your body again in another way. Holistic (whole body, integrated) health is about balance. It's not about taking handfuls of supplements for the rest of your life. Now, in order to heal yourself you may very well have to take a lot of supplements, for a number of years even (depending on how ill, or out of balance your body is). But know this: The point of this program is to help you to heal the root cause(s) of your dis-ease and lead a strong, healthy, natural life – where ongoing health is maintained via natural foods, exercise, and emotional and spiritual health, not by being reliant on handfuls of supplements, the way everyone else takes handfuls of pills. Don't necessarily look to supplement companies for guidance on this, as like pharmaceutical companies, they make their money from your illness or imbalance, so they have a vested interest in your ingesting their products on an ongoing basis. It's worrying that medical doctors (MDs) gain money/perks from getting us to use certain medications. But likewise, many naturopathic doctors (NDs) sell products right from their clinics – while I realize this practice helps to keep the actual visit with the naturopath affordable, this arrangement hardly fosters an unbiased view of supplement use.

> The point of this program is to help you to heal the root cause(s) of your dis-ease and lead a strong, healthy, natural life – where ongoing health is maintained via natural foods, exercise, and emotional and spiritual health, not by being reliant on handfuls of supplements, the way everyone else takes handfuls of pills.

Make Sure Products Meet Label Claims

If a product that I've recommended is not available at your local health pharmacy, consult Appendix C for the relevant contact information so you or your pharmacy can order the product in. Also, keep in mind that when buying products from a health pharmacy (particularly liquid or chewable products) you can usually take the product back if you don't like the taste of it. Ask about the store's refund policy before purchasing and be sure to keep your receipt. You also need to make sure that the supplement you're buying actually meets its label claims. Up to 80% of the supplements on the market today do not contain what they claim; in fact, many of them only contain 15 – 20% of their label claim. Therefore, it's important to purchase products from reputable companies who carry out independent testing/confirmation of their label claims. Some reliable supplement manufacturers at this time include Nature's Way, Eclectic Institute, Enzymatic Therapy, Allergy Research Group, and AOR (Advanced Orthomolecular Research). However, health companies are bought and sold all the time and new owners may not adhere to the same standards of quality. You can ask the health store personnel which companies carry out independent testing to confirm product quality, or, you can contact the supplement companies directly and ask them to fax you the independent lab assay confirming their product meets their label claim.

Now, having said all that, I have also put together an online Holistic Health Shoppe in response to readers telling me of their frustration, difficulty and hassle in finding all the recommended products. I got so many emails from readers saying, "I can't find any of "X", can you just tell me where to go to get some??" So, if you wish, you can go to: *www.LTYGshoppe.com* and there you will find – all in one place – all of the products that I recommend in my programs. I have also done the homework for you in vetting the reliability of manufacturers, making sure the products actually meet label claims. This online natural health store ships worldwide, so no matter where you are, if you're having trouble finding the appropriate products, you can order from the Holistic Health Shoppe. For those of you that prefer to source your own products, or have your local health store order them in, I've provided detailed contact information for every recommended product manufacturer in Appendix C at the back of the book.

> ☼ Remember, you can order almost every product recommended in this program from my online health store, we're open 24 hours a day, 7 days a week, and we ship worldwide:
>
> **LTYG HOLISTIC HEALTH SHOPPE**
> www.LTYGshoppe.com
> Toll free: 1.888.866.7745
> Tel: +1.360.384.8632
>
> Even if you don't want to use the Holistic Health Shoppe, feel free to view the listings for products that have been chosen and approved by me – so as to not aggravate your sensitive system – then you'll know exactly which brands to get at your local health store.

Products I've Formulated

I have personally formulated three of the products recommended in this program: Absorb Plus, MucosaHeal and FissureHeal. I'm approached every so often by people/companies wanting me to formulate a product (especially probiotics!) but my response is very simple: Is someone already doing a top quality product of that type? If the answer's yes, then I'm not really motivated to add just one more of the same to the marketplace. However, I do get really excited about formulating products for which there is a clear need, but nothing decent available. I also like to innovate, to take something and make it ten times better. The story of how I came to formulate Absorb Plus is available online at their website *(www.absorbplus.com)* so I won't repeat it here. The story of how FissureHeal came to be is quite funny, so I will relate it here.

My motivation for developing FissureHeal suppositories came from myself. I would repeatedly get rectal fissures and there was nothing available to heal them aside from steroid suppositories (which I would not use) and some herbal suppositories for hemorrhoids that might have worked; but once I got a look at the size of them, there was no way I was going to insert them into my narrowed, already wounded rectum! So I put on my thinking cap, and after numerous experiments, came up with my own formula that I melted down and poured into drinking straws as the mold. Perfect width and I could make them really long to reach a fissure that may be higher up in the rectal canal, if I wished. However, getting them out of the drinking straws was a very difficult endeavour; involving much struggle, mess and breakage. Nevertheless, I was happy because at last I had a suppository that would heal up my fissures very quickly. Of course, word spread once I started giving a few suppositories to people who were really desperate. But no one wanted to cook them up in their kitchen as I was doing. As one guy said after I gave him the recipe to make his own, "I can hardly cook, there's no way I'm gonna be able to make these! Can't you do them for me and I'll pay you?"

Then a local midwife and some postpartum mothers asked me for some as they all had rectal fissures that wouldn't heal since giving birth from 2 – 6

> I get really excited about formulating products for which there is a clear need, but nothing decent available.

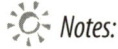
Notes:

years ago! How could I turn down people in pain like that? Well, the night I found myself struggling to remove suppositories from drinking straws at midnight, I turned to my husband and said, "This is ridiculous. We've got to find someone who'll manufacture these properly and then I can just tell everyone to go buy them from there!" My husband is a former advertising executive and he's the salesman and dealmaker in our family, so he went to work. The result is that FissureHeal suppositories – which took six months to find a way to mass-produce and are still made by hand – are now available to anyone who wants them and I'll never have to squeeze them out of a drinking straw mold again!

The company that makes FissureHeal *(www.fissureheal.com)* also manufactures an intestinal/mucosal lining product I formulated called MucosaHeal. There are other products in this category already on the market (Robert's Formula being the most well-known) but MucosaHeal is my ideal formula, designed to minimize the risk of any adverse reactions (always a concern with multiple-herb products), whilst containing the substances that I feel are most beneficial. When you read the list of ingredients and what they do (in the sections below) you'll see why I feel it's currently the best product in its class.

What If I'm Not Seeing Results?

Herbal therapies can be very effective. However, I've found that dosages and concentrations that are fine for most people are not always fine for people with sensitive digestive tracts. Keep these factors in mind when you're trying a new remedy. Go slowly – maybe starting at half the normal/prescribed dose – and watch closely for any adverse reactions. I've received countless emails from readers who are following the guidelines and supplements in this program, but not experiencing the desired relief. When I ask them for a complete list of all the supplements they're taking, I discover they're also simultaneously ingesting supplements that directly aggravate the symptom they're trying to resolve!

I had a phone consultation once with a reader named Eric who had colitis. At the time he called me, he was bedridden from weakness and weight loss. Eric was having approximately forty bloody bowel movements per day, and could no longer even get up to go to the toilet. He wore diapers constantly, which his wife changed for him throughout the day and night. I had his wife go and get all the supplements, vitamins, protein powders, etc. that he was ingesting and we went through the ingredient list on each one. We discovered that Eric was ingesting four different supplements that cause diarrhea in people with sensitive digestive systems! Obviously, the supplements were not the sole cause of his extreme diarrhea, but they certainly were contributing to, and exacerbating the problem.

You'll see the best results from this program if you only take the supplements recommended here. Afterwards, if your naturopathic doctor recommends other supplements that you want to try, then test them one by one, making sure they're safe and compatible with your body. Also, keep in mind that many of the drugs your medical doctor prescribes will cause problems in your body that are just as bad, and often worse, than the symptom you're using them to suppress – pharmaceutical companies refer to this damage as 'side effects'. I'll discuss this more in detail in Chapter Five. For now just keep in mind that if you're not seeing the desired results from these supplements, you need to take a look at what else you're ingesting that might be interfering with their healing action.

Unfortunately, medical, naturopathic and homeopathic physicians do not always know what's safe for people with IBD/IBS. They will recommend a supplement that works well for most people, but unbeknownst to them, it will aggravate the sensitive gut of someone with IBD. For example, MSM (methylsulfonylmethane) is routinely used as an anti-inflammatory. However, as it is a sulfur-based compound, it often causes gas, bloating and sometimes spasming in people with IBD or IBS. Aloe vera is another problem remedy – most brands of aloe vera do not have all of the aloin removed. Now in most people aloin is very healing and contains many powerful and active components that greatly assist the body – hence the reason it's usually included in aloe vera products. However, for people with IBD, aloin is a very aggravating substance and can result in increased diarrhea and cramping. Therefore, when I recommend aloe vera juice, I

> In every single phone consultation I've had to date, the client has been ingesting herbal supplements that directly aggravate the symptoms they're trying to resolve.

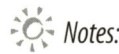 Notes:

stipulate that it *must* be George's 'Always Active' Aloe Vera Juice as this is the only brand I've found that removes 100% of the aloin, whilst leaving the rest of the highly beneficial healing compounds in place.

When I stipulate that you must buy a certain brand, I'm doing so for two reasons: Firstly, it's the only brand I know of that will give you the desired results, and secondly, other brands could be ineffective, or aggravate your condition. My recommendations are based on years of testing by thousands of people with IBD or IBS, so please do not try to substitute another brand where specified, or you may risk aggravating your condition and setting your healing back considerably. I do not receive financial compensation from the products I recommend and if a product suddenly changes quality or formulation, I will notify you as soon as I become aware of it.
To receive these updates, keep your email current with Caramal Publishing by emailing *service@listentoyourgut.com* if you change your email address, or, simply check the Listen To Your Gut – Book Updates page at *www.ListenToYourGut.com* regularly.

In every single phone consultation I've had to date, the client has been ingesting herbal supplements that directly aggravate the symptoms they're trying to heal. To help you avoid making this mistake, stick to only the supplements recommended in this program, and make sure any supplement you ingest does not contain any of the following:

- ▶ Methylsulfonylmethane (MSM)
- ▶ Fructooligosaccharides (FOS), inulin, or other prebiotics, or indigestible starches
- ▶ Bacterial Soil Organisms (SO's, SBO's, HSO's, etc.)
- ▶ Betaine HCL
- ▶ Peppermint (unless enteric-coated)
- ▶ Blueberries, cherries or citrus fruits
- ▶ Ascorbic Acid
- ▶ High levels of Magnesium

You must carefully read the labels on every single supplement you take, including vitamins and minerals. Or, you can simply buy your supplements at my online LTYG Holistic Health Shoppe, where I've already screened all the supplements for you, to ensure they're safe for people with IBD and IBS: *www.LTYGshoppe.com*.

HOW TO INTRODUCE SUPPLEMENTS

Herbs and other natural substances can be just as powerful as drugs, so you want to be sure you're effecting the appropriate action in your body and gut – and not simultaneously sabotaging your healing with an aggravating supplement. In light of these factors, I recommend you follow this regimen for putting together your herbal supplement treatment protocol:

1. Immediately stop taking ALL herbal and natural supplements (even if prescribed by a naturopathic physician, Chinese medicine doctor or herbalist). Allow one week to clear any effects.

2. Then, introduce the supplements recommended in this program, one at a time, leaving a few days to a week in between to check for any adverse reactions. The supplements recommended in this program are the safest and have been trial-tested by thousands with IBD. When you've introduced all the supplements you want to try from this program, stay on just these supplements for a month.

3. Next, introduce any other supplements you wish (or those recommended by other sources, physicians, etc.) but make sure you test them one at a time, leaving at least two weeks in between each one to test for adverse reactions or signs of intolerance. Be especially cautious when testing Chinese or Ayurvedic remedies that often contain a number of herbs or substances mixed together – these have the highest possibility for aggravation or intolerance.

When I stipulate that you must buy a certain brand, I'm doing so for two reasons: Firstly, it's the only brand I know of that will give you the desired results, and secondly, other brands could be ineffective, or aggravate your condition.

Notes:

Young Children Or Pregnancy

For very young children and babies, or if you're pregnant, it's very important to check with your naturopathic physician (or do some quality research online) before supplementing with these or any other herbs. I can't possibly advise you on whether a supplement is safe for your baby, or if you're pregnant, because I don't know what other conditions/complications you or your baby may have. Since babies are so precious, it's best to err on the side of caution. Before each *Symptom Treatment Summary* (below) I do tell you when I have personally used a supplement whilst pregnant or breastfeeding, or on my own babies/children. But keep in mind, I am only relating my own, personal experience and beyond that you will have to take responsibility and check with your naturopathic or holistic physician before using any supplement. There are no clinical trials that have been conducted on any of these herbal products on babies or pregnant women, so any examples I give you are strictly anecdotal. When in doubt about the appropriate dosage for children, either start really low and gradually work up to 1/4 of the recommended adult dosage to begin with, or use this simple formula to determine the appropriate dose:

Young's Formula

$$\frac{\text{Age in years}}{\text{Age} + 12} = \text{portion of the adult dose}$$

For example, the correct dose for a 6 year old child would be:

$$\frac{6}{6+12} = \frac{6}{18} = \frac{1}{3} \text{ of the adult dose}$$

Again, your naturopath will also be able to give you some guidelines on which herbs are safe for your child and a recommended dosage. For optimal absorption, it's best to ingest a smaller amount of the supplement, several times a day, rather than one dose all at once. However, if this is too much hassle for you, then take it only once or twice a day, or whatever works best for your schedule. It's better to take a supplement once a day than not at all.

Formulation Guidelines

When buying any herbal preparation or vitamin/mineral, make sure it's free of additives and fillers (yeast, starch, sugar, etc.). Look first for a brand that's certified organic, or harvested in the wild. If you're like me and can't or hate to swallow pills, check around because most herbal remedies are available in liquid form. Liquids are also easier to digest and absorb, as people with IBD can have very rapid transit times through the gastrointestinal tract. Therefore pills or capsules often do not have enough time to be broken down or absorbed properly. So even if you can swallow pills, I recommend you use liquid or powder preparations whenever possible. Some liquid herbs are only available in a high alcohol base and the alcohol can trigger intestinal bleeding. The solution is to put the herb in warm/hot water, which causes the alcohol to evaporate (let it sit for a few minutes), and then drink it. However, don't buy a liquid preparation of an herb or vitamin that also contains a lot of other ingredients (usually to make it taste better or improve absorption for normal people) as these other ingredients can often aggravate your sensitive gut. It's best to get either an herbal tincture (prepared in just alcohol or glycerin) or a straight powder (or capsules that you can open to release the powder) that you can then mix in water or apple juice. A very easy way to take your supplements is to whip them all in a blender in a protein or weight gain shake (more on this later in the chapter).

> Through trial and error, from myself and thousands of readers, we have sifted through those herbal treatments that produce positive results to find the *most* effective treatments with the lowest possible risk of intolerance.

SYMPTOMS & RECOMMENDED TREATMENTS

Following are the herbal treatments that I have found *most* effective, listed under the specific symptom or condition that they relieve. Through trial and error by myself and thousands of readers, we have sifted through those herbal treatments that produce positive results to find the most effective treatments with the lowest possible risk of intolerance. Those of you who have the first edition of this book will notice that there are a few remedies recommended in the earlier edition, that are no longer recommended here. This doesn't mean that those remedies don't work; it means that together we've narrowed it down to the remedies that work the best. And those are the remedies that are listed here in this Revised, Expanded Edition.

Herbal supplements can also be loosely categorized into those that primarily address the symptom, and those that address the root cause of the symptom. In general, supplements that alleviate symptoms tend to work very quickly and those that heal the root cause take much longer. Therefore, I've tried to provide a good balance of both of these healing tools for each symptom, so that you can still get quick relief whilst working on the root-level, long-term healing of your condition. Obviously, because these substances are healing by nature, there will be a fair amount of overlap between categories.

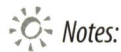 Notes:

To give you an example: For Heartburn (Acid Reflux), George's Aloe Vera Juice and DGL lozenges both provide very effective, quick relief (symptoms). And over time, both will provide some healing of the root cause of heartburn. But, *L. acidophilus* is what's needed to really heal the root cause of acid reflux, because until you balance the bacteria in your stomach and achieve the pH needed for proper digestion and acid production, you will always tend towards heartburn. However, although a proper implantation and colonization of good bacteria can take two to three months to establish, acidophilus will also provide varying degrees of immediate symptomatic relief as well (how much, how quickly, depends on the person).

So, at the end of the list of treatments for each symptom is a *Symptom Treatment Summary*; which gives you a quick-action plan for relieving that particular symptom. Please note that the points in these Symptom Treatment Summaries are listed in order of importance, or, according to which supplement I feel will deliver the most effective relief, or, in the shortest amount of time. I have also tried to point out (wherever applicable) the delineation between supplements that primarily address symptoms (and therefore provide the quickest relief) and those that may take longer to work, but are still crucial, since they address the root cause of the symptom.

❋ ANEMIA

This is a condition with a fair degree of controversy involved. Some researchers and naturopathic doctors say that it's very difficult for the body to absorb iron supplements and that taking extra iron actually promotes intestinal infection. They maintain that the only way to treat anemia is by improving absorption. However, your medical doctor and other naturopaths will still stick with iron supplementation as the best way to treat anemia. My own experience over the course of ten years with anemia has led me to a combined position: I've found you need to both take an iron supplement and improve absorption to see any significant results. You also need to make sure that the type of iron you're taking is one that can be easily absorbed by your body. However, before you begin any iron supplementation, have your doctor do a blood test to ascertain that your anemia is not just due to a vitamin B12 or B6 deficiency, which can be remedied simply with B6/B12 supplementation.

Inorganic iron derived from rock or 'iron salts' is not compatible with our bodies and therefore we can only absorb about 3% of this type of iron. This is why many forms of iron are hard on your body and cause constipation and iron toxicity. Some manufacturers add amino acids to these types of iron in an attempt to improve absorption, but this only increases the absorption ratio to about 10%. Alternatively, organic iron derived from plants and vegetables is much more readily accepted by our system. It sometimes comes in a complex of other minerals, amino acids, enzymes and vitamins and/or is already protein-bound for easy absorption and utilization by the body. This type of iron is also less likely to constipate you. Following is what I've found to be the most effective way of increasing your hemoglobin:

If you're taking an iron supplement and experiencing intestinal bleeding, stop. Large doses of iron can be irritating and unless you're quite healed it may re-open your wounds and trigger bleeding. This may be because iron is one of the more powerful free radical generators. If it is not used or absorbed properly, excess free radicals can cause tissue damage (and premature aging). Therefore, my recommendation is to adhere to the Healing Diets and take the recommended healing supplements until you've had no bleeding for one month. Then you can start to slowly re-introduce the iron supplement. You should also be drinking ¼ of a cup of George's

☼ Large doses of iron can be irritating and unless you're quite healed it may re-open your wounds and trigger intestinal bleeding

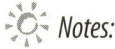 Notes:

aloe vera juice every day. Begin with one capsule or one teaspoon of liquid iron at lunch or supper every other day. Auxima Fera is the liquid brand I prefer, or Floradix brand with no alcohol and no preservatives is also good. However, the absolute best iron supplement I've ever found is Ferrasorb by Thorne Research Inc. (in Canada it's now called Ferra-Complex by Selekta). It comes in capsule form together with vitamin B12 and folic acid.

The powder in the capsules dissolves easily into liquid and is by far the most easily absorbed, non-irritating brand I've ever tried. I've used Ferrasorb to raise my hemoglobin 3 points in one month (3 – 4 capsules per day), and I've heard nothing but good reports from all my readers who have used it. It really is a fantastic product and I recommend you try it first.

The only difficulty with this product is that Thorne Research Inc. does not sell directly to consumers, they only sell to physicians and some herbal pharmacies that carry it require a prescription from a naturopathic or medical doctor before they'll sell it to you. If you have difficulty getting it, you can order it online from our LTYG Holistic Health Shoppe (*www.LTYGshoppe.com*). If you're worried about iron triggering bleeding, then drink your aloe vera juice first, followed by your iron, followed by your meal. It's best if your meal also contains certified organic liver or some other iron-rich food. Take one capsule or one teaspoon every other day, or, once every three days.

Pay attention to your body, if you see any streaks of blood in your stool or in the toilet bowl, stop taking the iron and see if the bleeding ceases fairly quickly. If it does, it may have been caused by the iron supplementation and you might want to give your body more time to heal and then try again in another month or two. If you're tolerating the iron well, continue on the dosage for a week or two and then increase it to one teaspoon or one capsule (25 mg.) every day. Again, monitor for signs of intolerance and either lower the dosage, or stop for a week or two and then begin again. The key is to listen to your body. If all goes well, keep increasing the dosage slowly until you're up to a tablespoon per day (or three 25 mg. capsules per day) or every other day – whatever dosage works best for you. Remember to keep taking the George's aloe vera juice for as long as you're taking the iron (if you're prone to bleeding).

At the same time as you're supplementing with iron, try to eat as much and as many iron-rich foods as you can tolerate (depending on where you're at in your healing process). These include red meat, spinach, green seaweed (particularly dulse), broccoli, blackstrap molasses, cow's liver, etc. Try to eat organic produce and hormone/drug-free meat and liver – if you can't get certified organic liver, then it's best not to eat it at all since the liver is a storehouse for all the animal's toxins.

You also simultaneously need to increase your absorption of iron. The following vitamins are absolutely necessary in order for your body to absorb iron:

- Vitamin C
- Vitamin B12
- Folic Acid
- B Group of Vitamins

If you go to a health pharmacy, you should be able to get folic acid and B12 together in a liquid and you just put a few drops under your tongue each day. Otherwise, get your doctor to give you a prescription for 4mg. pills of folate (folic acid), then go to a health store and get some sublingual B12 pills. Also get a vitamin B group capsule or liquid and 500-1000mg chewable tablets of vitamin C. If you find vitamin C gives you diarrhea, only take 500 mg, or make sure you take your vitamin C in mineral ascorbate form (e.g. vitamin C as calcium ascorbate). Vitamin C in mineral ascorbate form causes no diarrhea whatsoever unless it's in magnesium ascorbate form, in which case large amounts of magnesium may contribute to diarrhea. Numerous companies make a powdered Vitamin C that dissolves in water (some contain additional vitamins and minerals as well) so you can drink it along with your dinner for added absorption. A really easy and delicious way to take your vitamin C at dinner (or any other time) is by using Emergen-C drink packets by Alacer Corp. You just add water and it makes

☼ Iron-rich foods include organic red meat, spinach, green seaweed (particularly dulse), broccoli, blackstrap molasses (use in baking or on hot cereals in place of sugar) and organic cow's liver.

a really delicious drink. The vitamin C is in mineral ascorbate form so you may be able take up to 10,000 mg per day with no diarrhea. I've been using this product for years (my favorite flavors are raspberry, cranberry and cola) and I regularly take 2000 – 3000 mg per day (1000 mg per packet) and when I'm sick or stressed I increase it to 6000 mg per day. Try to sip these drinks slowly as vitamin C is absorbed very rapidly, but also goes through rapidly to urine if your body doesn't use it right away. Sipping slowly gives your body more time to actually utilise the vitamin C.

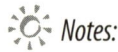
Notes:

If you're deficient in folic acid, then don't take it at the same time as vitamin C. Both folate and vitamin C are essential for iron absorption, however, they tend to interfere with the absorption of each other so don't ingest them at the same time. If you don't have a folate deficiency, then don't worry about this. To facilitate absorption further, liquid chlorophyll and homeopathic iron supplements work very well also, but are not essential.

Chlorophyll

Best absorbed in liquid form. This is an excellent blood-builder, it promotes energy and is an internal disinfectant. It also improves all blood disorders (including blood sugar disorders and anemia), cleanses the liver and the digestive tract. Because it has a cleansing action on the digestive tract, it may trigger diarrhea for some people. If you find yourself sensitive to this either reduce the dose or take it every third day. If your diarrhea continues, then stop taking the chlorophyll and save it for a later date when your system's had a chance to heal and calm down a bit more. Make sure you get a brand of chlorophyll that has no added flavors, preservatives, etc. It should be just pure chlorophyll and water. Follow directions on the bottle, but start with only ¼ – ½ of the recommended dose, and slowly increase according to tolerance. If possible, it's best to divide up the dosage so you're ingesting it 2-3 times a day (better for absorption than taking the whole dose at once). Continue taking until your hemoglobin levels are normal-high and you have plenty of energy, or until your intuition tells you to stop or take a break for a while. The taste is very mild, even pleasant – unlike wheatgrass (another source of chlorophyll), which is very strong-tasting and made me gag after a few doses. Don't use it if you're having intestinal bleeding or severe diarrhea and don't buy a brand that has other ingredients added (e.g., peppermint). Refrigerate after opening.

Homeopathic Iron

Homeopathic Iron (Ferrum phosphoricum) supplements are also very easily absorbed. They do not actually contain iron, but work energetically to facilitate the uptake of iron. Take five pellets, twice a day. Don't touch the pellets with your hands, shake out 5 pellets into the cap of the bottle and then drop them directly into your mouth, under your tongue, and let them dissolve. Take homeopathic remedies 20 minutes before or after you've had anything to eat or drink. Don't use strong essential oils (like peppermint, eucalyptus or wild oregano) or coffee whilst using homeopathic remedies. The pellets are quite palatable and just taste like sugar pills. The point is to allow the pellets to be absorbed directly by the blood vessels that are near the surface under your tongue (sublingual). Continue this process of supplementation until your hemoglobin levels are normal-high, you have plenty of energy, or until your intuition tells you to stop or take a break for a while.

> Both folate and vitamin C are essential for iron absorption, however, they tend to interfere with the absorption of each other so don't ingest them at the same time.

Intravenous Iron Infusion

If your anemia is extreme enough (around 6.0 g/l or lower) for your doctor to strongly recommend a blood transfusion, then suggest trying an intravenous iron infusion first (carries less risk than a blood transfusion). This procedure is usually done on an out-patient basis and requires 1 – 3 treatments lasting approximately four hours each. A down-side to this treatment is that some people can have an allergic reaction to the iron. For both blood and iron infusions, I've found it really helpful to prepare my body to receive the substance. I hold the bag of iron (or blood) in my hands and lay it on my body. I thank the iron/blood for its gift to my body, I tell it that it is welcome in my body and that we're looking forward to it becoming one with us. I then 'sweep out' any negative or harmful elements that may be present (or you can pray that these be removed), thank it again for its gift to me and then hand it to the nurse to be hooked up. Whether

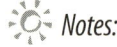 *Notes:*

this works because it actually effects change of some sort on an energetic level, or because it psychologically prepares my mind/body to accept the substance, I don't know. I just know that it works really well for me. If you have this treatment done, make sure you also follow the guidelines above for increasing iron absorption. During the infusion you may want to sip some liquid chlorophyll and vitamin C as well. Also, here are a few tips to make the IV needle insertion easier: Drink 1 – 2 glasses of water prior to your session and take a hot water bottle along with you. Lay the hot water bottle on top of your forearm (or wherever they want to insert the needle) for at least 5 – 10 minutes prior to insertion. The combination of the water ingested and the heat from the hot water bottle will cause your veins to swell up nice and big, so the nurse will be able to insert the needle quickly and easily. Take along a good book or a friend/spouse to chat to, as four hours sitting in a chair can be a long time!

Pregnancy/Breastfeeding/Babies: I have used Ferrasorb Iron, George's Aloe Vera and Emergen-C whilst pregnant and breastfeeding. I have also given all three to my kids as babies and toddlers (the Ferrasorb in very small amounts). A George's Aloe Vera distributor once told me about a customer who gave all three of her infants George's in a bottle or mixed with breastmilk/formula.

Symptom Treatment Summary – Anemia

- Take 1 – 4 capsules of Ferrasorb per day (in divided doses) with meals, accompanied by an Emergen-C vitamin C drink packet.
- Drink George's 'Always Active' Aloe Vera Juice before taking iron, if necessary.
- Make sure you're also taking a vitamin supplement that contains all the B vitamins, or, supplement separately with B complex.
- Use liquid chlorophyll or homeopathic iron to further facilitate absorption if needed.

☼ CONSTIPATION

You may find it easier to defecate if you place your feet on a child's stepping stool (or a couple of phone books). This raises your knees higher than your hips and more closely approximates a squatting position – the ideal position for opening the rectal canal and facilitating the quick passage of stool. Also, be sure and use the *Colonic Massage* method (in Chapter Six) before and during a bowel movement.

Probiotics

For a long term healing of constipation to take place, you need to improve the bacterial flora in your gut. The other remedies below will produce fairly quick results, but they are treatments that address the symptom, not the cause. Probiotics are one of the remedies that will heal the cause of your constipation. Ingesting good bacteria improves digestion, absorption and elimination of food. Certain strains of bacteria help produce digestive enzymes, peptides, amino acids and B vitamins for your body's use. They also inhibit or eliminate pathogenic microorganisms, like yeast, fungus, parasites, and bad bacteria. See the expanded section on *Probiotic Supplementation* later on in this chapter for more information and details. Currently, I only recommend Natren brand probiotics as they are the only company that currently meet basic, essential standards for quality and efficacy (see *Probiotic Supplementation* section for quality standards). You need to take the full spectrum of probiotics in either capsule (Healthy Trinity) or powder form (Megadophilus, Bifido Factor, Digesta-Lac). Ideally, take 1 capsule 1-2 times per day on an empty stomach. Or, take 1 tsp. of each powder mixed together in 8 ounces of room temperature filtered water three times per day on an empty stomach (20 minutes before food, or two hours after food) until you're no longer constipated. Then take one capsule once a day, or, the powders 1 – 2 times per day for the next three months. Then take as needed – let your bowel movements be your guide, if you start to get constipated again, start taking probiotics once a day (or more as needed). For faster treatment/results, kick off your probiotic regimen with a Probiotic Retention Enema (see *Probiotic Supplementation* section below for details) and then follow with the oral supplementation outlined here.

☼ Raising your knees higher than your hips more closely approximates a squatting position – the ideal position for opening the rectal canal and facilitating the quick passage of stool.

Psyllium

An effective remedy for constipation consists of using a psyllium-based fiber supplement mixed with half George's Roadrunner Aloe Vera Juice and half fruit juice. Take it first thing in the morning on an empty stomach. I recommend Aerobic Bulk Cleanse (ABC) from Aerobic Life Industries, which contains psyllium seed husks, licorice and hibiscus. Or, you can just buy straight psyllium seed powder from your health store (very inexpensive). If you don't like psyllium fiber supplements, then take apple pectin (500mg) instead. You may also want to experiment with herbal laxatives like senna leaf, but do not use them long-term. Equally important is to drink lots of spring or filtered water (10 glasses per day) and exercise regularly (at least do a daily stretching routine).

Vitamin C (Ascorbic Acid Form) & Magnesium

A quick and easy short-term remedy for constipation is to increase your vitamin C in ascorbic acid form (up to 10,000 mg/day) and/or magnesium (up to 1000 mg/day) intake, drink lots of water, and exercise (even if this just means walking around and stretching). Ascorbic acid and magnesium both have a laxative effect in higher doses. If you're still constipated after two weeks of that, then in an emergency, you can resort to an herbal laxative, like senna. For many people I suspect simply raising your intake of vitamin C and magnesium (up to 1000 mg/day) and drinking extra water (10 glasses/day) should alleviate your constipation. Remember though, for long-term permanent resolution of constipation, you need to ingest a full spectrum of Natren brand probiotics.

Pregnancy/Breastfeeding/Babies: I have used George's Aloe Vera, Natren probiotics and Emergen-C whilst pregnant and breastfeeding. I have also given them to my kids as babies (give babies ONLY Life Start – *B. infantis* – probiotic) and toddlers. A George's Aloe Vera distributor once told me about a customer who gave all three of her infants George's in a bottle or mixed with breastmilk/formula. There are no known contraindications for psyllium seed, but you would need to check with a naturopath before giving a baby high doses of mangnesium.

Symptom Treatment Summary – Constipation

▶ Take a full spectrum of Natren brand probiotic powders (Megadophilus, Bifido Factor, Digesta-Lac) 1 – 3 times per day until no longer constipated, or, take 1 Healthy Trinity capsule 1 – 2 times per day. Continue to take powders 1 – 2 times per day, or, capsule once a day for the next three months. Then take only as needed. Dosage consists of one capsule, or, 1 tsp. of each powder mixed in 8 ounces of room temperature filtered or spring water (no tap water!) on an empty stomach (20 minutes before food, or 2 hours after food).

▶ For quick relief, take Vit. C in ascorbic acid form (up to 10,000 mg per day) and magnesium (up to 1000 mg. per day) and drink 10 glasses of spring or filtered water per day.

▶ Take psyllium seed mixed with aloe vera juice and fruit juice.

Cramping/Spasming Intestines

Cramping and spasming in the intestines is usually due to the painful passage of gas and/or pain from intestinal inflammation or ulceration. For some reason, trapped gas hurts much more than trapped stool. See *Gas & Bloating* if you suspect your pain is due to copious or trapped gas. If you suspect your cramping is due to intestinal inflammation and/or ulceration, then see *Intestinal Inflammation, Ulceration, Bleeding* for remedies. When you solve the underlying problem, the pain will automatically disappear. Also, be aware of and look for emotional triggers that may need to be addressed. The fastest, most effective therapy for resolving emotional issues is EFT (see Chapter Six for more details). Don't underestimate the effect of emotions on the gut and keep in mind that pain pretty much always has an emotional component.

Pregnancy/Breastfeeding/Babies: EFT can be used very effectively on babies, toddlers and children (see Chapter Six for more details) and I've

---

☼ Cramping and spasming in the intestines is usually due to the painful passage of gas and/or pain from intestinal inflammation or ulceration. For some reason, trapped gas hurts much more than trapped stool.

used it with both my children. If you think the cramping/pain is due to trapped (or excessive) gas or stool, then please see my *BABY FART AEROBICS: And Other Natural Treatments for Colicky Babies* DVD. You can read all about it and watch a sample video clip of me demonstrating techniques on my 8-week-old daughter, Zara, by going to: *www.ColicInfant.com*

SYMPTOM TREATMENT SUMMARY – CRAMPING/SPASMING INTESTINES

▶ Pain always has an emotional component – use EFT (see Chapter Six) to resolve and release emotional issues from both the mind and body.

▶ If your cramping is due to abundant or trapped gas, then see GAS & BLOATING for remedies.

▶ If you think your cramping/pain is due to inflammation or ulceration, then see INTESTINAL INFLAMMATION, ULCERATION, BLEEDING for remedies.

DIARRHEA

Diarrhea can be caused by many, many factors. These can include any combination or singular occurrence of any of the following:

▶ Food allergies or intolerances

▶ A damaged mucosal lining

▶ Impaired digestion and absorption resulting in very rapid food transit times through the gastrointestinal tract

▶ Infection by pathogenic microorganisms – diarrhea is one of the mechanisms your body uses to expel pathogens or poisons as quickly as possible

▶ A colon that is incapable of absorbing water/fluid from stool

Notes:

- Result of prescription drug use
- Lack of 'good' bacteria in the gut
- Tense, spasming intestines

You can use the *Colonic Massage* method in Chapter Six whilst sitting on the toilet, to help you reduce bowel movement frequency. If your bum is getting sore from frequent bowel movements, then wipe your anus with 2-ply tissues (Kleenex) moistened with warm tap water after each bowel movement. Wear only 100% cotton underwear and natural fabric trousers, shorts, etc. Sleep bare-bum at night and make sure your sheets are 100% cotton. Be sure and follow the *Reduce Diarrhea Diet* in Chapter Three. Do not ingest any capsules or tablets if you're having more than four bowel movements per day – as they likely will not be absorbed properly. Open all capsules, mix the contents in liquid, and then drink.

Probiotics

For a long term resolution of diarrhea to take place, you need to improve the bacterial flora in your gut. The other remedies below will produce fairly quick results, but they are largely treatments that address the symptom, not the cause. Probiotics are one of the remedies that will address the cause of your diarrhea. Ingesting good bacteria improves digestion, absorption and elimination of food. Certain strains of bacteria help produce digestive enzymes, peptides, amino acids and B vitamins for your body's use. They also inhibit or eliminate pathogenic microorganisms, like yeast, fungus, parasites, and bad bacteria. See the expanded section on *Probiotic Supplementation* later on in this chapter for more information and details. Currently, I only recommend Natren brand probiotics as they are the only company I know of that currently meets the basic standards for probiotic quality and efficacy (see *Probiotic Supplementation* section for quality standards). You need to take the full spectrum of probiotics (Megadophilus, Bifido Factor, Digesta-Lac) in powder form only. Do not take the probiotics in capsule form as diarrhea indicates rapid transit time through the gut and the capsule may not have a chance to dissolve and disperse properly. Ideally, and for fastest relief, start probiotic supplementation with Jini's Probiotic

> ☼ Do not ingest any capsules or tablets if you're having more than four bowel movements per day – as they ikely will not be absorbed properly. Open all capsules, mix the contents in liquid, and then drink.

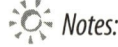 *Notes:*

Retention Enema (see *Probiotic Supplementation* section below) Then follow with oral supplementation: Take 1 tsp. of each powder mixed together in 8 ounces of room temperature filtered or spring water (no tap water!) 3 times per day on an empty stomach (15 – 20 minutes before food, or 2 hours after food) until you no longer have diarrhea. Depending on your whole-body health, you'll see improvements fairly soon, but complete elimination of diarrhea may take a year or more of supplementation, or it can be as quick as a couple of months. Then take 1 – 2 times per day for the next 3 months. Then take as needed – let your bowel movements be your guide, if your stools start getting loose again, start taking probiotics once a day (or more as needed).

While waiting for your gut flora to improve, you can also use the remedies below for quick relief – but keep in mind that you don't want to just take L-Glutamine or Bentonite Clay for the rest of your life. The goal is to heal the root cause(s) of diarrhea so that you can pass normal stool without having to use a supplement for years and years.

Dry Curd

This is simply cottage cheese without the surrounding milky liquid and it works well for mild diarrhea. Try to eat some for breakfast and you'll notice it begin to take effect within 24 – 48 hours. It's quite dry so a good way to eat it is with a well-ripened banana (which will also help alleviate diarrhea). If you have a lactose intolerance, you can still eat this dairy product as it contains virtually no lactose.

L-Glutamine

This is one of the best remedies for quickly alleviating diarrhea that I have found. However, while it resolves the symptom, it does not completely address the cause of diarrhea, for that, you also need to take the probiotics. I initially heard about L-glutamine from a health pharmacy owner and then discussed it with my naturopath, who said he'd been having real success with some IBD clients using it. I've since heard from hundreds of readers who've also had good results from using L-Glutamine. Here's an overview for your information or experimentation, and I really encourage you to give it a try.

Glutamine is very well known to athletes and body builders as a key to the metabolism and maintenance of muscle. It can be considered (along with numerous other amino acids) as a primary fuel, or energy source, for the entire immune system. It is essential for DNA synthesis, cell division and cell growth; which are all necessary for wound healing and tissue repair. L-glutamine is of particular interest to people with digestive disorders because it's also the primary nutrient for the cells that line the gastrointestinal tract. It's an important nutrient for the large bowel and helps maintain normal functioning of the mucosal cells that line the colon. One of L-glutamine's primary effects is the increased transport of water from the inside of the colon back into the body. This diminishes the loss of electrolytes and water from the intestines that usually occurs with diarrhea. However, it's important to keep in mind that L-glutamine only has this effect when taken on an empty stomach. When it's mixed with other foods (including protein shakes and elemental diet shakes) it functions more as a protein (amino acid) that particularly nourishes the mucosal lining and does not produce the anti-diarrhea effect. Therefore, for people who tend towards constipation, L-glutamine is perfectly safe and beneficial to ingest when mixed with food or added to shakes.

Several trials conducted on patients with Short Bowel Syndrome found that with the supplementation of L-glutamine, people who had been on intravenous feeding for six to eleven years were able to make the transition to a modified diet. They also had two to three semi-solid bowel movements per day, instead of numerous bouts of watery diarrhea. In another trial conducted at the Mayo Clinic, patients with recurring pouchitis put ¼ teaspoon of L-glutamine in their pouches twice a day and showed a much greater reduction in inflammation than the control group. Also, the patients using glutamine were able to eat without incurring infection or requiring long-term antibiotic therapy.

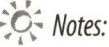 *Notes:*

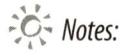 Notes:

Here are two of my favorite anecdotes from the book, *The Ultimate Nutrient Glutamine* by Judy Shabert MD, RD and Nancy Erhlich:

> "The baby had had colic and bloody diarrhea since she was five months old. Crohn's disease, the doctors had said, making her the youngest patient diagnosed with this ailment in the country. Steroids had been prescribed, and they helped, but the baby did not grow. By the time the child was six years old, her now-desperate mother took matters into her own hands. She had heard from other patients about the importance of glutamine for bowel growth, so at night, she gave her child a liquid feeding containing glutamine. During the day, she added glutamine powder to the child's cold drinks. After five months of glutamine, the child's bowel symptoms reversed, and the physician reduced the steroid medication. Unlike the five previous times when the anti-inflammatory drugs had been reduced, the child's symptoms did not recur. The steroids were stopped, but the glutamine was continued. The child has had only minor gastrointestinal symptoms and has been off steroids for one and a half years. Additionally, she has had a significant growth spurt." [1]

> "The patient, who needed to get his food in liquid form because he had a gastrointestinal problem, had developed a heart condition. He had cardiac arrhythmias (irregular heartbeats), and he needed a medication called quinidine. But quinidine can cause diarrhea, and in this patient, the consequences were disastrous. The doctors tried switching the patient's liquid diets, but the diarrhea got worse and worse. Then, the doctors gave the patient a liquid feeding that contained glutamine. Within thirty-six hours, the diarrhea decreased by two-thirds. The patient continued the glutamine-supplemented feedings, and he was able to take the heart medication and resume his normal life." [2]

Recommended Dosage: The book recommends anywhere from 1 – 6 teaspoons of glutamine per day (typical concentration is ¼ teaspoon equals 1 gram of glutamine), mixed in cold or room-temperature water. You can buy it in powder form, and the great news is it's practically tasteless and odorless. You can also mix the glutamine with cold or room-temperature, non-acidic juice if you like (e.g., apple or pear juice). Again, it's best to break the dosage down as much as possible (e.g., 1 teaspoon, 6 times per day). Take it on an empty stomach. Store your glutamine in a cool, dry place, but do not refrigerate.

Let me add one word of caution here: If you've had diarrhea for a long time, your rectal canal and other parts of your colon will have grown used to only soft, watery stool passing through. I found the glutamine took effect very quickly and within a few days (at a dosage of one and a half teaspoons per day) my stool was formed and semi-solid. This actually was not such a good thing as it caused pain in my colon as the harder, larger stool passed through a colon that had grown used to only soft, mushy stuff passing through. It also opened up some anal fissures as my rectal canal was quickly stretched much wider than it was accustomed to, in order to pass the larger, firmer stool. Also, the number of my bowel movements increased initially as the glutamine caused a lot of the water that was normally in my colon to be re-absorbed. I think my peristaltic mechanism (rhythmic contractions of the intestinal wall) had gotten used to lots of water helping it do its job, and then had to readjust to moving the stool along by itself. This resulted in more frequent bowel movements of just a small amount of formed stool each time. Basically, expect a bit of an uncomfortable period as your colon learns to adjust to a new type and process of passing stool. It's best to take it slowly, and give your colon plenty of time to adjust gently to the changes.

My recommendation is to start with only ¼ teaspoon of glutamine per day in half a glass of cold or room-temperature water, on an empty stomach, for the first two weeks. If your colon is handling that dosage well, then increase it to ½ teaspoon per day; if not, stay at ¼ teaspoon until your bowel has adjusted. Gradually increase the dosage by ¼ teaspoon at a time as your colon adjusts to the firmer stool, until you're up to a dosage that works well for you. I reached my maximum at 2 teaspoons per day (any more began to constipate me), you may need more or less, just follow your body. Also, I noticed when I took a dose right before bed I would need to get up

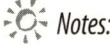 *Notes:*

several times during the night to urinate, but who knows, your body may respond differently. Take it on an empty stomach, mixed with cold or room-temperature water. L-glutamine purchased at a body-building supplement store can be a lot cheaper (sometimes half the price) than glutamine purchased at a health food store/pharmacy. However, the more expensive L-glutamine powder (pharmaceutical grade) is usually more finely ground and dissolves better in water.

If you have chronic renal failure (kidney disease) or liver disease, you should not take L-glutamine. If you have problems with constipation, make sure you don't take glutamine on an empty stomach, but always mix it with other foods or put it in a protein or elemental (pre-digested) diet shake.

Psyllium Seed

You can buy finely ground (powdered) Psyllium Seed in a health store. Some grocery stores carry it in their bulk bin section as well and it's very cheap. Or you can buy a commercial product that contains Psyllium Seed (like Metamucil) but make sure it has no artificial ingredients or sweeteners. Start with 1 tsp. mixed in 4 ounces of non-acidic juice, like apple, pear or mango (I find the taste is too strong to just mix in water) and then increase dosage as needed, up to 3 times per day. People with Short Bowel Syndrome sometimes find Psyllium works better for them than L-Glutamine. Best if taken on an empty stomach, just before a meal.

Bentonite Clay

Some people find they prefer Bentonite Clay to Psyllium Seed and some find the reverse to be true. The easiest thing is to test both and see which works best for you. The Bentonite has the blander taste of the two – I find it's easily drinkable just mixed in water and it's certainly my preference, taste-wise.

Bentonite Clay is a volcanic ash containing many minerals and it also has the added benefit of being a good detoxification agent. Good quality Bentonite Clay should be grey/cream in color. It has a very fine, velveteen feel and is odorless and non-staining. The value of montmorillonite (the active ingredient in Bentonite) lies in its ability to adsorb (not absorb) many times its own weight and volume in a liquid medium. It has a predominantly negative charge that is capable of attracting many kinds of positively charged particles. Bentonite Clay's structure assists it in attracting and soaking up toxins and contaminants on its exterior wall and then drawing them into the interior center of the clay where they are held and then excreted out in your stool. It is this sponge-like quality of the Clay that makes it a good anti-diarrhea substance whilst detoxing your body!

However, the only drawback is that montmorillonite has been shown in studies to also draw bacteria out of the intestines. So, if your bacterial flora is unhealthy, this is a good thing. But, if you're supplementing with probiotics, trying to implant a healthy bacterial flora, then you certainly don't want to be ingesting a substance that's going to pull all these good bacteria out of your gut as well! Therefore, I would only use Bentonite Clay short-term and then get yourself on the high dose probiotic supplementation that will address the root-cause of your diarrhea.

Start with one teaspoon mixed in 4 ounces of spring or filtered water once a day on an empty stomach. Increase the dosage and/or frequency as needed. If you've been on drugs or been living a toxic lifestyle (i.e. a normal western diet and environment!) then go slowly as you don't want to detox too quickly or you'll make yourself sick (nausea, headaches, bloating, etc.). If you're simultaneously taking probiotics, then take the Bentonite Clay first. For example, upon waking, take the Bentonite Clay, wait 15 – 20 minutes and then take the probiotics, wait 15 – 20 minutes and then have breakfast.

Pregnancy/Breastfeeding/Babies: I have used George's Aloe Vera, Natren probiotics, L-Glutamine and Emergen-C whilst pregnant and breastfeeding. I have also given them periodically to my kids as babies (give babies ONLY Life Start – *B. infantis* – probiotic) and toddlers. A George's Aloe Vera distributor once told me about a customer who gave all three of her infants George's in a bottle or mixed with breastmilk/formula with good results.

 *Notes:*

There are no known contraindications for Psyllium Seed or Bentonite Clay. Avoid giving babies any cow's milk products.

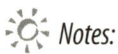 Notes:

Symptom Treatment Summary – Diarrhea

- ▶ Take the full spectrum of Natren brand probiotics (Megadophilus, Bifido Factor, Digesta-Lac) in powder form only. Begin with *Jini's Probiotic Retention Enema*. Following this, mix 1 tsp. of each powder in 8 ounces of room temperature spring or filtered water (no tap water) and take 3 times per day on an empty stomach until stool is formed and sits on the bottom of the toilet. Then take 1 tsp., 1 – 2 times per day on an empty stomach (15 minutes before food, or 2 hours after food) for the next three months. Then, take as needed – let your bowel movements be your guide. For detailed guidelines and information, see the *Probiotic Supplementation* section later in this chapter.

- ▶ Take ¼ teaspoon of L-glutamine powder per day in half a glass of cold or room-temperature water, on an empty stomach, for the first two weeks. If your colon is handling that dosage well, then increase it to ½ teaspoon per day; if not, stay at ¼ teaspoon until your bowel has adjusted. Gradually increase the dosage by ¼ teaspoon at a time as your colon adjusts to the firmer stool, until you're up to a dosage that works well for you. Take it on an empty stomach (15 minutes before food, or 2 hours after food), mixed with cold or room-temperature filtered water.

- ▶ Take 1 – 3 tsp. of Psyllium Seed powder mixed with apple juice, 1 – 3 times per day, on an empty stomach, just before food. If you have Short Bowel Syndrome, try Psyllium before trying L-Glutamine. You may also prefer Bentonite Clay, 1 tsp. – 1 tbsp.

mixed with water, 1 – 3 times per day, but go slowly to avoid rapid detoxification, and don't use for longer than two weeks.

☀ Fistulas

Fistulas are cracks or fissures that penetrate right through the intestinal wall. They can tunnel through one section of intestine and then into an entirely new section of intestine – thereby bypassing a loop of intestine (for example) that would normally be used for the passage of food. Or, fistulas can tunnel through the rectum and exit into either the vagina, or, outside the body in the tailbone region (for example).

Fistulas are usually formed as a result of chronic infection. Whenever there is infection in the body, the body will need to find a drainage hole for the pus and fluid containing the infectious microorganisms. The most common place you see this mechanism at work is with a cold. When you have a cold (whether caused by bacteria or virus), the body will produce mucus to trap the infectious microorganisms and then it will cause you to expel the mucus via the nose and throat. This is why you must never suppress a moist, chesty cough – the body needs you to cough up that mucus from the lungs and expel it. If you don't, and you suppress the body's natural drainage/elimination mechanism, you risk developing a serious bronchial infection. Likewise, the fluid and pus from a deep, chronic infection within the GI (gastrointestinal) tract must be somehow drained or expelled from the body and if the infection is not resolved, the body will create a drainage hole for itself. It's quite an amazing mechanism really, that the body can tunnel through tissue, muscle and even bone to create a drainage hole, rather than risk death via infection.

Keeping this in mind, it doesn't do any good to just heal the tissue, or surgically close the fistula path/hole. Because if the underlying infection is not resolved, the body will just create another drainage hole (or two or three). To heal infection naturally, without resorting to drug antibiotics or antifungals, see the section below on *Natural Antibiotics / Antimicrobials*.

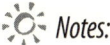 *Notes:*

LISTEN TO YOUR GUT

Many people use *Jini's Wild Oregano Oil Protocol* both topically and orally to help heal their fistula infection. I'd like to offer you an additional experimental procedure that you may want to try. If you don't have a fistula yet, but you have a rectal abscess that your doctor is afraid is going to develop into a fistula, find out whether the abscess is still accessible from (open to) your rectum, and approximately how high up your rectum it is. If you can still access your abscess via your rectum, you may want to try syringing diluted Wild Oregano Oil (see the section on *Wild Oregano Oil* for dilution instructions) up your rectum, to the area of the abscess. One of the main problems with a rectal abscess or fistula is that it's very hard for the antibiotics to reach it, hence medical treatment is often ineffective. However, if you can regularly (three times per day, or as much as you can manage) syringe diluted Wild Oregano Oil up into the area of your abscess, you have a very good chance at killing off the infection. Syringes (with a plastic tip – the longer, the better – not a needle) can be obtained from any pharmacy.

Now, if your abscess has been walled off from your rectum (the body commonly does this) into an isolated pocket, then you have two options. Firstly, depending on the size of your fistula hole, you can try inserting the syringe into your fistula and then depressing the plunger to release the Wild Oregano Oil as far up into the abscess pouch as you can. Or, if you've had surgery already to drain the fistula (or are planning on it) then post-surgery the doctor will usually leave a drainage tube inserted in your fistula. You can then syringe the diluted Wild Oregano Oil up this drainage tube to ensure the infection is eliminated completely and does not recur.

For both procedures – syringing an abscess or a fistula – dilute the Wild Oregano Oil according to the instructions in the *Wild Oregano Oil* section below (15:1 or 10:1). However, then try to increase the concentration of the dilution, one drop at a time, to see if you can get the concentration of Oregano Oil stronger, without causing pain. Keep increasing the concentration until you reach your own pain/tolerance threshold, as the stronger you can get it, the more effective it will be at eliminating the infection. Continue to take the Wild Oregano Oil orally as well for the

---

It's quite an amazing mechanism really, that the body will tunnel through tissue, muscle and even bone to create a drainage hole, rather than risk death via infection.

duration of the Protocol. As these syringing procedures are experimental and have not been trial-tested by many people yet, you may want to consult with your doctor before proceeding.

Fistulas require a multi-pronged approach to treatment as you need to first eliminate any infection, then heal the mucosal lining and the intestinal wall and simultaneously restore proper bacterial flora throughout the gut. Again, you *must* maintain a healthy, balanced bacterial flora to prevent future infection and damage to the intestinal lining.

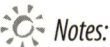 Notes:

Elemental Diet

The fastest method for healing fistulas may be employing the other remedies listed here whilst on an elemental diet. An elemental diet can aid in the healing of fistulas because it reduces food matter and fecal waste to a watery minimum. Therefore, there is no bulky food or waste to push through a fistula hole, keeping it active or open. However, make sure there is no infection present in your fistula or region before beginning the elemental diet, as this will prevent the body from healing. The body will not seal up a drainage hole (the fistula) for infection, it will not seal infection inside the body as this could endanger your life.

Also, keep in mind that while some people find the liquid diet and liquid bowel movements help their fistula to heal, other people find it aggravates their fistula. I once had a consultation with a reader who told me that if his bowel movements were formed, then none of the feces came out the fistula hole. However, if his bowel movements were liquid, then some of the stool would exit through the fistula and aggravate it. So, obviously for him, an elemental diet would not be a good idea.

Another reader with a fistula that exited in his tailbone region followed the IBD Remission Diet and used the FissureHeal suppositories in the manner recommended here. However, he had a long-running infection present in the surrounding tissue and pus would often drain from the fistula hole. He suffered numerous unpleasant side-effects from antibiotics, so he didn't want to go on a course of antibiotics to clear up the infection. As this was several years ago, I had not yet developed *Jini's Wild Oregano Oil Protocol*. At that time, he hoped that being on the Diet, using Tea Tree Oil topically and taking Epsom salt baths would look after the infection. Unfortunately, it didn't work sufficiently and after six weeks on the elemental diet, his fistula was only 80% healed. He couldn't bear the liquid diet any longer and was desperate for real food, so he ended it and then eventually went for surgery. I talked to him a few months after the surgery and he felt it had been successful. However, because he didn't resolve the underlying infection that caused the fistula in the first place, within 18 months he had a severe flare, could no longer work and was facing surgery, or long-term prescription drug use again.

There are more aggressive and highly effective natural ways to combat infection without resorting to antibiotics (Grapefruit Seed Extract, Olive Leaf Extract, Wild Oregano Oil, high doses of probiotics, etc.). About one year after the reader mentioned above used Tea Tree Oil and Epsom salt unsuccessfully to try and clear his infection, I discovered Wild Oregano Oil and within another year and a half had used it for numerous yeast, fungal, bacterial and viral infections on myself and family members.

I then felt experienced enough in its use to develop *Jini's Wild Oregano Oil Protocol* offered here (see *Natural Antibiotics / Antimicrobials* section) where I combine Wild Oregano Oil with probiotics. It's best if you can use this protocol or another antimicrobial treatment (some prefer Olive Leaf Extract) to first heal the infection. Depending on your overall state of health, you can use *Jini's Wild Oregano Protocol* in conjunction with the IBD Remission Diet (do this if you're very sick, or malnutritioned, or have had active IBD for two years or more), or you can use a natural antibiotic/antimicrobial treatment on its own combined with other remedies listed below. If your health is quite compromised, I recommend you first start on a natural antibiotic/antimicrobial treatment (see *Natural Antibiotics / Antimicrobials* section) and then in Week Three of *Jini's Wild Oregano Oil Protocol*, or, similar appropriate point in whichever other antibiotic/antimicrobial treatment you may choose, begin the IBD Remission Diet. Once you've ascertained that there is no remaining infection, and it has completely cleared up, then the IBD Remission Diet combined with the other remedies listed here may offer your best chance of healing fistulas. See Chapter Three for more information on an elemental (liquid, pre-digested) diet, or see my book, *The IBD Remission Diet* (www.IBDremissionDiet.com).

FissureHeal Suppositories

Remember: You MUST be completely free of any infection before beginning the treatments below.

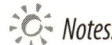 *Notes:*

This healing protocol is to be used by people whose fistulas exit either into their vagina, or, outside their rectal/tailbone area.

Once your infection is cleared up, if your fistula still hasn't healed, massage Doctor Burt's Res-Q Ointment (available from Burt's Bees Inc. in health stores or at *www.LTYGshoppe.com*) all over the wound and surrounding tissue. Rub in as much as possible. Then leave the wound open to the air for as long as possible (sleep with your bum naked overnight). If you get leakage then sleep on a big towel or washable mattress pad, but make sure it's 100% cotton so the wound can breathe adequately. Comfrey is the most fantastic wound healer I've ever encountered and both Dr. Burt's Res-Q Ointment and FissureHeal suppositories contain good amounts of Comfrey.

In conjunction with the topical Comfrey treatment, get a supply of FissureHeal herbal suppositories from *www.LTYGshoppe.com* (or see Appendix C for order details) to help heal the fistula from inside the body as well. Insert the suppository and push it up far enough so the suppository is as close to the area of the fistula as possible. The suppositories contain effective wound healers like Comfrey, Slippery Elm, Marshmallow Root and Cocoa Butter. This will help to heal your fistula from the inside while you sleep. I've used them myself on two separate occasions for rectal fissures and they work very well. If you have a fistula that exits into your vagina, then insert a FissureHeal suppository into your rectum and another into your vagina and position both in the area of your fistula. The suppositories contain Cocoa Butter which is a very rich emollient, so if you get vaginal itching due to too much moisturizer, then discontinue vaginal use and just insert the suppository into your rectum. Also, the Cocoa Butter can damage condoms so switch to another method of birth control if that's what you're using – or better yet, just abstain from intercourse to give your fistula the best chance for undisturbed healing. If you've used the FissureHeal suppositories vaginally and they've resulted in severe or chronic itching, then chances are the area has become infected. If this is the case, then douche using the Wild Oregano Oil as described in *Jini's Wild Oregano Oil Protocol* (see *Natural Antibiotics / Antimicrobials* section) until there is no more itching. This will not hinder your healing as Wild Oregano Oil is also an anti-inflammatory and wound-healing agent.

Heal The Mucosal Lining & Intestinal Wall

The following supplements are all effective for healing the mucosal lining and the intestinal wall: MucosaHeal, George's Roadrunner 'Always Active'Aloe Vera juice, N-Acetyl Glucosamine (NAG), Essential Fatty Acids (EFA), and L-Glutamine. See the sections on *Inflammation, Ulceration & Bleeding* and *Diarrhea* for detailed descriptions of each of these supplements. If you're using MucosaHeal, you don't need to take N-Acetyl Glucosamine (NAG) because it's already contained in MucosaHeal. If you're simultaneously on the IBD Remission Diet (elemental diet) then you don't need to take L-Glutamine because you automatically get 1000 mg of L-Glutamine per serving of Absorb Plus. And you'll also already be getting your Essential Fatty Acids (EFA) from adding the Udo's or flax oil to your shakes. If you're not on the IBD Remission Diet, then I recommend you use MucosaHeal and George's Aloe Vera juice – a tablespoon of Udo's oil per day and/or fish oil would also be great if you can manage it.

Probiotics

For long term healing of fistulas and the conditions that create them, you must improve the bacterial flora in your gut. Having a healthy bacterial flora will also help to prevent future or recurrent infection of the GI tract. Ingesting good bacteria also improves digestion, absorption and elimination of food. Certain strains of bacteria help produce digestive enzymes,

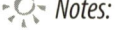 Notes:

peptides, amino acids and B vitamins for your body's use. They also inhibit or eliminate pathogenic microorganisms, like yeast, fungus, parasites, and bad bacteria that wound or burrow through the intestinal wall – possibly the beginning of fissures and fistulas. See the expanded section on *Probiotic Supplementation* later on in this chapter for more information and details. Currently, I only recommend Natren brand probiotics as they are the only company that meets the basic standards for quality and bio-availability (see *Probiotic Supplementation* section for quality standards). You need to take the full spectrum of probiotics (Megadophilus, Bifido Factor, Digesta-Lac) in powder form only. Do not take the probiotics in capsule form as you want to reap the benefits of the probiotics beginning in your mouth and esophagus and on down from there. Take 1 tsp. of each powder (Megadophilus, Bifido Factor, Digesta-Lac) mixed together in 8 ounces of room temperature filtered or spring water (no tap water!) 3 times per day on an empty stomach (15 – 20 minutes before food, or 2 hours after food), until your fistula is healed. Then take 1 tsp. of each powder (or you can now take the capsule if your bowel movements are not loose or watery), 1 – 2 times per day for the next three months. If you're going on the IBD Remission Diet, then make sure you stay on this probiotic supplementation throughout the course of the Diet. For ongoing probiotic supplementation, please see the section on *Probiotic Supplementation* below.

Pregnancy/Breastfeeding/Babies: I have used George's Aloe Vera, Natren probiotics, L-Glutamine, Udo's Oil, FissureHeal and Emergen-C whilst pregnant and breastfeeding. I have also given them periodically to my kids as babies (give babies ONLY Life Start – *B. infantis* – probiotic) and toddlers. A George's Aloe Vera distributor once told me about a customer who gave all three of her infants George's in a bottle or mixed with breastmilk/formula with good results. I have used Wild Oregano Oil on my daughter from 4 months topically, and very sparingly internally from 1 year old. I used it with my son internally (when necessary) from 3 years of age. See the *Wild Oregano Oil* section (later in this chapter) for more guidance on Wild Oregano Oil usage for children.

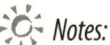 Notes:

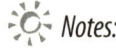 Notes:

Symptom Treatment Summary – Fistulas

- Heal all infection present using a natural antibiotic/antimicrobial treatment (see *Natural Antibiotics / Antimicrobials* section), then go on an elemental diet, if needed. See Chapter Three, or my book, *The IBD Remission Diet* for more information on elemental diets.

- Whilst on the IBD Remission Diet, supplement with MucosaHeal and George's Aloe Vera juice – the rest of the supplements to rebuild the intestinal wall and lining you'll automatically be ingesting by following the IBD Remission Diet. If you don't follow the Diet, then take MucosaHeal, George's 'Always Active' Aloe Vera juice, and flax or Udo's oil. Make sure you take probiotics whilst on the Diet and following.

- If your fistula exits in your rectal/tailbone area or vagina, then follow the instructions above for using FissureHeal suppositories to speed tissue healing.

- Take the full spectrum of Natren brand probiotics in powder form only. Mix 1 tsp. of each powder (Megadophilus, Bifido Factor, Digesta-Lac) in 8 ounces of room temperature spring or filtered water (no tap water) and take 3 times per day on an empty stomach until fistula is healed. Then take either in powder or capsule form (whichever you prefer), 2 times per day on an empty stomach (15 minutes before food, or 2 hours after food) for the next three months. For ongoing probiotic supplementation, see the *Probiotic Supplementation* section later in this chapter.

Gas & Bloating

Excess gas in the gut is due to food not being digested or absorbed properly and the rotting/fermenting food gives off a lot of gas. Often, the undigested food passes into the colon where it feeds the unhealthy bacteria and other pathogenic (disease-causing) microorganisms and this causes bloating as even more gas is produced. The cornerstone treatment for healing gas and bloating is probiotic supplementation. Sometimes, probiotics alone can resolve the problem in as little as a week. However, depending on the state of your gut flora and also whether you have intestinal inflammation or ulceration present, it can take considerably longer. In the meantime, use the *Colonic Massage* technique (see Chapter Six) to move the gas around and out and minimize the pain of trapped gas. Also follow the *Minimize Gas & Bloating Diet* in Chapter Three to reduce or eliminate trigger foods until your intestine is healed enough and your bacterial flora is healthy enough to digest and absorb these foods properly. Personally, I don't recommend the use of digestive enzymes or products like Beano since they merely treat the symptom, not the underlying malfunction. Also, I intuitively wonder if taking digestive enzymes may actually encourage the body not to produce its own enzymes, or, suppress natural enzyme production over time. As far as I know, there have been no long-term studies on this.

Probiotics

Improving the bacterial flora in your gut will ultimately heal gas and bloating since it results in the suppression or elimination of bad bacteria (which cause a lot of gas) and it improves the digestion and absorption of nutrients – resulting in less/no undigested fermenting or rotting food in the GI tract. Certain strains of bacteria help produce digestive enzymes, peptides, amino acids and B vitamins for your body's use. They also inhibit or eliminate pathogenic microorganisms, like yeast, fungus, parasites, and bad bacteria. See the expanded section on *Probiotic Supplementation* later on in this chapter for more information and details. Currently, I only recommend Natren brand probiotics as they are the only company I know of that currently meets the basic standards for probiotic quality and efficacy (see *Probiotic Supplementation* section for quality standards). You need to take the full spectrum of probiotics *(L. acidophilus, B. bifidum, L. bulgaricus)* in powder or capsule form. If you tend towards diarrhea, then take the powder form only (Megadophilus, Bifido Factor and Digesta-Lac). If your bowel movements are normal or tend towards constipation, then you can take the capsules (Healthy Trinity), if you prefer. Take 1 capsule once a day, or, mix ½ – 1 tsp. of each powder in 8 ounces of room temperature spring or filtered water (no tap water) and take 2 – 3 times per day on an

The cornerstone treatment for healing gas and bloating is probiotic supplementation.

empty stomach, until gas/bloating subsides. Then take 1 capsule once every other day, or, 1 tsp. of the powders once before bed, on an empty stomach (15 minutes before food, or 2 hours after food) for the next three months following. Then, take as needed – let your digestion, gas/bloating, and bowel movements be your guide. While waiting for your gut flora to improve, use the other treatments below for relief.

Pregnancy/Breastfeeding/Babies: I have used Natren probiotics whilst pregnant and breastfeeding and also given them periodically to my kids as babies (give babies ONLY Life Start – *B. infantis*) and toddlers. If you have a baby with lots of gas and bloating, you will also find my DVD, *BABY FART AEROBICS: And Other Natural Treatments for Colicky Babies* invaluable. Go to: www.ColicInfant.com to see a free clip of the video and a detailed description of the contents. Avoid giving babies any cow's milk products.

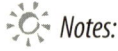 Notes:

Symptom Treatment Summary – Gas & Bloating

▶ Take the full spectrum of Natren brand probiotics (*L. acidophilus, B. bifidum, L. bulgaricus*) in powder or capsule form. If you tend towards diarrhea, then take the powder form only. If your bowel movements are normal or tend towards constipation, then you can take the capsules, if you prefer. Take 1 capsule once per day, or, mix ½ – 1 tsp. of each powder in 8 ounces of room temperature spring or filtered water (no tap water) and take 2 – 3 times per day on an empty stomach, until gas/bloating subsides. Then take 1 capsule once every other day, or, 1 tsp. of each powder once before bed, on an empty stomach (15 minutes before food, or 2 hours after food) for the next three months following.

▶ Perform *Colonic Massage* (Chapter Six) to move gas around and out of the colon.

▶ Follow *Minimize Gas & Bloating Diet* (Chapter Three) to reduce/eliminate trigger foods.

☼ Heartburn (Acid Reflux)

Doctors used to think that heartburn (acid reflux/GERD) was caused by too much acid in the stomach and this acid would wash up into the esophagus; causing the burning sensation that came to be called 'heartburn'. However, doctors now say that heartburn is actually caused by *not enough acid* present in the stomach to digest food properly and therefore the food sits in the stomach for too long and/or the esophageal valve is not functioning properly and so fails to keep the contents of the stomach from rising up into the esophagus. Then, you have to go one step further and ask yourself: What's causing my esophageal valve to malfunction and what can I do about that? And, why am I not producing sufficient stomach acid to digest my food properly?

The remedies below will provide both immediate and long-term healing for both these issues. However, you must discontinue any heartburn medication (either prescription or over-the-counter – that means not even Tums are allowed) since all these anti-acids impair or shut down stomach acid production. Shutting down your stomach acid production is never going to heal your condition, all it's going to do is impair your digestion. It's a classical medical/pharmaceutical approach of suppressing the symptom, whilst deepening and worsening the root problem. Also do not take any natural acid supplements, like Betaine HCL, for example. Naturopaths often prescribe acid supplements to improve the acidity of the stomach, however, for people with IBD this can easily trigger intestinal bleeding and I suggest you avoid it.

☼ Antacid use embodies the classical medical/pharmaceutical approach of suppressing the symptom, whilst deepening and worsening the root problem.

Lactobacillus Acidophilus

This is an extremely effective remedy for heartburn. There is mounting evidence that acid reflux is caused by a lack of good bacteria in the stomach and/or too much bad bacteria. Drugs like Zantac or Prilosec (and even Tums) that suppress stomach acid production also contribute to unhealthy stomach flora – since good bacteria need an acidic environment and many species of bad bacteria flourish in an alkaline (non-acidic) environment. Take *L. acidophilus* whenever you tend to get heartburn. For example, if you get heartburn after every meal, then take *L. acidophilus* 15 – 20 minutes before every meal. If you only get heartburn at night when you go to bed, then take it just before bed. The only restriction is that you have to take *L. acidophilus* on an empty stomach (otherwise it's destroyed by digestive stomach acid). Only use Natren Inc.'s Megadophilus (*L. acidophilus* DDS-1) in powder form, ½ tsp. mixed in 6 – 8 ounces of room-temperature spring or filtered water, *sipped slowly*, 15 – 20 minutes before meals, and/or before bed on an empty stomach. For more information on how probiotics like *L. acidophilus* benefit your body, see the section on *Probiotic Supplementation* later in this chapter.

DGL Chewable Lozenges

Deglycyrrhizinated licorice (DGL) in chewable lozenge form provides quite effective relief for acid reflux. I'm not sure of the exact mechanism by which DGL provides relief, but here's what DGL does for the body in general: It reduces muscle spasms (perhaps it relaxes the esophageal valve, allowing it to function properly and prevent acid from washing back up into the esophagus). It promotes adrenal gland function, soothes inflammation and fights bacterial, viral and parasitic infection (there is evidence that acid reflux is caused by a lack of good bacteria in the stomach and preponderance of bad bacteria). DGL also increases the number of mucus-secreting cells in the intestine which improves the quality of the mucosal lining, lengthens intestinal cell life and enhances microcirculation in the gastrointestinal tract. The fact that the licorice root is deglycyrrhizinated means that there's no risk of it increasing your blood pressure (as can happen with regular licorice root), so it's safe for pregnant women and those with high blood pressure problems.

Experiment to find the best time to chew/suck the lozenges. Try slowly chewing or sucking one lozenge before a meal, and then again after you've eaten. Depending on how long you've had acid reflux and whether you've been on a prescription drug (e.g., Zantac, Prilosec, etc.) that's shut down your natural stomach acid production (and thus exacerbated your unbalanced stomach bacteria problem), you may need to chew the lozenges more or less frequently than someone else. Also, keep in mind that even over-the-counter heartburn drugs (like Tums, etc.) alter the pH balance in your stomach making it overly alkaline and thus favorable for bad bacterial growth and inhibiting the growth of good bacteria, which only makes heartburn worse over time. Make sure your DGL lozenges don't have flavoring agents added (like peppermint). If you're diabetic, then make sure they're unsweetened as well.

Craniosacral Therapy

Sometimes heartburn is simply caused by an esophageal valve that is stuck or malfunctioning due to tissue adhesions or visceral strain in the region. Also, your diaphragm can (for various reasons) push up in your chest cavity, causing pressure and malfunction with your esophageal valve. In these cases, craniosacral therapy can be very effective at quickly and easily solving the problem. Whenever I used to get heartburn (except when I was pregnant), ten minutes of craniosacral completely cured the condition. Look for either an osteopathic doctor, or, a massage therapist with certification in craniosacral therapy. They must be at least Level II or higher, certified by the Upledger Institute. For a listing of therapists in your area, go to *www.upledger.com*.

Pregnancy/Breastfeeding/Babies: I have used Natren probiotics whilst pregnant and breastfeeding. Herbal literature states that DGL is also safe for pregnant/breastfeeding women, while regular licorice is not (it can elevate blood pressure). I have also given Natren probiotics to my kids as babies (give babies ONLY Life Start – *B. infantis* – probiotic) and toddlers. I have also taken both my children for craniosacral therapy from newborn to present – it is an invaluable tool for assisting children to be able to grow and develop unhindered. See my DVD, *BABY FART AEROBICS: And Other Natural Treatments for Colicky Babies* for an entire section on how/why craniosacral treatments are good for your kids and also to see a live demo on my daughter, Zara (available at *www.ColicInfant.com*).

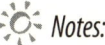 *Notes:*

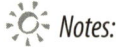 Notes:

SYMPTOM TREATMENT SUMMARY – HEARTBURN

The most effective treatment for heartburn that I've discovered involves a multi-pronged approach:

- Take Natren's Megadophilus *(L. acidophilus)* in powder form, ½ tsp. mixed in 6-8 ounces of room-temperature spring or filtered water, 15 – 20 minutes before meals, and/or before bed on an empty stomach. Sip it slowly.

- If you can't take the *acidophilus*, or you still need additional relief, chew slowly or suck a DGL Lozenge (15 – 20 minutes after you've taken your *acidophilus*) right before you eat, and then again after your meal. Experiment with how many lozenges you need to chew and how often, to provide the relief you need. George's 'Always Active' Aloe Vera Juice is also helpful when sipped slowly before eating, or before bed.

- Do not eat less than two hours before bedtime and don't lie down after eating – remaining upright uses gravity to help your system digest properly.

- Follow the guidelines in the *Reduce Diarrhea Diet* (see Chapter Three); this will eliminate the citrus, acidic and tomato-based foods that are primary triggers of heartburn. Also avoid peppermint, spearmint, coffee, chocolate and high fat meals (particularly before bed).

- Visit a craniosacral therapist to have your diaphragm released and to un-stick and heal your esophageal valve (see Chapter Six for more details). Follow up with self-massage to your solar plexus, stroking downward towards your navel.

☼ Hemorrhoids

Hemorrhoids are swollen blood vessels in and around the anus and lower rectum that stretch and bulge out under pressure, similar to varicose veins in the legs. Hemorrhoids often result from straining to have a bowel movement, or, from chronic diarrhea or constipation. Other contributing factors include pregnancy, heredity, aging and toxicity. Hemorrhoids are either inside the rectum (internal) or under the skin around the anus (external). External hemorrhoids are often painful, but internal hemorrhoids rarely hurt at all. If you don't have any pain but find yourself straining to poo (even though the bowel movement may be soft or liquid), or, you have your bowel movement and there's no blood whatsoever and then all of a sudden at the end there's anywhere from ½ a teaspoon to several tablespoons of blood, it's likely you have a bleeding internal hemorrhoid. With internal hemorrhoids, you may also feel a pressure in your rectum (almost like there's a large stool coming through), and then a gush of blood. You may also feel a 'popping' type of sensation and then the blood appears. The blood from an internal hemorrhoid will be bright red and can be loose in the water, streaked along the sides of the stool, and/or on the toilet paper when you wipe.

☼ External hemorrhoids are often painful, but internal hemorrhoids rarely hurt at all.

It's a good idea to experiment with different positions whilst defecating to discover which positions increase or lessen the pressure on your hemorrhoids. For example, I found that if I sat straight up, or leaned forward, the stool would almost always tear open my hemorrhoid(s). However, if I leaned all the way back and did not push at all (just used deep breathing and colonic massage to move the stool along) then the hemorrhoid would not bleed – unless I was *really* stressed. Remember that stress causes tissue to tense up or become rigid. You may find it easier to defecate if you place your feet on a child's stepping stool (or a couple of phone books). This raises your knees higher than your hips and more closely approximates a squatting position – the ideal position for opening the rectal canal and facilitating the quick passage of stool. If this makes your stool move *too* quickly though, and thus tears your hemorrhoids(s), then try another position.

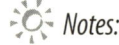 *Notes:*

Liver Tonic

According to Chinese and naturopathic medicine, hemorrhoids are a sign of liver congestion which in turn can lead to weak blood vessels. Milk Thistle (Silymarin) is an excellent herb for flushing and strengthening the liver, however, people with IBD need to proceed *very* slowly with liver support measures since their systems are so weakened and their livers are usually weak or damaged from prescription drugs. Start with only 3 – 5 drops of Milk Thistle tincture in a bit of warm water once a day (Herb Pharm is my favorite brand), and gradually increase from there as your system can tolerate it, up to the recommended dose on the bottle. An excellent tonic for relieving liver congestion is to juice together:

- 2 carrots
- 1 bunch of kale
- 2 beets
- 1 stalk of celery

If you need the juice to be sweeter, then add more carrots. This is a very potent tonic though, so only drink ¼ – ½ cup per day. Freeze the rest immediately to keep it fresh. I like to pour the juice into empty ice cube trays and once frozen transfer the cubes to a ziplock freezer bag. Then it's easy to just defrost 1 – 2 cubes in a glass each day – either put the cubes in a glass bowl or cup in the fridge overnight, or, just let them sit at room temperature until thawed and then drink. Do not thaw the juice by heating it, or you'll lose the health benefits. Again, start slowly and gradually build up the amount as you can tolerate it. If all you can tolerate is a tablespoon per day, this will still really benefit you. If it gives you diarrhea, even at a low dose, then leave it until your system's healed and you're stronger, and then try again. Remember that beets turn your stool (and sometimes your urine) pink or red, so don't confuse this with bleeding.

Rutin & Horse Chestnut

Horse Chestnut is a very effective herb for strengthening blood vessels (works really well for varicose veins as well) – take 300 mg twice a day, standardized to contain 16 – 20% aescin. Bioflavonoids (Rutin, Hesperidin,

Quercetin) also strengthen vein and capillary walls so they don't tear and bleed so easily. Rutin is one of the most effective for hemorrohoids, so you can either take just Rutin, or, you can take a mix of all three. Take 500 mg of Rutin, or a mixed bioflavonoid, twice a day. They're not a quick cure though so allow 1 – 2 months of supplementation to see results. Research shows that taking bioflavonoids can also reduce leg and back pain, promote circulation, treat and prevent cataracts, stimulate bile production, and lower cholesterol levels. By strengthening your blood vessels, you will not only heal your hemorrohoids, but you will be addressing the root cause and thereby prevent recurrence.

 *Notes:*

FissureHeal Suppositories

The other remedy you can try for internal hemorrhoids is FissureHeal suppositories *(www.fissureheal.com)*. FissureHeal contains comfrey, which is an excellent wound-healer, and the cocoa butter base is a very rich emollient so it will help the rectal tissue to be more supple. This is a symptom-based treatment though, so while it will help stop the bleeding quickly and help your rectal canal to stretch for the next bowel movement, it won't heal the root cause (weakened, swollen blood vessels). Be cautious when using them though as you don't want insertion of the suppository to open up the hemorrhoid. Insert them very slowly and gently, allowing your body heat to melt the cocoa butter and lubricate your rectum. Take deep breaths to relax the tissue during insertion. Also, only use once or twice per day to avoid aggravating the hemorrhoid.

Pregnancy/Breastfeeding/Babies: I have used FissureHeal whilst pregnant and breastfeeding and used FissureHeal suppositories on my daughter at 6 months for a few days. Bioflavonoids in the appropriate dose should be fine for toddlers/children, but check with your naturopath for guidelines before supplementing toddlers with Milk Thistle or Horse Chestnut.
Milk Thistle is probably not good to use whilst pregnant (especially during the first trimester) since your liver is already working hard – unless under the supervision of a physician. Likewise, use the Liver Tonic sparingly whilst pregnant.

 Notes:

SYMPTOM TREATMENT SUMMARY – HEMORRHOIDS

- ▶ use FissureHeal suppositories once or twice a day to lubricate and soften rectal tissue and speed wound healing.
- ▶ Take Horse Chestnut extract – standardized to contain 16 – 20% aescin (300 mg, twice a day) and/or Rutin/bioflavonoids (500 mg, twice per day) to strengthen blood vessels.
- ▶ Drink Liver Tonic (see recipe above) but discontinue or reduce amount ingested if it causes diarrhea. Or, take Milk Thistle tincture, 3 – 5 drops in warm water per day and increase as tolerated.

✷ Immune System Strengtheners

Most people's understanding of the immune system seems to be that of an efficient army that attacks and defeats invaders. This is correct, but it is only one component of the immune system. The other, equally important function of the immune system is to monitor and manage the attack on invaders. If our immune system was in "attack" mode all the time our body could actually kill itself, so a very important component of the immune system is its suppressive mechanism. When these two facets get out of balance, disease manifests in the body. So, when I talk about immune system boosters or strengtheners, I'm not just referring to the body's ability to produce antibodies, but also to its suppressive ability. By strengthening the immune system we are supporting the body's wisdom to find and return to its optimum state of balance or health.

Astragalus*

This is a Chinese herb, a really good overall immune booster and anti-inflammatory and stronger than Echinacea. Astragalus also aids adrenal gland function and digestion. It's quite potent, so depending on what preparation you get, experiment with the dosage until it feels right – just listen to your intuition and you'll know what's right for you. I like Herb Pharm's tincture as they test to ensure purity of product – free from pesticides or other toxins. This is my favorite immune booster and it works really well with my body. I use 20 drops in warm water, twice a day for a maximum of 2 – 3 weeks. Take a break of a few days or week, and then start again if needed. Excellent if you feel a cold, flu or mouth ulcers coming on. May produce spontaneous sweating – this is not harmful, unless you're dehydrated.

Maitake*

This is an extract from the Japanese maitake mushroom and is probably the most powerful immune strengthener listed here (and the most expensive). Don't take this herb at night as you may have trouble sleeping due to the energy it gives you. I really like this herb because the energy you feel is not the frantic type of energy that you get from caffeine or guarana, but rather a steady, foundational type energy. Maitake and Reishi mushrooms contain a substance called Beta-Glucan, which is proving very effective in clinical trials for cancer treatment.

Coenzyme Q10

The main function of CoQ10 is as a powerful antioxidant. Grape Seed Extract and Pycnogenol (French Maritime pine bark) are also very powerful antioxidants, so if possible, take at least one of these as well as CoQ10. It was first isolated and extracted from mammalian tissue in 1957 by Dr. F.L. Crane and his initial research concluded that CoQ10 could add or remove oxygen from a biologically active molecule. This is significant because a lack of oxygen can produce a decline in cellular energy, while an excess of oxygen will result in the formation of toxic elements. Studies have demonstrated a marked CoQ10 deficiency in thymic tissue and pronounced suppression of immune response in aged mice. Partial improvement in immune response was accomplished with CoQ10 therapy. The healing and repair of the gastric mucosa are very energy dependent and presumably would depend upon antioxidants like Coenzyme Q10. Early research in Japan showed that CoQ10 protects the stomach lining and duodenum. Healing of gastric ulcers has been demonstrated in animals but not humans – further studies are in progress. Cellular health is crucial to the balanced

> When I talk about immune system boosters or strengtheners, I'm not just referring to the body's ability to produce antibodies, but also to its suppressive ability. By strengthening the immune system we are supporting the body's wisdom to find and return to its optimum state of balance or health.

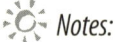 *Notes:*

and healthy functioning of your body and antioxidants (including Selenium, Vitamins A, C, E, Grape Seed Extract, Pycnogenol, and Coenzyme Q10) play a vital role in cellular energy, respiration and reduction of free radicals. People participating in clinical studies (for breast cancer) have taken up to 200 mg. of CoQ10 per day with no harmful side effects, but 30 – 60 mg. per day should be sufficient for maintenance. Absorption is substantially increased if you take it with a cold-pressed oil containing Omega-3 or Omega-6 essential fatty acids and many preparations now come in capsules where the CoQ10 is already mixed with an EFA (essential fatty acid) and vitamin E oil.

Vitamin C

An antioxidant required for at least 300 different metabolic functions in the body, including adrenal gland function, tissue growth and repair, protection against infection, and cancer prevention. Literally hundreds of clinical (including double-blind and placebo controlled) studies have been done on vitamin C to determine its safety and efficacy. It is one of the most beneficial substances you can take for your immune system. In one particularly memorable trial, researchers gave 60 patients with Polio intramuscular vitamin C shots (1 – 2 grams every 2 – 4 hours, depending on the age of the patient, for the first 24 hours, then 1 – 2 grams every 6 hours for the next 48 hours) and within 72 hours every single one of them was diagnosed "clinically well". [3] If a drug could accomplish what vitamin C does for our bodies, it would be all over the media, every doctor would prescribe it, and it would be part of nearly every hospital visit. Alas, as it's a natural, non-patentable substance, there's no exclusive, economic reward for promoting vitamin C and, more importantly, its widespread use would cause billions of dollars in lost revenue for drugs and vaccines.

Vitamin C in its common ascorbic acid form causes diarrhea. Therefore, make sure you get a vitamin C powder in mineral ascorbate form (e.g., calcium ascorbate, magnesium ascorbate, etc.). High doses of magnesium can also cause diarrhea so get a higher proportion of calcium ascorbate if the two are mixed, or just get vitamin C in calcium ascorbate form.

The mineral ascorbate form is also preferable as it's more readily absorbed – ascorbic acid has to first be converted to mineral ascorbates by the body prior to absorption. However, some people with IBD do report increased diarrhea from the mineral ascorbate form as well, so test it and see how you respond. Another delicious way to get your daily vitamin C in mineral ascorbate form (for ongoing use) is by using Emergen-C (by Alacer Corp.) handy single-serving packets, naturally flavored in your choice of tangerine, cranberry, raspberry, lemon-lime, etc. Emergen-C is a common product in any health store or see Appendix C for order details. If you're taking vitamin C regularly, or in high doses, make sure you don't just suddenly stop taking it, or you'll experience a rebound effect where your immune system becomes depressed. If, for some reason, you want to stop taking it, then wean off gradually to prevent this rebound effect.

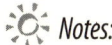 *Notes:*

If you don't like or can't tolerate oral vitamin C supplementation, then see your Naturopathic Physician for intravenous vitamin C. Start with 10 grams and then increase to 25 – 50 grams per session. Intravenous vitamin C is also great if you have any other kinds of immune system malfunction; lupus, herpes, AIDS, etc. I've had it done myself and it is very safe with no side effects.

*Astragalus and Maitake are medicinal herbs and therefore should not be taken non-stop. Just like drugs, if you use them long-term, your body may develop dependencies on them and they may gradually lose their effectiveness. Remember that health is a state of balance. Use these herbs to help your body regain its state of balance, but remember that using them non-stop or long-term can throw your body out of balance in another way. A good naturopathic physician could guide you in how much for how long, or, you could just listen to your body and when you feel you've had enough, stop taking it and then resume when/if you feel you need it again.
I generally use the Astragalus or Maitake for a maximum of 2 – 3 weeks at a time, then I take a break of a week or so before resuming use (if needed). To prevent the onset of a cold or flu, ingesting 20 – 30 drops in warm water twice a day for three to four days is usually sufficient, or, you can take it while you have a cold or flu to reduce the duration of illness. Mix herbal

tinctures with warm or hot water whenever possible as it facilitates their action and evaporates the alcohol.

Pregnancy/Breastfeeding/Babies: I have used Astragalus sparingly and CoQ10, Pycnogenol, Grape Seed Extract and Emergen-C whilst pregnant and breastfeeding. I have also given all of them to my children periodically from 1 year onwards. Herbal literature states that DGL is safe for pregnant/breastfeeding women, whilst regular licorice is not (it can elevate blood pressure).

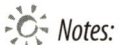
Notes:

Symptom Treatment Summary – Immune System Strengtheners

▶ take Astragalus or Maitake extract. Herb Pharm makes excellent quality tinctures, take 20 – 30 drops in warm or hot water, or in your favorite herbal tea, two to three times per day.

▶ Some companies make a liquid tincture mix of Astragalus, Maitake and Reishi mushrooms, and deglycyrrhizinated licorice (DGL), which is very good. Take as directed on the bottle.

▶ Take CoQ10 with either Pycnogenol or Grape Seed Extract, to a combined maximum of 200 mg per day.

▶ Take as much vitamin C daily, in mineral ascorbate form, as you can tolerate, or, see your naturopath for intravenous vitamin C.

Intestinal Inflammation, Ulceration & Bleeding

If you have intestinal inflammation, ulceration and/or bleeding (i.e. Crohn's, colitis, or any other inflammatory bowel disease!) you can be pretty sure one of the foundational factors of your condition is an unhealthy or unbalanced bacterial flora in your gut. Whether a bad bacterial flora is the *cause* of IBD or the *result*, doesn't matter. For your digestive system to become healthy again, it is a vital component that must be addressed/balanced. In severe cases – and any IBD indicates a severe case – balancing the bacterial gut flora requires two steps: First, you need to eliminate pathogenic microorganisms (yeast, fungus, bad bacteria, parasites, viruses, etc.) and heal the infection. Then, you need to repopulate the gut with good, healthy bacteria to ensure ongoing good digestion and prevent recurrence of infection with pathogenic microorganisms.

This can be accomplished using a natural antibiotic/antimicrobial treatment (see *Natural Antibiotics / Antimicrobials* section below) to clear any infectious microorganisms, followed by high doses of probiotics. However, if you have heavy bleeding or hemorrhaging, I believe it's best to first get the bleeding stopped before starting a natural antibiotic/antimicrobial treatment. If your colonic bleeding is very light and infrequent, or, if your bleeding is just from a fissure in your rectum, then you can begin a natural antibiotic/antimicrobial treatment right away, combined with the other remedies in this chapter that address your particular symptom profile. Remember that if you're experiencing intestinal bleeding and/or diarrhea, you're losing a lot of fluids and electrolytes. It is absolutely vital that you remain adequately hydrated during this time or your body may go into shock. Drink lots of water, Emergen-C, and diluted apple or pear juice during times of bleeding. If your bleeding is moderate to severe, then you need to be drinking these fluids continually until you get the bleeding stopped – to avoid dehydration and electrolyte imbalance. See the section below on *Danger Signals* for what to do if your body does go into shock.

One of the most confusing things in treating intestinal bleeding can be discerning where the blood is coming from. There are some guidelines to use, which I will give you, but other times the only way to know for sure is by trying different remedies and seeing what works. If your stool is black or green, the bleeding is coming from your stomach or small intestine. However, certain foods (like blueberries) and iron supplements can also turn your stool green or black, so don't confuse the two. Bleeding from your colon (large intestine) or rectum will be bright red. This is where things can get very confusing. You may think you're having colonic bleeding but it may only be from a rectal fissure or internal hemorrhoid (or both!). If you have some pain in your rectum or anus upon defecating, then it's likely you

> ☼ If you're experiencing intestinal bleeding and/or diarrhea, then you're losing a lot of fluids and electrolytes. It is absolutely vital that you remain adequately hydrated during this time or your body may go into shock.

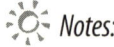 *Notes:*

have a fissure that's getting torn open by the bowel movement and bleeding. If you don't have any pain (or only mild pain) but find yourself straining to poo (even though the bowel movement may be soft or liquid), or, you have your bowel movement and there's no blood whatsoever and then all of a sudden at the end there's anywhere from ½ a teaspoon to a couple tablespoons of blood, it's likely you have an internal hemorrhoid. External hemorrhoids cause pain, but internal hemorrhoids rarely hurt at all. With internal hemorrhoids, you may also feel a pressure in your rectum (almost like there's a large stool coming through), and then a gush of blood. You may also feel a 'popping' type of sensation and then the blood appears. Alternatively, depending on where your hemorrhoids are, the blood can be both mixed in with the stool and loose – this is what makes it confusing. If you're not sure whether your blood is coming from your rectum or colon, the only way to find out is to see which treatment stops the bleeding. Also, keep in mind that if your bleeding is colonic, you'll likely have other signs of more serious illness, such as fatigue, pain or cramping, anemia, gas/bloating, etc., and the blood loss will likely be larger. If you feel perfectly fine otherwise, have fairly normal bowel movements, plenty of energy, etc. then there's a good chance the bleeding is merely due to a fissure or hemorrhoid(s) in your rectum. If this is the case, then see the relevant sections for *Hemorrhoids* and/or *Rectal Fissures* for healing guidelines.

Danger Signals

If your body goes into shock from blood or fluid loss (dehydration and/or electrolyte imbalance) you'll need to go into the hospital to get rehydrated via an intravenous saline and electrolyte solution. When you're in shock, your body will start shaking uncontrollably (even mild convulsing) and you'll feel freezing cold. Do not get into a hot bath to warm yourself up if this happens, but go straight to the hospital where they will warm you whilst simultaneously rehydrating you with fluids and electrolytes. Your body becomes cold because it has pulled the blood from your extremities to your internal organs – as a life-saving device. Taking a hot bath, or some other similar action, that causes the blood to be pulled back out to the surface of your skin could have dire consequences (even death). So if you get really cold and blankets and a hot water bottle can't warm you up, and/or you start shaking/convulsing, you need intravenous rehydration. Drinking a lot of water and electrolyte fluids at that point, is probably too late, you need to receive them intravenously – directly to the bloodstream.

The other warning signals you need to look out for are signs of intestinal rupture or perforation. In this case you will experience a fever, very rigid abdomen, severe shaking or shivering and constipation – where you're not passing any gas or stool. Intestinal rupture or perforation are very dangerous conditions requiring immediate surgery, so if you find yourself with these symptoms, then call an ambulance and get to the hospital right away – delaying treatment could result in death (similar to a ruptured appendix).

As long as you're not experiencing either of these severe and dangerous conditions (shock or intestinal rupture/perforation) you can treat yourself using the holistic methods outlined below and in the rest of this program. Also, remember that just because you're admitted to the hospital, does not mean you have to consent to intravenous steroids or colonoscopies, etc. I've been admitted twice and just received intravenous saline and electrolytes and then gone back home the same day to continue with my natural healing protocols. On one occasion my hemorrhaging had been so severe (this was before I developed the IBD Remission Diet) that my hemoglobin was only 3 out of 14 (or 30 out of 140), so I agreed to a blood transfusion along with fluids, but nothing else. Remember, you are 100% in charge of your body. Doctors cannot force you to do anything, so don't give your power away. In cases of extreme pressure or intimidation, just threaten to sue them and that should cause them to back off. You can also try saying something like, 'Well, if you're right and I'm wrong, I can always come back! But I'm going to try this holistic method first.'

Elemental Diet

An elemental (liquid, pre-digested) diet is as effective as steroids (Prednisone) in inducing remission. My second book, *The IBD Remission Diet* combines an elemental diet, with a targeted supplementation plan and

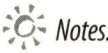 *Notes:*

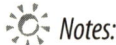 Notes:

probiotic therapy to completely heal the gastrointestinal tract, repopulate with good bacteria, and ensure ongoing, long-term health. If your bleeding is moderate to severe I highly recommend you follow this program as it is the fastest route to complete healing. You should also combine the elemental diet with a natural antibiotic/antimicrobial treatment (see *Natural Antibiotics / Antimicrobials* section below). If you have moderate to severe bleeding, then start the IBD Remission Diet first and don't begin a natural antibiotic/antimicrobial treatment until your bleeding has stopped or is only intermittent and very light. Otherwise, start a natural antibiotic/antimicrobial treatment first and then in Week Three, begin the IBD Remission Diet simultaneously along with ongoing probiotic supplementation. See Chapter Three for more detailed information on elemental diets. You can also read Chapter One of my book, *The IBD Remission Diet* online at www.IBDremissionDiet.com.

Probiotics

If you follow *Jini's Wild Oregano Oil Protocol*, or, go on the IBD Remission Diet, both provide instructions for probiotic supplementation. If you don't do either, then it is imperative you follow the instructions here for supplementing with probiotics to assist your gut in healing inflammation and ulceration. I recommend you don't begin probiotic supplementation until you have no bleeding, or, only light, infrequent bleeding. See the section on *Probiotic Supplementation* below for reasons why and how to test/slowly introduce probiotics following bleeding. Certain strains of bacteria help produce digestive enzymes, peptides, amino acids and B vitamins for your body's use. They also inhibit or eliminate pathogenic microorganisms, like yeast, fungus, parasites, and bad bacteria. Currently, I only recommend Natren brand probiotics as they are the only company I know of that meets the basic standards for probiotic quality and efficacy (see *Probiotic Supplementation* section for quality standards). You need to take the full spectrum of probiotics *(L. acidophilus, B. bifidum, L. bulgaricus)* in powder or capsule form. If you tend towards diarrhea, then take the powder form only (Megadophilus, Bifido Factor and Digesta-Lac). If your bowel movements are normal or tend towards constipation, then you can take the capsules (Healthy Trinity), if you prefer. Take 1 capsule 1 – 2 times per day, or, mix 1 tsp. of each powder in 8 ounces of room temperature spring or filtered water (no tap water) and take 3 times per day on an empty stomach, until you have no more inflammation or ulceration. Then take 1 capsule once per day, or, 1 tsp., 1 – 2 times per day on an empty stomach (15 minutes before food, or 2 hours after food) for the next three months. Then, take as needed – let your digestion and bowel movements be your guide. It is also a good idea to do *Jini's Probiotic Retention Enema* once per month, for three months, if you can, since you'll see the fastest results that way (see *Probiotic Supplementation* section for instructions). While waiting for your gut flora to improve, use the other treatments below for relief and to help heal the mucosal lining and intestinal wall.

Aloe Vera Juice

You must only use George's 'Always Active' Aloe Vera Juice (available in most health stores or www.warrenlabsaloe.com) because it has 100% of the laxative component removed and also has no carrageenan (used in large quantities to induce ulcerative colitis in guinea pigs and primates) or additives. Do not buy a brand that's flavored or contains citric acid or sodium benzoate (carcinogenic preservative), make sure it has the laxative component (aloin – contained in the 'middle' leaf) completely removed, has no carrageenan, and no other additives. The juice should be clear and taste pretty much like distilled water – if it tastes bitter, then it's probably going to have a laxative effect. If you can only find it in gel form (make sure it conforms to all the specifications listed above), dilute the gel with plenty of filtered or spring water before you drink it. Aloe vera juice soothes inflammation, heals open or raw wounds, increases tissue suppleness and has antiviral properties. George's Aloe Vera Juice is especially excellent if you're having any intestinal bleeding as it helps to heal it up really fast (drink ¼ – ⅓ cup 3 times per day on an empty stomach). If you have mouth ulcers, swirl it around and hold it in your mouth for a while before swallowing to soothe and speed healing of the ulcers. It is also effective in soothing and preventing heartburn. I sometimes just use it for maintenance

Notes:

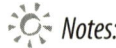 Notes:

as well, about ¼ cup/day or every other day (whenever I feel I need it). Refrigerate after opening as this will maintain its tastelessness.

Coenzyme Q10

The main function of CoQ10 is as a powerful antioxidant. Antioxidants reduce free radical damage and promote tissue repair. Coenzyme Q10 was first isolated and extracted from mammalian tissue in 1957 by Dr. F.L. Crane and his initial research concluded that CoQ10 could add or remove oxygen from a biologically active molecule. This is significant because a lack of oxygen can produce a decline in cellular energy, while an excess of oxygen will result in the formation of toxic elements. Studies have demonstrated a marked CoQ10 deficiency in thymic tissue and pronounced suppression of immune response in aged mice. Partial improvement in immune response was accomplished with CoQ10 therapy. The healing and repair of the gastric mucosa are very energy dependent and presumably would depend upon antioxidants like Coenzyme Q10. Early research in Japan showed that CoQ10 protects the stomach lining and duodenum. Healing of gastric ulcers has been demonstrated in animals but not humans – further studies are in progress. Cellular health is crucial to the balanced and healthy functioning of your body and antioxidants (including Selenium, vitamins A, C, E, Grape Seed Extract, Pycnogenol – pine bark extract, and Coenzyme Q10) play a vital role in cellular energy, respiration and reduction of free radicals. People participating in clinical studies (for breast cancer) have taken up to 200 mg. of CoQ10 per day with no harmful side effects, but 30 – 60 mg. per day should be sufficient for maintenance. Absorption is substantially increased if you take it with a cold-pressed oil containing Omega-3 or Omega-6 essential fatty acids and many preparations now come in capsules where the CoQ10 is already mixed with an EFA (essential fatty acid) and vitamin E oil.

Essential Fatty Acids (EFA)

Fish oil supplements contain Omega-3 essential fatty acids which are anti-inflammatories. You've probably heard quite a bit about their efficacy in healing/treating IBD. In a double-blind, placebo-controlled study, researchers gave 39 Crohn's Disease patients with a high risk of relapse fish oil capsules daily for one year. By the end of the study, 59% (23 patients) experienced full remission, compared with only 25% (10 patients) in the control group[4]. However, there has also been some controversy regarding the source and toxicity of fish oil and many people can't deal with the fishy odor. If you purchase fish oil capsules, buy them only from a reputable health store that can also give you some information about the source of the oil and ongoing testing carried out by some sort of certified/registered body to determine that the oil is toxin-free. However, a pristine fish oil with hardly any fishy odor or taste was tolerated well by even a pregnant reader with colitis – as you know, pregnancy often increases nausea and intolerance. Nordic Naturals is an excellent brand of fish oil that tests to ensure purity and is available in many health stores.

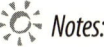
Notes:

Another way to get your Omega-3s is by eating canned or fresh sardines, herring, mackerel or wild salmon, two or three times per week. Cold-pressed Flax seed oil also contains Omega-3s and hemp seed oil contains both Omega-3 and Omega-6 essential fatty acids. The only restriction is that you can't heat these oils, they must be ingested cold – either swallowed straight or as salad dressings, over grilled vegetables (after you've taken them off the grill), drizzled over cooked fish, etc. Flax seed oil has a fairly mild, benign taste and hemp seed oil has a more intense, nuttier flavor. You need approximately a tablespoon per day to equal the fatty acids of two fish oil capsules. Your local organic grocer probably carries some salad dressings using these oils and you should also be able to get the flax seed oil in capsule form if you prefer. Flora manufactures an excellent blend of these oils along with vitamin E, evening primrose oil and numerous other beneficial cold-pressed oils called Udo's Choice Ultimate Oil Blend that I highly recommend (available in capsule or liquid form in most health stores).

Some health professionals maintain that if you have active inflammation or bleeding, you should not ingest Omega-6 (only Omega-3) and that fish is a much more bioavailable source than flax. Personally, I've been very successful using flax oil and Udo's Oil (which contains Omega-6) as an anti-inflammatory and hundreds of readers have confirmed this. However, as information and knowledge improves, so can treatment methods. If you've researched this topic and wish to avoid Omega-6 oils during active inflammation, by all means do so. And if you are equally happy ingesting fish oil supplements, then please go ahead – they can only benefit you. You can always begin using flax and Udo's Oil once your body is more balanced and your inflammation is resolved, if you wish.

My personal view on this whole topic is that if you regularly eat the suggested fish, and use hemp oil, flax oil, or Udo's Choice oil either mixed in with your food or as a daily supplement, you'll be just fine for ongoing health. For healing active inflammation and ulceration, you'll need to ingest higher amounts of essential fatty acids and may wish to ingest fish oil rather than flax. You may also wish to avoid any oils containing Omega-6 (like hemp seed oil, sunflower oil, or Udo's Oil). You can safely consume up to eight tablespoons per day of Udo's or flax oil. Depending on your level of health (liver function, antioxidant capability, etc.) you'll be able to consume more or less of these oils. Take as much as you can according to your particular tolerance level – even the smallest amount is better than none. A lot of the foods and spices recommended in *The Healing Diets* are also natural anti-inflammatories, as is the aloe vera juice.

Here's a recipe for a delicious salad dressing for regular, daily use, that will give you your Omega 3, 6 and 9 essential fatty acids. However, all the oils must be certified organic cold-pressed oils (Omegaflo and Spectrum Naturals are both good brands):

Jini's EFA Salad Dressing

¼ cup sunflower oil (if you can't get it cold-pressed, then use cold-pressed sesame oil)
¼ cup extra virgin olive oil
¼ cup hemp seed or flax seed oil
½ cup Bragg's Aminos (non-fermented soy sauce substitute) or soy sauce (organic, no wheat, no sugar)

¼ cup fresh organic lemon juice (leave this out if you're supposed to avoid citrus)
1 tablespoon sesame seeds (no seeds if you have diverticulosis)
½ teaspoon ground ginger

If you want to make up a sample of this dressing first, then just use 1 tablespoon for the oils and lemon juice with 2 tablespoons of Bragg's or soy sauce. This dressing also tastes great on cooled, steamed spinach or seaweed.

N-Acetyl Glucosamine (NAG)

Consists of an amino sugar that is normally formed in our bodies from glucose. It is the starting point for the synthesis of many important molecules of which tissues are composed. NAG is bound with other molecules to produce glycomsaminoglycans which are then attached to oligosaccharide chains to produce proteoglycans. Proteoglycans are part of several tissues including cartilage, ligaments, mucous membranes, skin and tendons. Therefore, NAG is particularly beneficial in restoring and healing the intestinal mucosa. You can take up to 10 capsules per day (500 mg each) but six per day is sufficient. If you have diarrhea, then you need to empty the capsules, as they may not have enough time to dissolve properly due to a rapid transit time through the gastrointestinal tract. Break open the capsules and mix the powder with water, it tastes like powdered sugar. I find it easiest to shake the powder from the capsule directly into my mouth, then take a sip of water, swish it around and swallow. In order for the NAG to go directly to your intestinal lining you need to take the capsules on an empty stomach (½ hour before a meal, or 1 – 2 hours after a meal depending on what you've eaten). It's best to take one capsule at a time, for example, 1 capsule 4 – 6 times a day. Like the L-Glutamine (listed below), NAG can also have an anti-diarrhea effect, although far less than L-Glutamine. It's an excellent therapy and I know of one person who was able to get himself off Prednisone using NAG supplementation. If you're taking MucosaHeal, then you don't need to supplement separately with NAG as MucosaHeal contains NAG already.

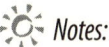 *Notes:*

Jini's Healing Implant Enema

This enema mixture is excellent for wound healing if you're experiencing bleeding primarily from your colon, and it works very quickly. It will stop your bleeding the fastest of any remedy listed. It can even stop severe, steady hemorrhaging in as little as two applications. Once you've got your hemorrhaging stopped, you can then do *Jini's Probiotic Retention Enema* to further prevent recurrence (see *Probiotic Supplementation* section below).

Because *Jini's Healing Implant Enema* is an implant enema (rather than a cleansing enema), the goal is to keep the enema mixture inside your colon for as long as possible. Therefore, you'll have best results if you administer it first thing in the morning (after your morning bowel movement) or last thing at night, or whenever your bowel is likely to be the most clear of stool. You can buy disposable enema kits from any medical supply shop (or your naturopath/doctor may have some in-house). The disposable kits have a much smaller nozzle than the regular, re-usable ones, so they're more comfortable and don't aggravate your rectum as much. The disposable kits can also be used more than once if you rinse thoroughly with hot water and clean the tip well. If you have difficulty finding the powdered herbs, you can order them from LTYG Holistic Health Shoppe *(www.LTYGshoppe.com)*.

The enema mixture consists of: 1 tsp. Comfrey Root powder, 1 tsp. Marshmallow Root powder and 1 tsp. Slippery Elm (inner bark) powder, mixed in ½ litre (2 cups) of filtered or spring water. If you find you can't retain two cups of liquid, then you can cut the water to only one cup, until you can tolerate, or retain, two cups of water. An herb pharmacy should have all the ingredients, but they must be in powder form. The powders mix best if you put the whole mixture in a blender and whip it for 30 seconds. If you don't have a blender then just mix them as best you can in the water by using a whisk, or squashing the lumps with a spoon. Heat the mixture on the stove until it reaches body temperature or, if you're whipping it in the blender, just use hot water. When the mixture is body temperature, or about the temperature of milk in a baby's bottle, pour it into the enema bag. You'll probably need someone to assist you in administering the enema, at least for the first few times.

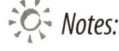 Notes:

Using the clamp on the enema tube stops the flow of liquid, as does holding the end of the tube higher than the bag. So let the mixture flow down almost to the end of the tube and then clamp it about a foot and a half from the end to shut off the flow. You want the mixture right at the end of the tube so that when you insert it and release the flow into your colon you don't get a lot of air going in as well. You may find it easy to insert the tube into your anus, but I'm going to give you instructions that will make it as easy as possible for even the most sensitive of rectums.

Start by rinsing a washcloth in hot water, wring it out, then press it against your perianal area. The heat and moisture will cause the tissue to soften up. Next, use your fingers to apply vitamin E oil (available in capsules, just puncture the end with a needle and squeeze out the oil) or a Comfrey salve all round and inside your anus. Also apply it to the tip of the enema tube and about 2 inches along the length. You can use KY jelly instead, but I prefer the vitamin E oil or Comfrey salve as they're also excellent wound healers that will prevent or help to heal any anal/rectal fissures. Lying on your right side, insert the enema tube gently into your rectum (about 3 inches should be sufficient) and then have your assistant slowly release the clamp, allowing the mixture to flow in at a comfortable rate. You may have to keep the flow quite slow for the first few times and stop it every now and again before you're able to continue. But as you get used to the enemas you'll be able to accept the liquid faster. When all the mixture has gone in, re-clamp the tube and withdraw the tip from your rectum.

Here are some tips that will really improve the ease and efficacy of the implant enema:

1. Lie down on your right side with one or two pillows (covered with a towel) under your bum/hips. Having your bum raised up enables you to use gravity to assist the flow of the enema mixture into your colon. Lying on your right side draws the liquid into the rest of your colon, reducing the pressure on your rectal canal.

2. Be sure to breathe deeply and relax your abdomen throughout (fear or apprehension causes us to tense up). Visualize the mixture flowing in

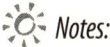 *Notes:*

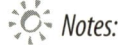
Notes:

around the whole length of your colon, imagine your colon welcoming it and helping it along.

3. After the mixture is inside your colon and you've withdrawn the enema tube, begin gently massaging the mixture around in your colon so it gets into all the folds and ridges of the intestinal wall. However, be sure to massage and stroke in a counter-clockwise direction; up the left side (descending colon), across the top (transverse colon) from left to right, and down the right side (ascending colon) towards the ileocecal valve and the small intestine. This is the reverse order of the *Colonic Massage* technique outlined in Chapter Six, because you don't want to cause a bowel movement, you want to prevent one, by massaging away from the rectum, not towards it.

4. The point of an implant enema is to hold the mixture inside your colon for as long as possible – ideally until all the liquid has been absorbed. Therefore, it's best if you can stay lying down with your bum raised on the pillows for as long as possible. You may also want to lie first on your right side for half an hour, then on your back for half an hour, then on your left side for half an hour, allowing the mixture to saturate the different parts of your colon.

The first time I tried this enema, I was able to hold it in for one hour, the next time, an hour and a half. By the fourth time, I could hold it till all the liquid was absorbed and then didn't have a bowel movement until three hours later. If you're bleeding from your colon, it's best if you can do this enema once (or even twice) a day. Once the bleeding stops, do it every second day for a week, then every third day for another week, then once a week for a month. If you find your anus/rectum getting sore from the tube then you may want to discontinue or administer it less. As long as your bleeding's stopped, *Jini's Healing Implant Enema* is no longer crucial and you can move onto other colonic healing remedies like MucosaHeal or George's 'Always Active' Aloe Vera Juice, if you wish. Again, it's your body; do what you feel is best.

I know there's been a fair amount of controversy in the popular media regarding Comfrey being harmful to the liver. With all due respect, this appears to me to be another example of a pharmaceutical/medical-backed hysteria over a product that's shown itself to be very safe over thousands of years of use. Why isn't the media trumpeting the 7,000 deaths in the U.S. from Aspirin every year and demanding its use be discontinued? Always look for the financial motivation.

I have consulted several respected naturopaths and herbalists and the consensus is that Comfrey taken internally in this manner is safe as long as it's not continued long-term. Therefore, don't use *Jini's Healing Implant Enema* for longer than six months at a time. You can use it for six months, take a break of a month or two to allow your liver to cleanse and then you can resume usage. Obviously, it's highly unlikely that anyone is going to administer daily enemas for six months continuously anyway! However, if you still have reservations about using the Comfrey powder, you can replace it with 1 tsp. Plantain powder and 1 tsp. Calendula powder – it will still be effective, but it will take quite a bit longer to heal your colon.

MucosaHeal

If your bleeding or inflammation is primarily in your stomach or small intestine, you should experience particularly good, quick results from using a product called MucosaHeal (available online at *www.mucosaheal.com*). The herbs contained in this product will also benefit your colon, but it will probably take a bit longer to see results. *Jini's Healing Implant Enema* is still your best course of quick healing if bleeding is present primarily in your large intestine. However, MucosaHeal is still an excellent product for overall healing of the mucosal lining of the entire gastrointestinal tract. Follow dosage instructions on the bottle as the dosage varies according to whether you're experiencing active bleeding and inflammation, or not. If you're taking a high dosage of MucosaHeal, then you don't need to supplement separately with NAG (listed above), as there's enough in the MucosaHeal. Unfortunately, at the time of writing, the product is only available in capsules, so I like to empty the capsules into diluted apple juice and drink it

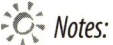 Notes:

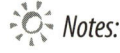 Notes:

that way – the taste isn't great, but it's fairly mild and certainly tolerable. If you have frequent bowel movements, or diarrhea, then you must open the capsules, mix with water or apple juice and drink it down. Don't swallow the capsules as they may not have enough time to dissolve properly before you defecate. Below is a list of the ingredients in MucosaHeal and how each one helps to heal your gut.

Deglycyrrhizinated Licorice – reduces muscle spasms, promotes adrenal gland function, soothes inflammation and fights bacterial, viral and parasitic infection. Increases number of mucus-secreting cells in intestine which improves the quality of the mucosal lining, lengthens intestinal cell life and enhances microcirculation in the gastrointestinal tract. The fact that the licorice root is deglycyrrhizinated means that there's no risk of increasing your blood pressure (as can happen with regular licorice root).

Slippery Elm – good for diarrhea and ulcers when taken internally. Soothes inflamed mucous membranes of the stomach, intestines and urinary tract.

Marshmallow – soothes and heals mucous membranes, skin and other tissues. Aids the body in expelling excess mucus and fluid.

N-Acetyl Glucosamine (NAG) – an amino sugar that forms the basis of complex molecular structures that are key parts of the connective tissue and mucous membranes of the body – tendons, ligaments, cartilage, bone matrix, skin, synovial (joint) fluid, and intestinal lining. To maintain healthy absorption and digestion of food, the body needs a healthy mucosal lining to lubricate and protect the digestive tract. To keep this lining healthy the body uses the natural amino acids and sugars L-Glutamine and N-Acetyl Glucosamine. It is also an immune system modulator with anti-tumor properties.

Pregnancy/Breastfeeding/Babies: I have used Natren probiotics, CoQ10, Udo's Oil, George's Aloe Vera Juice, and FissureHeal whilst pregnant and breastfeeding. I have also given Natren probiotics to my kids as babies (give babies ONLY Life Start – *B. infantis* – probiotic) and toddlers and they have also ingested George's Aloe Vera, CoQ10, and Udo's Oil periodically from one year onwards. I used FissureHeal suppositories on my daughter at six months of age, for a few days. A reader in Canada went on the IBD Remission Diet whilst pregnant rather than use Prednisone during a flare and she also added raw vegetable juices to the diet (we thought it would be good for the fetus to receive phytochemicals and other key vegetable nutrients if she could tolerate it – she could). Her baby was born healthy and has developed well with no complications. Herbal literature states that MucosaHeal and *Jini's Healing Implant Enema* should be safe to use whilst pregnant/breastfeeding, or with babies/toddlers. Wild Oregano Oil is contraindicated (i.e. do not use) for pregnant or breastfeeding women, and see the Natural Antibiotics / Antimicrobials section below for more information on its use with babies/children. If you have a baby who's been diagnosed with any sort of bowel malfunction, please see my DVD, *BABY FART AEROBICS: And Other Natural Treatments for Colicky Babies* for lots of really great techniques for relieving your infant's pain and discomfort. The techniques are very easy to learn and I demo everything on my daughter, Zara, who was eight weeks old at the time (available at *www.ColicInfant.com*).

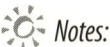 *Notes:*

Symptom Treatment Summary – Inflammation, Ulceration & Bleeding

For Active Bleeding Or Hemorrhaging

If bleeding is from your stomach or small intestine (blood will be green or black – iron therapy also turns your stool green or black so don't confuse the two):

- For quickest healing, immediately go on the elemental diet, see Chapter Three for more details, or read my book, *The IBD Remission Diet (www.caramal.com)*. Once bleeding has stopped or is only very light/intermittent, then begin *Jini's Wild Oregano Oil Protocol* (see *Natural Antibiotics / Antimicrobials* section).

- George's 'Always Active' Aloe Vera Juice, ¼ cup, 2 – 3 times a day on an empty stomach.

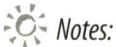 Notes:

- MucosaHeal, follow label instructions for Severe Symptoms, open capsules and mix with water or diluted apple juice. If you don't take MucosaHeal, then supplement with NAG, up to 3000 mg per day.

- Once bleeding is stopped or only intermittent, begin taking the full spectrum of Natren brand probiotics (Megadophilus, Bifido Factor, Digesta-Lac) in powder form. However, start with JUST one species of bacteria first and see how your body responds to that. Some people find they can tolerate *acidophilus* initially, but not *bifidum*. Others find the reverse order to be true. Go with your gut, experiment and see what works best for you. If you can't tolerate any of the probiotics, then wait a couple of months whilst continuing to use the other healing remedies that apply to your condition, and then try again. Please see the *Probiotic Supplementation* section later in this chapter for detailed guidelines and information on how to introduce/test probiotics slowly and gradually increase to full dosage. Or, if you're on *Jini's Wild Oregano Oil Protocol* and/or the IBD Remission Diet, then follow the dosage instructions there.

- Essential Fatty Acids (particularly Omega-3) in either fish oil or flax oil form, at least 1 tablespoon or 2 – 3 capsules per day. You can safely ingest up to 8 tablespoons of Udo's or flax oil per day; take as much as you can according to your tolerance levels. You don't need to take this if you're on the IBD Remission Diet as you'll already be adding Udo's or flax oil to your shakes.

- CoEnzyme Q10, up to 200 mg per day – likewise, if you're following the IBD Remission Diet, you'll already be adding this to your shakes.

If bleeding is primarily from your large intestine *(blood will be bright red or dark red)*:
- *Jini's Healing Implant Enema*, twice a day until bleeding stops, administer when colon is most likely to be and stay empty for a period of time (e.g., after morning bowel movement and last thing before bed at night). Follow with FissureHeal suppositories if anus/rectum is also bleeding.

- For quickest healing, immediately go on the elemental diet, see Chapter Three for more details, or read my book, The *IBD Remission Diet (www.caramal.com)*. Once bleeding is stopped or only light/intermittent, then begin *Jini's Wild Oregano Oil Protocol* (see *Natural Antibiotics / Antimicrobials* section).

- George's 'Always Active' Aloe Vera Juice, ¼ cup, 2 – 3 times a day on an empty stomach.

- MucosaHeal, follow label instructions for Severe Symptoms, open capsules and mix with water or diluted apple juice. If you don't take MucosaHeal, then supplement with NAG, up to 3000 mg per day.

- Once bleeding is stopped or only intermittent, begin taking the full spectrum of Natren brand probiotics (Megadophilus, Bifido Factor, Digesta-Lac) in powder form. However, start with JUST one species of bacteria first and see how your body responds to that. Some people find they can tolerate *acidophilus* initially, but not *bifidum*. Others find the reverse order to be true. Go with your gut, experiment and see what works best for you. If you can't tolerate any of the probiotics, then wait a couple of months whilst continuing to use the other healing remedies that apply to your condition, and then try again. Please see the *Probiotic Supplementation* section later in this chapter for detailed guidelines and information on how to introduce/test probiotics and gradually increase to full dosage. Or, if you're on *Jini's Wild Oregano Oil Protocol* and/or the IBD Remission Diet, then follow the dosage instructions there.

- Essential Fatty Acids (particularly Omega-3) in either fish oil or flax oil form, at least 1 tablespoon or 2 – 3 capsules per day. You can safely ingest up to 8 tablespoons of Udo's or flax oil per day, take as much as you can according to your tolerance levels. You don't need to take this if you're on the IBD Remission Diet as you'll already be adding Udo's or flax oil to your shakes.

- CoEnzyme Q10, up to 200 mg per day – likewise, if you're following the IBD Remission Diet, you'll already be adding this to your shakes.

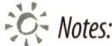 *Notes:*

Notes:

For Just Inflammation Or Ulceration *(no bleeding)*

- For quickest healing, immediately go on a natural antibiotic/antimicrobial treatment (see *Natural Antibiotics / Antimicrobials* section) and if needed, start the IBD Remission Diet in Week Three of treatment. See Chapter Three for more details on an elemental diet, or read my book, *The IBD Remission Diet* (www.IBDremissionDiet.com).

- Take the full spectrum of probiotics (Megadophilus, Bifido Factor, Digesta-Lac) in powder or capsule form. Ideally, begin with *Jini's Probiotic Retention Enema* (see *Probiotic Supplementation* section below for details), then follow with oral supplementation. If you tend towards diarrhea, then take the powder form only (Megadophilus, Bifido Factor and Digesta-Lac). If your bowel movements are normal or tend towards constipation, then you can take the capsules (Healthy Trinity), if you prefer. Take 1 capsule 1 – 2 times per day, or, mix 1 tsp. of each powder in 8 ounces of room temperature spring or filtered water (no tap water) and take 3 times per day on an empty stomach, until you have no more inflammation or ulceration.

  Then take 1 capsule once per day, or, 1 tsp., 1 – 2 times per day on an empty stomach (15 minutes before food, or 2 hours after food) for the next 3 months following. Then, take as needed – let your digestion and bowel movements be your guide. For detailed guidelines and information, see the *Probiotic Supplementation* section later in this chapter, or, if you're on *Jini's Wild Oregano Oil Protocol* and/or the IBD Remission Diet, then follow the dosage instructions there.

- George's 'Always Active' Aloe Vera Juice, ¼ cup before bed on an empty stomach.

- MucosaHeal, follow label instructions for Moderate Symptoms, open capsules and mix with water or diluted apple juice if you tend towards frequent bowel movements. If you don't take MucosaHeal, then supplement with NAG, up to 3000 mg per day.

- Essential Fatty Acids (particularly Omega-3) in either fish oil or flax oil form, at least 1 tablespoon or 2 – 3 capsules per day. You can safely ingest up to 8 tablespoons of Udo's or flax oil per day, take as much as you can according to your tolerance levels. You don't need to take this if you're on the IBD Remission Diet as you'll already be adding Udo's or flax oil to your shakes.
- CoEnzyme Q10, up to 200 mg per day – likewise, if you're following the IBD Remission Diet, you'll already be adding this to your shakes.

 Notes:

JOINT PAIN & SWELLING

Acupuncture often provides fairly swift relief from swelling and excess fluid accumulation. For a long-term cure, you'll have to look at the factors that may be causing this condition. Most likely culprits are a food allergy, drug reaction or 'side effect', or allergy to bowel microorganisms. Ralph Golan, MD, addresses this last factor in his book *Optimal Wellness*:

> "To make matters worse, you can become allergic to bowel microorganisms. In bombarding these bacteria with antibodies, your immune system can mistakenly attack your own healthy tissues and produce chronic illness in many systems of the body. Intestinal bacteria – *Proteus mirabilis*, for example, an organism recently implicated in rheumatoid arthritis – share some antigenic determinants with the body. This means that certain aspects of the proteus cell wall resemble aspects of the synovial membrane of our joints. If conditions in the intestine cause *proteus* to overgrow, overwhelm secretory IgA defenses, and invade the intestinal wall, the antibodies attempting to attack it will inadvertently attack the joints as well. The same kind of link has been made between another bacteria *(Klebsiella pneumoniae)* and alkylosing spondylitis, a severe form of arthritis affecting the spine. There have also been reports of intestinal bacteria actually translocating to joints and causing arthritis." [5]

> If conditions in the intestine cause *proteus* to overgrow, overwhelm secretory IgA defenses, and invade the intestinal wall, the antibodies attempting to attack it will inadvertently attack the joints as well.
>
> Ralph Golan, MD

If you suspect an allergy of this sort, you should see good results from probiotic supplementation. Probiotics (good/friendly bacteria) will inhibit or eliminate pathogenic bowel microorganisms and also improve the mucosal lining, thereby preventing or eliminating leakage of allergens into the bloodstream. If you suspect a food allergy, the best way to identify food allergies is by performing a food clearance (going on the elemental diet, for example) for a week and then introducing foods one at a time to check for signs of food intolerance. See Chapter Three for more information on testing and food reintroduction.

Following is an email I received from a reader that I want to include because she addresses not only joint swelling, but also inflammation in the eyes. The best natural remedy I've tried, specifically for the eyes, (other than the holistic anti-inflammatories listed in this program) is Euphrasia eye drops. These are a homeopathic remedy and often used for hay-fever related eye problems, or for when eyes are sore or damaged, resulting from accident or injury. Euphrasia eye drops are widely available in health stores. If you think you might be experiencing inflammation in your eyes as well as your joints, then this reader's email gives a good outline of what to watch out for:

> "I also need to thank you for saving my life! My "Crohns" attacked my eyes & several of my joints. I was at the point with my eyes that I was running out of time with my prednisone eye-drops (if you take them for too long they cause serious damage) and my collection of Doctors (I had seven all together – from an Internal Medicine Doc to an Ophthalmologist – one specialist for each "hot spot") all wanted me to start taking the "new" immune suppressants – they were really exited about them. Well, I'm lucky enough to come from an alternative health family, and there was no way I would accept the gastroenterologists' Curse that I would be, "Taking this medication all my life, and would probably spend time in the hospital periodically, and most likely require surgery sometime down the road.
>
> This is where you saved my life – your books gave me the tools I needed to start *healing*. I immediately started with the diet monitoring and modifying, the supplements (L-glutamine wiped out 3 months of

diarrhea in 2 days!!), the Aloe, and I found a wonderful Cranio-Sacral therapist. I'm on 6 weeks no eye-drops, my joint inflammation has decreased to the point I am able to start doing Belly Dance & Tai Chi again (no Kung Fu yet-but I'll get there). And I'm totally off the Asacol – and my gut's feeling better all the time!! I don't know if I would have literally died if I had followed the standard medical model, though I doubt I would have lived to my genetic potential, but I do know that my quality of life was so terrible when I was so sick – I was dead. Thank you so much Jini – not only has your hard work healed me, it also let me be the wife, sister, daughter, friend, and most importantly mom (I'm lucky enough to have four sweet children) I want to be. Thank you, thank you!

 *Notes:*

P.S. I was wondering why you didn't talk about the eye side effects in your books. Are they that uncommon? Mine got better as my gut got better, but I wondered if you knew of any therapies specifically for the eyes? I used the standard herbal & supplemental therapies for inflammation – and this helped me through until my gut healed enough to stop making me swell up. I also think it's important for people with IBD to know that their eyes may be affected. I thought my painful, swollen eyes were due to some kind of allergy. My eye-doctor said that if I had waited a day or two longer my eyes would have been permanently damaged, as it is, some of my Iris cells in one eye tore-off onto my lens, slightly impairing my vision in that eye. Please help get the word out that any feeling of pressure, sensitivity to light, swelling, or redness that may occur should be checked out when you are having an inflammatory response in other parts of your body."

Pregnancy/Breastfeeding/Babies Guidance: I have used Natren probiotics and acupuncture whilst pregnant and breastfeeding. I have also given Natren probiotics to my kids as babies (give babies ONLY Life Start – *B. infantis* – probiotic) and toddlers and my infant son had a 'no-needle' acupuncture treatment. Acupuncture is considered safe for babies and toddlers.

Notes:

SYMPTOM TREATMENT SUMMARY – JOINT PAIN & SWELLING

▶ Go for acupuncture immediately to reduce swelling and pain caused by fluid retention (see Chapter Six for more details on different kinds of acupuncture)

▶ You need to take the full spectrum of probiotics *(L. acidophilus, B. bifidum, L. bulgaricus)* in powder or capsule form. If you tend towards diarrhea, then take the powder form only (Megadophilus, Bifido Factor and Digesta-Lac). If your bowel movements are normal or tend towards constipation, then you can take the capsules (Healthy Trinity), if you prefer. Take 1 capsule 1 – 2 times per day, or, mix 1 tsp. of each powder in 8 ounces of room temperature spring or filtered water (no tap water) and take 2 – 3 times per day on an empty stomach, until you have no more joint pain or swelling. Then take 1 capsule once per day, or, 1 tsp. of each, once before bed, on an empty stomach (15 minutes before food, or 2 hours after food) for the next three months following. Then, take as needed – let your bowel movements or joint symptoms be your guide. For detailed guidelines and information, see the *Probiotic Supplementation* section later in this chapter.

▶ If you suspect a food allergy, first eliminate the most likely culprits, one at a time, in the following order: Dairy, wheat, corn, soy, potatoes. If none of these foods are the culprit, then go on a food clearance and gradual reintroduction program to test thoroughly for food allergies – see Chapter Three for more information.

❈ MALNUTRITION

People with IBS or IBD often become malnourished and underweight. It's very hard to eat enough food to gain weight when:

▶ Most things you eat make you feel sick

▶ Your appetite is poor

- Even though you eat enough calories, your body cannot extract or absorb the nutrients from the food you're eating
- You're stressed, exhausted and find it difficult to eat properly, or have the time/energy to prepare nutritious meals
- You're breastfeeding a baby/child who's taking a significant number of calories from your body each day

The first time in my life I had to focus on gaining weight resulted from a convergence of events that caused my weight to drop from my usual 135 pounds down to only 102 pounds. The first thing that happened was I discontinued using the birth control pill and immediately shed about 15 pounds (a common occurrence when you go off the Pill). Then I took a course of Chinese herbs that caused me to "cleanse and detox" to the tune of about seven pounds. The final blow was that I then caught a nasty flu bug, ulcers erupted all over my gums, tongue and throat and I couldn't eat anything but Cream of Wheat and tapioca pudding for two weeks – goodbye to another 11 pounds. As you can imagine, at 5'7" and only 102 pounds, I was a pretty sorry sight.

I knew I needed help, so I called my mum up and asked her if she could fly over and cook for me for a couple of weeks, to help me gain some weight – she arrived the next day. The next thing I did was go to see my doctor who ordered a comprehensive battery of stool and blood tests. I'd recently come back from Florida and she wanted to make sure I hadn't picked up a parasite. All the test results came back normal (except for my hemoglobin levels which were quite low), so she suggested I focus on gaining weight and increasing my hemoglobin.

She then recommended a common pharmacy-stocked liquid weight gain/meal replacement product. I asked my mum to pick up this liquid supplement and a few of the other mass-marketed weight gain and liquid meal replacement products the pharmacy stocked so I could take a look at them. Unfortunately, whilst they provide calories, the nutritional make-up of these products is far from ideal. Most of the calories are supplied by sugar and oil and some products even contain the same amount of oil as they

> It's very hard to gain weight when you have no appetite – and everything you eat makes you feel sick, or results in multiple bowel movements.

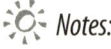 Notes:

do protein – which is not a good ratio! In addition, many of the products also contain carrageenan (a seaweed derivative used as a thickening agent). Sugar is a proven depressant of the immune system and large amounts of carrageenan, in repeated trials, have been used to induce ulcerative colitis in guinea pigs and primates. Granted, extremely high doses of carrageenan were used to induce the colitis, but until further studies are done I prefer to err on the side of caution. In addition, most people with digestive sensitivities will find it hard, if not impossible, to tolerate the amount and type of oil in these products. The result will be severe gas, cramping and diarrhea. And what kind of weight are you going to gain from consuming mostly oil and sugar anyway? True, solid and healthy weight gain should put meat/muscle on your bones, not fat.

The second time I needed to gain weight was following a bout of severe hemorrhaging, that left me weighing only 99 pounds. The malnutrition combined with the traumatic blood loss and ulceration of my colon required that I go on an elemental diet and consume only liquid, pre-digested food to regain my weight and health. You can read the complete story of this episode and how I came to formulate my own elemental shake product (Absorb Plus) as a result, in the *Bowel Rest Elemental Diet* section in Chapter Three. Again, I had to formulate my own product since the hospital/pharmaceutical elemental diet products available all had the same drawbacks as the meal replacement formulas above; toxic ingredients, way too much oil and sugar, and most had quite low quality and/or allergenic protein sources as well.

Two Ways To Gain Weight

There are two main ways to gain weight when you have IBS or IBD. Suprisingly, the fastest way to gain weight is to stop eating regular food altogether and go on a strictly elemental (pre-digested) diet using liquid shakes. This is because it's much easier and simpler to drink 3000 calories per day, than to eat it. Also, people with IBS/IBD tend to be intolerant of many foods, which also makes it hard to eat enough food each day to gain weight. The third complication is that even if you consume 3000 calories of food per day, if your digestive system is compromised or malfunctioning, you may actually absorb and utilize only half the calories you chew and swallow. All of these problems are resolved by forgoing regular food altogether and going on a pre-digested, elemental diet – where everything you drink goes pretty much instantly into your bloodstream. Pharmaceutical, elemental diet products do not typically help people gain weight, for the reasons listed above. If you try and consume large amounts of low quality, toxic food, even though it's pre-digested, you won't be able to tolerate it and your body will not make much use of it. Even when these products are pumped directly into the stomach (via a shunt) people don't gain much weight on them. However, when you ingest a high quality, 100% natural elemental diet product, your body is happy to absorb and utilize all the nutrients and calories ingested and weight gain is quite rapid. I used Absorb Plus (the product I formulated, available at *www.absorbplus.com*) to gain 36 pounds of solid muscle in only seven weeks. I combined its use with healing broths and targeted supplements that also assisted weight gain and rapidly healed my ulceration and restored a healthy bacterial flora to my entire gastrointestinal (GI) tract. You can read lots more about how I did this in my book, *The IBD Remission Diet* (available at *www.IBDremissionDiet.com*, and you can read Chapter One for free online). I also talk more about this in the *Bowel Rest Elemental Diet* section in Chapter Three of this book.

> Suprisingly, the fastest way to gain weight is to stop eating regular food altogether and go on a strictly elemental (pre-digested) diet using liquid shakes.

The second way to gain weight is to consume an easily digested liquid food shake in conjunction with your regular diet. Depending on the amount of weight you want to gain, you can drink 1 – 3 shakes per day in addition to your regular food intake. If your digestion is quite compromised and you suspect you're having difficulty absorbing nutrients, then you should drink Absorb Plus (*www.absorbplus.com*) in addition to your food.

If your digestive and absorptive abilities are functioning fairly well, then you can use a whey protein isolate supplement (or vegetable protein) combined with your choice of liquid (rice milk, yoghurt, water), 1 tsp. – 1 tbsp. of flax oil (adjust oil according to tolerance) and your choice of fruit (a well-ripened banana, canteloupe, papaya, mango, pear, etc.).

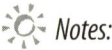 Notes:

It's best if you can add the flax oil because the oil is quite high in calories (1 tbsp = 120 calories) and the omega-3 fatty acids are natural anti-inflammatories. You can use protein shakes in conjunction with any of *The Healing Diets* in Chapter Three. Cold-extracted whey protein isolate is the best form of protein in terms of bioavailability and uptake into the bloodstream. Be sure to use a whey protein that does not contain any casein, as casein is the protein in milk that most people with a milk allergy are allergic to. Also make sure the whey protein you choose is lactose-free. Many people with IBS and IBD that are intolerant or allergic to milk or dairy products are able to consume whey protein isolate with no problems if it contains no casein or lactose. If you can't tolerate whey protein, then try rice or hemp protein – but your weight gain will take longer since vegetable protein is not as bioavailable as whey isolate. See *Soy Products* in Chapter Three for why you should not use soy protein or soy milk. Make sure the product is not sweetened with Aspartame, and the flavor should be from natural sources. At the time of writing, Proteins+ by ehn company (available in most health stores) is an excellent quality whey protein. For myself, even though my digestion is great, I still use Absorb Plus (even though it's more expensive than mixing protein shakes with fruit) because it's simpler to mix, tastes good and it also contains a healing, free-form amino acid blend, 1000 mg of L-Glutamine per serving, and an extensive vitamin/mineral panel (including trace minerals). I have my Absorb Plus shake (blended with water and 1 tbsp. of Udo's oil) for breakfast along with any extra supplements I want to take blended into the shake as well.

Keep track of the number of calories you're consuming each day and aim for around 3000 – 4000 per day (more or less depending on your size). It takes 3600 calories to create one pound of body weight. If you're not getting enough calories from your regular food, then use the liquid shake supplement to bring your total consumption up to your target each day. Listen to your body, begin slowly and give yourself a week or two to build gradually up to your ideal calorie count. Protein is a key element in tissue repair and weight gain, so make sure you're getting enough. Ideally, you want 40% of your daily calories coming from protein. Normally, a good *maintenance* ratio for an active person is one gram of protein per day for every one kilogram (2.2 pounds) of body weight. However, if you're trying to *gain* weight, you can supplement with up to 3 grams of protein per kilogram of body weight. For example, if you weigh 110 pounds, your maintenance protein intake would be 50 grams/day. To gain weight, you could ingest up to 150 grams of protein/day.

Weight Training

These supplements will work best if you begin a weight training regimen at the same time. Don't worry if you're at a very low weight and don't have any energy – just start with 15 minutes of weight training per session.
Or while you're doing your weight routine, rest for five minutes between each set. Take it slowly and honor your body at all times. Your body will gain muscle much more rapidly if you create a demand for that muscle. If you're just sitting around, not doing much of anything, why would your body need to gain weight? You need to exercise the following muscle groups to get a good, full body workout and to create the demand for your body to gain healthy, solid weight:

▶ Biceps (the bulging muscle on the upper front part of your arm)

▶ Triceps (the opposing smaller muscle on the upper back part of your arm)

▶ Quadriceps (also known as the thigh muscle)

▶ Hamstrings (the back of the thigh)

▶ Calves

▶ Abdominals (working these will also strengthen your lower back)

If you're not familiar with weight training, just take this list of muscle groups to an instructor at your gym and have them show you the machines or free weights you can use to exercise each one. Do two sets of each exercise, with 10 repetitions of the exercise per set. I like to do just one set of each muscle group and then do the whole circuit again a second time. For example, rather than doing two sets of bicep curls in a row, I'll do:

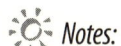 *Notes:*

- one set of 10 bicep curls
- one set of 10 tricep extensions
- one set of 10 leg extensions (quadriceps)
- one set of 10 leg presses (also quads)
- one set of 10 hamstring curls
- one set of 10 calf raises
- one set of 25 crunches (abdominals).

I'll then start all over again at the beginning of that sequence and do the second set of each exercise. This gives each muscle group a chance to rest while you're working the other muscles. To establish the amount of weight you should lift with each exercise, experiment until you find the amount of weight that makes it really hard to complete the tenth repetition of the exercise. This indicates the right threshold for your body. When it becomes easy to perform the tenth repetition, you need to increase the threshold. You can do this by either increasing the number of repetitions (up to 60 repetitions per set), or by leaving the reps the same and increasing the amount of weight you're lifting. Increasing the repetitions of each exercise will result in lean, streamlined muscles. Increasing the weight lifted per exercise will result in bigger, bulkier muscle, so do whichever meets your personal goals or preference for your body.

Work your whole body every other day, or twice a week, whichever you can manage. You need to have a day's rest between sessions to allow your body to build the new muscle tissue; working the same muscles every day would defeat the purpose.

Also, make sure you stretch your muscles thoroughly after each weight training session for at least 10 to 15 minutes. Stretching prevents pooling of lactic acid, which can make you feel sluggish and result in muscle pain. Controlled trials have also shown that stretching after a workout results in increased strength. Stretching or yoga is wonderful for improving circulation, blood flow and toxin flushing. Again, if you don't know any stretches, ask an instructor at the gym to show you a simple routine. Many

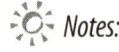
Notes:

gyms have posters with all the stretches illustrated so you can follow the figures each time in case you forget between workouts. Sometimes I'll stretch out certain muscles between exercises and then at the end of both sets I like to do about 20 – 30 minutes of continuous stretching.

Again, when you're first beginning, start out really slowly and if all you can do is a few of the exercises, then that's great! You may also want to proceed slowly with the abdominal exercises as your tummy area is likely to be quite tender – just start with 3 – 5 crunches to begin with and increase as it feels comfortable. Putting in the effort to learn weight training will pay dividends for the rest of your life. It's an ideal form of exercise that can be used whether you're healthy, ill, pregnant, injured or elderly – again, because weight training increases bone density, it's a particularly ideal workout for people aged 50 and older, or those at risk of osteoporosis.

If you're not inclined to join a gym, devise an exercise routine for yourself at home. Use simple weight-bearing exercises like squats, push-ups (start with wall push-ups if you're not strong enough), crunches, leg extensions etc. Go to a fitness supply store and just buy one 5-pound or 10-pound free weight to use for bicep curls at home. Any fitness magazine or book will have exercise routines and detailed descriptions of individual exercises along with their proper form that you can learn from.

To get the maximum mileage out of your protein shake, take it half an hour to an hour before or after your workout. Weight training has the added benefit of stimulating your appetite, which will help you gain weight faster as well. Arrange your schedule so that you can eat a big, delicious meal immediately following your weight training session.

Having had to both lose and gain weight in my life, I will say that I've found it just as hard to gain weight as to lose it. So don't get discouraged if it takes you a while to gain those desired pounds. Focus on stimulating and increasing your appetite for fresh food, take a good quality protein shake (as discussed above), go to the gym for weight training at least twice a week and let your body take care of the rest. You will gain the weight, slowly but surely. Don't weigh yourself more than once a week or you'll end up

> Your body will gain muscle much more rapidly if you create a demand for that muscle. If you're just sitting around, not doing much of anything, why would your body need to gain weight?

obsessing over your weight, which won't help you. The better you feel about yourself and the more positivity you can maintain, the more weight you'll gain. If your weight is really low and you want to gain weight as quickly as possible, then see the *Bowel Rest Elemental Diet* section in Chapter Three. Remember that going on a completely liquid diet, consisting of all the essential nutrients in a pre-digested form, is actually the quickest way to gain weight.

A quick note to those of you who are trying to LOSE weight due to steroids or for some other reason: Follow the same workout regimen outlined above, but, instead of doing high weights with low reps, go for low weights with high repetitions. Reduce your weights to 3 – 5 pounds for your arms and 20 – 30 pounds for your legs and try to do two sets of around 60 – 100 rapid (but controlled) repetitions of each exercise (or as many as you can manage). Do abdominal exercises, like crunches, between each exercise – don't bother counting them, just do as many as you can and then go on to the next machine/exercise. You'll find that following this regimen turns your weight training into a cardiovascular routine which will also help you to lose weight. Doing low weights with a high number of repetitions creates lean, streamlined muscles which are smaller and thinner but with a high capacity for endurance. The cardiovascular component of the regimen along with the added muscle fibre will burn up fat much more quickly than if you just did aerobics or went jogging. Don't forget to stretch all your muscles for at least 10 – 15 minutes at the end of your session.

Mouth Ulcers

Mouth ulcers, like lip canker sores and herpes, are most likely viral in origin. Therefore, the quickest, most effective way to heal mouth ulcers is by eliminating the infectious agent that's causing them.

Wild Oregano Oil

The best way to eliminate infectious agents is by using Wild Oregano Oil. Wild Oregano Oil is the MOST potent antiviral, antibacterial, antifungal, antiparasitic (anti-everything it seems!) that I have come across in 20 years of searching and testing natural medicines. I am very enthusiastic about this herb and once you've used it, you'll know exactly why. Wild Oregano Oil can be unpleasant to use because it creates a very strong heat sensation whenever it's applied to mucous membranes (nose, mouth, genitals, etc.) – it's like a very hot chili pepper, but unlike a chili pepper the heat sensation completely disappears after about two minutes. The results are so fast and effective though, that it's worth persevering through the heat sensation (and this from someone who's allergic to chilies and never eats them!).

 *Notes:*

Take a sip of water, hold it in your mouth and add five drops of Wild Oregano Oil to the water. Swish the oil and water mixture around your mouth (especially where your ulcers are) for as long as you can tolerate it. Then swallow. If you can, leave the residue in your mouth for as long as possible (the heat sensation will last about two minutes), but if you can't tolerate the heat sensation, then drink water till it subsides. Alternately, if you prefer, you can put a drop of Wild Oregano Oil onto your finger and apply it directly to each mouth ulcer, massage it in and leave it as long as you can (intense heat sensation will last about 2– 3 minutes). The longer you can leave the Wild Oregano Oil in your mouth, the more effective it will be at healing your ulcers. You should see results/partial healing after only one application of Wild Oregano Oil. Continue with treatment until mouth ulcers are completely gone (usually 2 – 3 applications).

My elderly Aunt was visiting me one winter and she had not been able to eat properly for months due to ongoing mouth ulcers. Her son and his wife are both pharmacists and so had given her every drug remedy under the sun, and nothing had provided any relief or healing. She was quite wary of trying the Wild Oregano Oil rinse since she'd recently had surgery for Trigeminal Neuralgia and was scared of anything that might somehow re-trigger the pain. However, upon my repeated assurances and encouragement to listen to her own gut, she tried a half dose (two drops) of the Wild Oregano Oil before bed and didn't swallow it either. She couldn't believe the improvement when she woke up the next morning (more than 50% healed) and insisted we immediately go out and buy a bottle of Wild

Oregano Oil for her to take back to London! Needless to say, she's used it ever since, and being able to chew and eat properly again has changed her life.

Become tuned to your body and you'll probably notice that prior to mouth ulcers erupting, your tongue, gums and lining of your mouth become quite tender and sore. Your taste buds may even change with the result that nothing tastes the way it should. When you notice these warning signs, immediately gargle/rinse your mouth with Wild Oregano Oil (as instructed above) and you'll probably avoid an outbreak altogether.

> The quickest, most effective way to heal mouth ulcers is by eliminating the infectious agent that's causing them.

DGL (Deglycyrrhizinated Licorice Extract) Chewable Tablets

This is the second most effective remedy available for soothing and healing mouth ulcers (after Wild Oregano Oil). Licorice extract has both anti-inflammatory and anti-viral properties. Unfortunately, you have to like licorice to be able to take these. Don't get the ones flavored with peppermint as that will aggravate heartburn. Just suck on one tablet at a time (take as often as you need to) and hold the juice in your mouth and swirl it around for as long as you can before swallowing the juice. Continue this process until the tablet is completely dissolved. If you like licorice enough to pursue this treatment, you'll get an instant soothing and lessening of pain and the mouth ulcers will heal up a lot faster than usual. If you have mouth and/or throat ulcers, you should also follow the *Reduce Diarrhea Diet* as it eliminates all tomato-based and acidic foods (which greatly aggravate ulcers) and also go easy on spices, salt and sugar – basically, the blander the better. Licorice has also been dubbed 'nature's steroid', so you may also want to check with your naturopathic doctor about supplementing with the tablets, capsules or liquid tincture as an anti-inflammatory, particularly if you're weaning yourself off Prednisone or Imuran or a similarly potent drug. DGL increases the amount of mucous-secreting cells in the digestive tract. This improves the quality of mucous, lengthens intestinal cell life and enhances microcirculation in the gastrointestinal lining. For these reasons, DGL should work particularly well for those with ulcerative colitis.

Probiotics

Beneficial bacteria can also heal and control future outbreaks of mouth ulcers. Clinical trials show *L. acidophilus* to be particularly effective. Use Natren Inc.'s Megadophilus powder amd mix ½ tsp. with a small amount of water (2–4 ounces). Take a sip and then swish it round your mouth and gums and hold it in your mouth for as long as you can before swallowing. Take another sip and continue in this manner until you've finished the dose. As with all probiotics, take it on an empty stomach.

Pregnancy/Breastfeeding/Babies Guidance: I have used Natren probiotics whilst pregnant and breastfeeding. I have also given Natren probiotics to my kids as babies (give babies ONLY Life Start – *B. infantis* – probiotic) and toddlers. I have used Wild Oregano Oil topically with my daughter from 4 months of age and very sparingly internally from 1 year old. I have used Wild Oregano Oil internally with my son from 3 years old. Herbal literature states that DGL should be safe to use whilst pregnant/breastfeeding, whilst regular licorice is not (may elevate blood pressure). Wild Oregano Oil is contraindicated (i.e. do not use) for pregnant or breastfeeding women, however, if you just rinse your mouth and then spit it out without swallowing it, that should be okay – check with your naturopathic physician to be sure.

SYMPTOM TREATMENT SUMMARY – MOUTH ULCERS

- Rinse/gargle with Wild Oregano Oil – 5 drops in a mouthful of water and then swallow it. 1 – 3 applications should completely heal mouth ulcers.
- Suck DGL lozenges (and swish DGL/saliva around mouth) as often as you can until mouth ulcers subside.
- Rinse your mouth often with Natren's Megadophilus powder (*L. acidophilus*), 1 – 6 times per day
- Follow *Reduce Diarrhea Diet* (see Chapter Three) to eliminate acidic foods

---

Notes:

☼ RECTAL FISSURES

Anal or rectal fissures are tears in the tissue of the anus or rectal canal. Sometimes a mild fissure will heal on its own with no additional help, but for deeper tears you need to assist the damaged tissue.

FissureHeal Suppositories

An absolutely fantastic product for healing anal and rectal fissures, or hemorrhoids, is an all-natural herbal suppository called FissureHeal. I created FissureHeal suppositories and I've used them myself to heal both minor and severe anal fissures and they work very well. I've also heard from readers who've used them to heal fissures they've had for 5 – 6 years continually and nothing else worked until they tried FissureHeal. A friend of mine who suffers from hemorrhoids (as a result of birthing two children) uses them every time her hemorrhoids flare and usually one or two suppositories is all she needs. The suppositories are very thin – as thin as a regular-sized drinking straw – so no matter how sore your anus/rectum is, they will insert easily. They've also made them extra long (2") so they can reach a fissure even high up in your rectal canal – or you can break them off at the length you need. They contain Comfrey Root, Slippery Elm, Marshmallow Root and Cocoa Butter, so the ingredients are very effective and healing. At the time of writing, FissureHeal is only available online at *www.fissureheal.com* (or by calling 1-800-460-8606). Of course, they're also available at the LTYG Holistic Health Shoppe *(www.LTYGshoppe.com)*. Insert them at night – or whenever you're likely to have your longest stretch without a bowel movement – so your anus/rectum has the maximum amount of time to heal undisturbed.

Fresh Aloe Vera

Alternatively, you may want to consider getting an Aloe vera plant to use for rectal suppositories. Cut off a piece of the leaf, then cut away the green leaf and inside yellowish layer (bitter and astringent), leaving only the clear inside meat of the plant. Insert this fresh Aloe vera (cut to desired length and width) into your rectum and leave it there until your next bowel

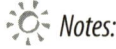
Notes:

movement when it will come out naturally. You may need to wrap the cut Aloe vera in cellophane wrap and freeze it first to firm it up and make it easier to insert. If you insert this suppository before bed then the Aloe vera has all night (hopefully) to work its healing action. If using the fresh plant doesn't appeal to you, you can always use a pure Aloe vera gel or salve, coat your finger with it and insert it into your rectum. Try to massage the gel or salve into the tissue gently. Re-apply after every bowel movement, or as often as you can. Make sure you've washed your hands with soap and water before application and never stick the same, soiled finger back into your pot of salve.

Comfrey Salve

Another good healing salve for anal/rectal fissures is one made primarily from the Comfrey plant. Other good ingredients to look for include Plantain, Aloe Vera and vitamin E. Most comfrey salves will contain some or all of these other ingredients as well. Again, coat your finger well with the salve and insert into your rectum, massaging the salve into the tissue. Re-apply after every bowel movement, or as often as possible. Make sure you've washed your hands thoroughly before application and never stick the same, soiled finger back into your pot of salve.

Pregnancy/Breastfeeding/Babies Guidance: I have used Natren probiotics, Aloe vera, Comfrey and FissureHeal whilst pregnant and breastfeeding. I have also given Natren probiotics to my kids as babies (give babies ONLY Life Start – *B. infantis* – probiotic) and toddlers and they have also ingested George's Aloe Vera Juice from one year onwards. I used FissureHeal suppositories on my daughter at six months of age, for a few days and have used Comfrey with both children when necessary since infancy.

> Sometimes a mild fissure will heal on its own with no additional help, but for deeper tears you need to assist the damaged tissue.

Symptom Treatment Summary – Rectal Fissures

▶ If you get the FissureHeal suppositories, that's likely all you'll need to heal even deep anal or rectal fissures. Use at night, right before bed, and once or twice during the day if you feel you need it. Follow insertion directions on the package.

▶ Otherwise, try the other remedies listed as you wish.

☀ STRICTURES

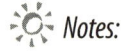
Notes:

Chronic inflammation of the intestinal wall can cause scarring of the intestines. This scar tissue is then not as flexible as healthy tissue and as the tougher scar tissue builds up, it results in a narrowed, or constricted area in the intestine. These constricted areas are called strictures. Strictures range from mild to severe, depending on how much they block the contents of the bowel from passing through the narrowed area. You may not even be aware that you have a stricture until it shows up on an x-ray, or, you may experience pain, cramping and bloating from a severe stricture as it obstructs the passage of food. If a stricture becomes so narrow that it completely obstructs the passage of food, then the intestine can rupture as a result. Current surgical procedures for strictures (including removal of the affected section of intestine, or strictuloplasty) do not usually prevent recurrence and in my opinion should be reserved for cases of absolute emergency. Strictures require a multi-pronged approach to treatment as you need to heal the underlying conditions in the body and immune system that are causing inflammation, heal the mucosal lining, heal the intestinal wall, and restore proper bacterial flora throughout the gut to prevent recurrence.

I also suspect that some of the drugs used in IBD directly contribute to or cause strictures, because, essentially, *any* drug that disrupts the bacterial flora of the gut can be considered a direct contributor to strictures. Recent reports have shown that a lack of good bacteria and overgrowth of bad bacteria in the small intestine are associated with strictures:

> "A variety of clinical conditions are associated with Small Intestine Bacterial Overgrowth (SIBO): …Small bowel diverticulae, Strictures, Fistulas, Chronic atrophic gastritis, Pancreatitis, Immune deficiency, Malnutrition…" [6]

The IBD Remission Diet

The fastest method for healing acute strictures and avoiding surgery may be employing the other remedies listed here whilst following the IBD Remission Diet. An elemental diet aids in the healing of strictures because it reduces food matter and fecal waste to a watery minimum. Therefore, there is no bulky food or waste to aggravate an inflamed intestine or stricture, and the supplements recommended in the Diet are designed to heal inflammation, balance the immune system, heal the mucosal lining and then restore proper bacterial flora to the gut.

You would also be well advised to eliminate any pathogenic/infectious microorganisms first (see *Natural Antibiotics / Antimicrobials* section below) and then begin the IBD Remission Diet. Or you can begin both simultaneously, if you prefer, or if your situation is acute. When you have an overgrowth of bad bacteria in your intestines (which directly contributes to strictures), Wild Oregano Oil or Olive Leaf extract are the quickest ways to eliminate the bad bacteria (and other pathogenic microorganisms). Combining this with high doses of probiotics is your best chance for avoiding recurrent strictures. See Chapter Three for more information on an elemental (liquid, pre-digested) diet, or see my book, *The IBD Remission Diet* (www.IBDremissionDiet.com – read Chapter One free online).

If your stricture is severe and/or strictures are an ongoing, recurrent problem for you, then you can get rid of all infection using the natural antibiotics/antimicrobials first and then begin the IBD Remission Diet immediately after, or in the last two weeks of antibiotic/antimicrobial treatment, if you still need to. However, if your stricture is severe enough to require immediate surgery, then begin the natural antibiotics/antimicrobials treatment and IBD Remission Diet together, simultaneously – and you have a good chance of avoiding surgery altogether. Remember though, that both these treatments require you to ideally be off all drugs – see Chapter Five for more information on drugs and weaning yourself off them.

If your stricture(s) is mild to moderate, then you may be able to heal it using just the natural antibiotic/antimicrobial treatments (see *Natural Antibiotics/*

> ☼ Strictures require a multi-pronged approach to treatment as you need to heal the underlying conditions in the body and immune system that are causing inflammation, heal the mucosal lining, heal the intestinal wall, and restore proper bacterial flora throughout the gut to prevent recurrence.

Antimicrobials section) followed by high doses of probiotics (see *Probiotic Supplementation* section), and going on the IBD Remission Diet may not be necessary.

Craniosacral Therapy

The medical community is not educated in effective bodywork treatments available to soften and relax scar tissue, hence they are not aware of it and do not recommend it as a viable treatment option. Find a massage therapist who is certified in craniosacral therapy from the Upledger Institute – at least Level II or higher. To find a therapist in your area, search the practitioner listings at *www.upledger.com*. If you can find a therapist who is also trained in myofascial or visceral release, they will be even more effective at releasing and softening scar tissue. Over the years, on numerous occasions, I've had all the symptoms indicating the presence of a severe stricture in my intestine. But I don't go for an x-ray to have it confirmed, instead I go to my bodywork therapist to have the area released. This therapy, combined with all the other remedies listed here, has thus far always worked for me and restored proper digestive function. I was able to have 'hard proof' of the efficacy of this therapy recently when I saw my bodywork therapist, Lori Main, to address a stricture in my rectum.

My rectum was narrowed to the point where my stool was the width and shape of a flattened pencil. If my stool was ever solid and hard, it would tear the stricture and I would have rectal bleeding. I let this condition go on for years as I had been quite traumatized about anyone inserting anything into my rectum following my initial diagnostic colonoscopy, which was very violent and abusive. Eventually though, I was ready to go the next step in healing this trauma and rectal damage. When I first started working with Lori on my rectal stricture, I could insert only the tip of my pinkie finger (without causing stress or bleeding) into my rectum. After four treatments, Lori could painlessly insert her index finger past the second knuckle (about ¾ inch diameter), with no bleeding or trauma to my rectum. Scar tissue (or a stricture) does not have to be permanently rigid and inflexible.

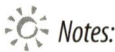 Notes:

There are effective therapies available for releasing and softening scar tissue, strictures and other areas of obstruction and restriction. Follow the kinder, gentler methods first and your body will begin to trust you and respond accordingly. For detailed information on bodywork therapies (including craniosacral) please see Chapter Six.

Heal The Mucosal Lining & Intestinal Wall

The following supplements are all effective for healing the mucosal lining and the intestinal wall, thus preventing ongoing inflammation and scarring: George's 'Always Active' Aloe Vera Juice, MucosaHeal, N-Acetyl Glucosamine (NAG), Essential Fatty Acids (EFA), and L-Glutamine. See the section on *Inflammation, Ulceration & Bleeding* for detailed descriptions of each of these supplements. If you're using MucosaHeal, you don't need to take N-Acetyl Glucosamine (NAG) because it's already contained in MucosaHeal. If you're simultaneously on the IBD Remission Diet (elemental diet) then you don't need to take L-Glutamine because you automatically get 1000 mg of L-Glutamine per serving of Absorb Plus. You'll also get your Essential Fatty Acids (EFA) from adding flax oil to your shakes. Essential Fatty Acids, or 'good fats' are also invaluable in softening scar tissue, so try to ingest Udo's oil, flax, or fish oil daily.

Basically, if you're not on the IBD Remission Diet, you should take MucosaHeal (*www.mucosaheal.com*) and at least 1 tablespoon of flax oil, and/or fish oil per day. You can also take George's Aloe Vera Juice if you like.

Probiotics

For a long term healing of strictures and the conditions that create them (such as SIBO), you need to improve the bacterial flora in your gut. Having a healthy gut flora will prevent future infection/inflammation in the intestines and if your intestines are not chronically inflamed, they will not build up scar tissue or thicken. Ingesting good bacteria improves digestion, absorption and elimination of food. Certain strains of bacteria help produce digestive enzymes, peptides, amino acids and B vitamins for your

 *Notes:*

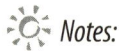 Notes:

body's use. They also inhibit or eliminate pathogenic microorganisms, like yeast, fungus, parasites, and bad bacteria that wound or burrow through the intestinal wall – possibly the beginning of inflammation and ulceration. See the expanded section on *Probiotic Supplementation* later on in this chapter for more information and details. Again, as I recommended above, you'll have the highest degree of success if you first follow a natural antibiotic/antimicrobial treatment (see *Natural Antibiotics / Antimicrobials* section) to eliminate the infectious microorganisms that are causing inflammation in your intestines, and then ingest high dosages of probiotics to repopulate your gut with good, healthy bacteria.

Currently, I only recommend Natren brand probiotics as they are the only company that currently meets standards for quality and efficacy (see *Probiotic Supplementation* section for quality standards). You need to take the full spectrum of probiotics *(L. acidophilus, B. bifidum, L. bulgaricus)* in powder form only. Do not take the probiotics in capsule form as you want to reap the benefits of the probiotics beginning in your mouth and esophagus and on down from there. Take 1 tsp. of each powder (Megadophilus, Bifido Factor, Digesta-Lac) mixed together in 8 ounces of room temperature filtered or spring water (no tap water!) 3 times per day on an empty stomach (15 – 20 minutes before food, or 2 hours after food), until your stricture is healed. Then take 1 tsp. of each powder (or you can now take one capsule once per day if your bowel movements are not loose or watery), 1 – 2 times per day for the next three months. If your strictures (or obstructions) commonly occur in your large intestine, then you may want to consider *Jini's Probiotic Retention Enema* for rapid repopulation of good bacteria in your colon. For details on how to administer *Jini's Probiotic Retention Enema* and for ongoing probiotic supplementation guidelines, please see the section on *Probiotic Supplementation* below.

Pregnancy/Breastfeeding/Babies Guidance: I have used Natren probiotics, Udo's Oil, George's Aloe Vera Juice, and FissureHeal whilst pregnant and breastfeeding. I have also given Natren probiotics to my kids as babies (give babies ONLY Life Start – *B. infantis* – probiotic) and toddlers and they have also ingested George's Aloe Vera and Udo's Oil periodically from 1 year onwards. I used FissureHeal suppositories on my daughter at six months of age, for a few days. A reader in Canada went on the IBD Remission Diet whilst pregnant rather than use Prednisone during a flare and she also added raw vegetable juices to the diet (we thought it would be good for the fetus to receive phytochemicals and other key vegetable nutrients if she could tolerate it). Her baby was born healthy and has developed well with no complications. Herbal literature states that MucosaHeal and *Jini's Healing Implant Enema* should be safe to use whilst pregnant/breastfeeding, or with babies/toddlers. Wild Oregano Oil is contraindicated (i.e. do not use) for pregnant or breastfeeding women, and see the *Natural Antibiotics / Antimicrobials* section below for more information on its use with babies/children. I have also taken both my children for craniosacral therapy from newborn to present – it is an invaluable tool for assisting children to be able to grow and develop unhindered. See my DVD, *BABY FART AEROBICS: And Other Natural Treatments for Colicky Babies* for an entire section on how/why craniosacral treatments are good for your kids and also to see a live demo on my daughter, Zara (available at *www.ColicInfant.com*).

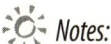 *Notes:*

Symptom Treatment Summary – Strictures

- Follow the natural antibiotics/antimicrobials treatment (see *Natural Antibiotics / Antimicrobials* section) and then go on an elemental diet. See Chapter Three, or my book, *The IBD Remission Diet* (read Chapter One online at: *www.caramal.com*) for more information on elemental diets.

- Whilst on the IBD Remission Diet, supplement with MucosaHeal and George's Aloe Vera juice (you'll automatically be ingesting the rest of the supplements needed to rebuild the intestinal wall by following the IBD Remission Diet). If you don't follow the Diet, then take: MucosaHeal as directed on the bottle, and at least 1 tablespoon of flax and/or fish oil per day. You can also take George's 'Always Active' Aloe Vera juice, if you wish.

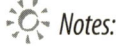 Notes:

- If you have a stricture in your rectum, then also follow the instructions in the *Rectal Fissures* section for using FissureHeal suppositories to speed tissue healing.

- Take the full spectrum of Natren brand probiotics *(L. acidophilus, B. bifidum, L. bulgaricus)* in powder form only. Mix 1 tsp. of each powder (Megadophilus, Bifido Factor, Digesta-Lac) in 8 ounces of room temperature spring or filtered water (no tap water) and take 3 times per day on an empty stomach until stricture is healed. Then take 1 tsp. 1 – 2 times per day in powder form, or, 1 capsule once per day (only if you defecate once or less per day), on an empty stomach (15 – 20 minutes before food, or 2 hours after food) for the next three months. Do *Jini's Probiotic Retention Enema* if you have strictures or obstructions in your colon. For ongoing probiotic supplementation, see the *Probiotic Supplementation* section later in this chapter.

- Simultaneously begin craniosacral treatments to release and soften scar tissue. You don't even need to know exactly where your strictures are as a good therapist will be able to discern this themselves. Make sure the therapist is certified by the Upledger Institute at Level II or higher. Go to: *www.upledger.com* to search for a practitioner in your area. See Chapter Six for more details.

NATURAL ANTIBIOTICS / ANTIMICROBIALS

If your doctor wants to put you on antibiotics or antifungals, for either a gut or secondary infection, there are several natural alternatives you can consider. These include: Garlic, Olive Leaf Extract, Grapefruit Seed Extract and Wild Oregano Oil. All of these substances also have varying levels of anti-viral, anti-yeast, anti-fungal and anti-parasitic activity. Of these, Wild Oregano Oil and Olive Leaf Extract are the most potent and powerful. The only drawback to Wild Oregano Oil is that it feels very 'hot' (like chili pepper hot) for about 2 – 3 minutes after you take it orally, therefore, it can be very difficult to use with children.

Grapefruit Seed Extract is also quite potent, but I don't recommend you use it if you have any tendency towards diarrhea, as it will exacerbate your condition. It is also extremely bitter and so may be quite difficult to get children to take. If you have no problems with loose stool or diarrhea, then you can take 10 – 15 drops in 5 ounces of filtered or spring water 3 times per day, on an empty stomach for best results – but it still works okay when taken with food. For kids under age 10, take 6 drops in 5 ounces of filtered or spring water 3 times per day. To maximize antibiotic therapy, also take Olive Leaf Extract at the same time. And remember to follow with probiotics during and/or at the end of treatment.

Garlic may also cause diarrhea and/or bloating in susceptible individuals, the only way is to try it and see. However, I would only use it on mild bacterial infections. For robust infections I don't think it would be strong enough, as "it exerts an antibacterial effect estimated to be equivalent to 1% of that of penicillin." [7] Garlic is also quite effective against yeast, fungus and viral infections. Therefore, it's excellent to consume garlic daily in your food. For therapeutic use, I recommend you use Kyolic from Wakunaga of America in either capsule or oil form – it is one of the most potent garlic products on the market and it is also odorless. Go to their website for lots of scientific articles on garlic's properties and abilities: *www.kyolic.com*. See your naturopathic physician for dosing guidelines for your particular condition.

Olive Leaf Extract is probably the most palatable of the remedies listed here. You can get it in powder (capsule) or liquid form. For children the powder can be mixed with applesauce or mashed banana and can also be mixed with an herbal salve and used as a poultice on topical infections. Dr Morton Walker, who wrote the book *Nature's Antibiotic: Olive Leaf Extract*, writes:

> "Seagate® Olive Leaf Extract offers a 450 mg capsule recommended to be taken preventively in a dosage of one or two to four capsules daily. For treatment of a microbial illness, the better dosage would be four to

☼ Remember to follow all antibiotic use – whether natural or pharmaceutical – with high dose probiotic supplementation. You can also use probiotics concurrently with antibiotics to minimize unpleasant side effects.

eight capsules daily for one week, but the daily dose must be spread out throughout the day. When the illness comes under control or disappears, the dosage may be reduced once again to one, two, three, or four capsules per day." [8]

In the same article, Dr. Walker also relates the story of a female patient infected with three different mycoplasma organisms, she suffered from chronic fatigue, fibromyalgia and IBS. She took 2 pills (of Seagate brand Olive Leaf Extract), 3 times a day (following meals) for three and a half months and then her lab reports came back completely clear of infection. She reported her condition as "excellent" and also that she was completely cured of IBS. Dr. Walker recommends you only use Seagate brand since it is a cold-extracted formulation of the whole leaf (not just an oleuropein extract) and therefore more effective than anything else he's tried. See www.seagateproducts.com for more information.

Olive Leaf is antibacterial, antiviral, antifungal and antiyeast. It is much more palatable than Wild Oregano Oil and so probably the best natural antimicrobial to use for children. Again, remember that anything that is an effective antibacterial needs to be followed with probiotics. If you're taking it long-term, I would also supplement simultaneously with probiotics.

Wild Oregano Oil is the antimicrobial that I've had the most experience with. I can confidently state that it is the most effective antimicrobial I've ever seen for topical or acute infections. However, for chronic infections such as *Candida albicans* (yeast), mycobacteria (bacteria/fungal hybrid), and mycoplasmas (prokaryote bacteria), it's very hard to make any kind of definitive statement on the efficacy of Wild Oregano Oil vs. Olive Leaf Extract. Wild Oregano Oil is relatively new and it does not have the longer history of anecdotal evidence that Olive Leaf Extract has. Having said that, Wild Oregano Oil does have a fair amount of data regarding its ability to kill pathogenic bacteria in the food industry in incredibly minute doses. Unfortunately, I am not able to offer completely definitive instructions on the use of Wild Oregano Oil for people with IBS or IBD at this time. What I can give you is a pretty good idea of what should work, a summary of the research I've done, my personal experience to date, and the feedback I've had from about thirty of my consultation clients who've been experimenting with it.

To further the education of all of us on this topic, please visit my blog at www.ListenToYourGut.com where I will post my ongoing feedback/thoughts on Wild Oregano Oil and other natural antimicrobials. Please post your experience with any of the antimicrobials that you try and be as specific and give as much detail as possible. If we all pool our knowledge and experience, over time we'll be able to extrapolate some solid guidelines for IBD and IBS usage. Perhaps you'll be able to find a naturopath in your area who is fluent in the usage of both Wild Oregano Oil and Olive Leaf and he/she could guide you.

Doug Kaufmann (who has a TV show called 'Know The Cause', which airs on Sky Angel, inspiration Network and Liberty Channel) and Dr. Dave Holland, MD have written a book called, *The Fungus Link*. I first heard about Doug Kaufmann when he invited me to be a guest on his TV show. Doug and Dave both recommend Olive Leaf extract (Seagate brand) for treating the underlying infection (bacterial/yeast/fungal) of IBD and IBS. Here is a fascinating excerpt from Chapter Three of their book, *The Fungus Link*:

> "We've seen thus far that, in just about every case of inflammatory bowel disease, conventional treatment involves the use of anti-inflammatories. Well, researchers at the Washington University in St. Louis took a bold step and did a study where they offered patients with Crohn's disease an immune stimulant instead. They used a medicine called Leukine--a naturally-occuring molecule called Granulocyte-Macrophage Colony Stimulating Factor (GM-CSF).
>
> And though they faced harsh criticism from scientists at other universities for doing this, they obtained amazing results: of the initial 15 patients in the study, 12 did "significantly" better overall, while eight went into complete remission! Every one of the half a million patients with Crohn's disease in America should know about this study.

> Typically, an anti-inflammatory medicine merely controls the symptoms of the disease – it doesn't cure it. That's because it rarely addresses the true cause of the disease.
>
> Doug Kaufmann, Dave Holland, MD
> *The Fungus Link*

> But they shouldn't feel they need to rush in to their doctor's office to get this expensive shot (it costs around $300 per milliliter--that's $1,500 per teaspoon). Rather, they should learn from this study: by giving an immune booster, these doctors were able to put 53 percent of the cases into total remission. That almost implies that an infection is at the root of the disease, and that by assisting the body's immune system the medication helped the body overcome the "infection," or the disease.
>
> Typically, an anti-inflammatory medicine merely controls the symptoms of the disease--it doesn't cure it. That's because it rarely addresses the true cause of the disease. In other words, if the wrong diet is constantly consumed, or if damage (i.e. yeast overgrowth) is never reversed from previous antibiotic use, a cure can almost never be achieved. In this case, we feel that the "infection" in the intestines of Crohn's patients is caused by fungi and their mycotoxins." [9]
> *(See Appendix D for the study referenced in this excerpt)*

As you can see, I'm certainly not the only one asserting that the infectious component of IBD and IBS must be addressed for complete and/or long-term healing to occur. Whether you want to use Olive Leaf Extract or Wild Oregano Oil (or perhaps a combination of the two) to address your infection, only you can decide.

If you're interested in finding out exactly which microorganisms you're infected with, you have to use a highly specialized lab to get reliable test results. A regular lab is not skilled enough, nor properly equipped to test for these bacterial/fungal organisms. One of the best labs I've come across is Immunosciences Laboratory in Beverly Hills, California: *www.immuno-sci-lab.com*, Tel: (310) 657-1077 Toll Free: (800) 950-4686. You get your doctor (MD or ND) to draw the blood samples needed, fill out the forms, and then courier the samples to Immunosciences Lab. If you need a lab in your own country, contact Immunosciences and see if they can refer you to a reputable lab in your area.

WILD OREGANO OIL

Wild Oregano Oil (*Oreganum vulgare*) is an anti-inflammatory in addition to being an extremely potent antiviral, antibacterial, antifungal, antiparasitic, (anti-everything!) agent. It is extracted from a particular species of oregano that grows wild in rocky regions of the Mediterranean and it has only been used in North America for about ten years. As such, it is a relatively 'new' herbal medicine in the U.S. and not many naturopathic physicians are even fluent in its uses and amazing efficacy. I expect it will gain momentum quickly in the coming years and like all really effective herbal medicines the FDA will probably try to ban it before too long!

Most of the scientific research on Wild Oregano Oil is currently coming from the Applied Microbiology field in the area of food preservation. Microbiologists have found that Wild Oregano Oil is so powerful that even minute amounts of it can kill common food-borne pathogens responsible for a lot of the food poisoning incidents with processed food. To give you just one example, scientists in The Netherlands found that Carvacrol (one of the active ingredients of Wild Oregano) at a dilution of only .25 mM led to cell death of the bacterial soil organism *Bacillus cereus*, "a spore-forming food-borne pathogen often associated with food products such as meat, vegetables, soup, rice, milk and other dairy products. Between 1 and 20% of the total number of outbreaks of food infection in the world is caused by *B. cereus*." The scientists summarized their results by saying, "From this study, it could be concluded that carvacrol interacts with the membranes of *B. cereus* by changing its permeability for cations like H+ and K+. The dissipation of ion gradients leads to impairment of essential processes in the cell and finally to cell death." [10] What this means for the layperson, is that even very small amounts of the phenolic compounds within Wild Oregano Oil (such as Carvacrol and Thymol) can disintegrate the cell walls of pathogenic microorganisms, resulting in their death.

> Even very small amounts of the phenolic compounds within Wild Oregano Oil (such as Carvacrol and Thymol) can disintegrate the cell walls of pathogenic microorganisms, resulting in their death.

My Personal Experience
I was first introduced to Wild Oregano Oil when my daughter developed a severe yeast infection in the folds of her skin at four months of age.

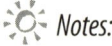 Notes:

I tried every natural substance I knew of to try and heal it and then finally consulted a naturopath who specialized in children. He immediately recognized it as a yeast infection and recommended a dilution of Wild Oregano Oil (diluted with olive oil 15:1). I applied it to her skin and within a day could notice a difference! Within three days, the lesions (which were several layers deep and weeping) had a complete covering of new healthy skin and within seven days her skin was completely healed and normal. None of us, including my physician father, had ever seen such a quick and total healing with any substance before – natural or pharmaceutical. We all jumped on this new wonder herb, began researching and reading about it, and started using it for everything that came up. Since that time, over the two years that followed, I and my family members have used Wild Oregano Oil with amazing results on the following conditions:

- Foot and Mouth Disease (viral)
- Herpes 2 (viral)
- Gum infections
- Mouth ulcers
- Flu and chest infection (bacterial and viral)
- Sore throats
- As a preventive, before and after plane journeys, or when exposed to someone with a cold or flu
- Skin infection (fungal)

I have also used it myself ongoing for about a year (alternating with probiotics), just 5 drops/day in the morning on an empty stomach, followed by a glass of water. That year was filled with lots of travel, sleep deprivation and difficulty eating proper meals, lots of stress financially and emotionally, and a crushing work load between my businesses and two young children. And yes, there were a few months where I was definitely using it as a crutch (like a drug) to keep myself going and buy myself some time to look at the root issues in my life that were resulting in such stress and exhaustion. At the time I took it, I had no overt symptoms of any gut disease, I would have been classed as "in remission". However, the difference was still remarkable: No more fuzzy-brain or depression, my memory got much sharper, my energy levels stayed strong and consistent throughout the day (instead of crashing around 4 – 5 pm) and I was less irritable and had more patience. All these symptoms are correlated with a compromised gut flora and thus I suspect that even though my health has been quite good, perhaps I have had a low-grade gut infection (yeast, mycobacteria, etc.) for years that has flared up or intensified during times of stress.

Infection & Inflammation In The Gut

Therefore, based on my own experience, what I've researched to date, and the experience of a few of my consultation clients who've experimented with Wild Oregano Oil, I'd like to offer you the following treatment protocol as a *starting point* for using Wild Oregano to heal gut infection. Please post your resulting experience and experiments at: www.ListenToYourGut.com as the more information we can gather, the better we can make this protocol for all of us. Again, this protocol is based on inflammatory bowel disease being an infectious disease (or having an infectious component). I have already written quite a bit about this in the sections above and I will offer even more evidence of this phenomenon in the *Probiotic Supplementation* section directly following this section. Regardless of where you stand on this theory, certain facts are inescapable: Inflammation is usually a response to infection, or, the body's attempt to get rid of something undesirable. If you get a splinter and it's not removed quickly, the body will launch an inflammatory response to push out the splinter. If you cut yourself and the wound gets infected, the body responds with inflammation; the wound swells up, pus forms and the body seeks to trap the infectious agent, kill it, and push it out of the body. The presence of inflammation in the gut likewise is probably signaling the presence of an undesirable or infectious agent that the body is trying to get rid of.

Many gastroenterologists work from the premise that IBD is an auto-immune disease, whereby, for some unknown reason, the body attacks itself, thus causing ulceration, lesions, bleeding, fistulas, etc. However,

> Inflammation is usually a response to infection, or, the body's attempt to get rid of something undesirable.

what if the body were actually attacking pathogenic microorganisms that have just not been identified yet? There is a relatively new breed of microorganisms that have evolved that are actually bacterial-fungal hybrids called mycobacterium. Another new type of bacteria called mycoplasma can actually enter and reside in the plasma of cells making both detection and elimination quite difficult. In identifying a certain type of mycobacterium called *Mycobacterium avium* (sub-species paratuberculosis) scientists have found the only reliable test to be one which tests for the DNA of *Mycobacterium avium*, rather than the physical organism itself. Personally, I suspect there is both an infectious and an auto-immune component to inflammatory bowel disease and you will have the highest degree of success if you treat for both (if you follow the protocols in this program, you will address both components).

There are two ways to eliminate infectious microorganisms: Antimicrobial drugs or substances, or high doses of probiotics. This protocol is unique in that it combines the two methods for maximum effectiveness in both eradicating infectious microorganisms, maintaining a healthy bacterial flora *during* antimicrobial supplementation, and maintaining a healthy gut environment ongoing, for continued long-term health.

The following 3-Phase protocol should eliminate infectious microorganisms (like mycobacterium, fungi, bacteria, yeast, viruses, parasites, etc.), provide a moderate level of detoxification, and restore beneficial gut flora. By healing the infection we also heal inflammation. Other supplements referred to often in this program (such as MucosaHeal, George's 'Always Active' Aloe Vera Juice, L-Glutamine, etc.) are then used to heal ulceration, bleeding, and repair the intestinal wall and mucosal lining. Supplementation with probiotics restores a healthy, balanced gut flora to prevent future recurrence. Once you've finished the Protocol outlined here, consult the *Probiotic Supplementation* section below for guidance on ongoing probiotic maintenance, or, preventive supplementation. If you are infected with *Mycobacterium avium* paratuberculosis (MAP), which is a sort of hybrid bacteria/fungus, then you may need to repeat this Protocol every 3 – 4 months for up to two years to completely eradicate these pathogenic microorganisms. MAP has a dormant/active lifecycle that surges again in as little as 3 – 4 months after treatment with aggressive antibiotics and antifungals. Doctors experimenting with eradicating this pathogen have found it takes up to two years to completely eradicate it. See the section on *Probiotic Supplementation* below for more details on MAP.

The dosage of Wild Oregano Oil recommended here in Phase 1 is the equivalent of Vancomycin (a potent antibiotic reserved for superbugs). However, depending upon the type of microorganisms and parasites you're infected with, and how widespread that infection is, your length of time on Phase I is going to vary. Again, all of this is still largely experimental, so you really need to follow your own gut, since each person is going to have different levels and types of infection present. Therefore, a moderate dosage protocol that may work for one person, is not strong enough for another person who has more rampant, or multiple infections present. And likewise, a powerful protocol that works for one person, may be far too strong and produce undesirable 'rebound' effects in someone with only a mild infection.

Again, like every recommendation in this program: Please follow your gut! Remember that you know your body better than anyone, and if you get a feeling you should change the dosage (longer, shorter, more, less, etc.) then please do so, but keep in mind that these substances are as powerful as drugs and must also be used intelligently. Remember, it's always better to take longer to accomplish a task, yet stay balanced.

Likewise, you may feel you need to slowly ease your way into the Protocol and may prefer to start with just 5 drops once or twice a day and see how that goes before beginning Phase 1. If you have a strong or rampant infection, you may find the Phase 1 dosage causes the pathogens to die off too quickly and you get sick with the symptoms of the die-off effect (headaches, nausea, bloating, diarrhea, cold, flu, etc.). This is also known as the Herxheimer Reaction and it occurs when the body detoxifies rapidly as a result of a quick, massive die-off of pathogenic microorganisms. If this is the case, then you may want to ease into the Protocol by starting with

☼ If you are infected with MAP, which is a sort of hybrid bacteria/fungus, then you may need to repeat this Protocol every 3 – 4 months for up to two years to completely eradicate the infection.

just 5 drops once or twice per day for two weeks (combined with probiotic supplementation), and then begin Phase 1. This will help you to avoid a rapid die-off of pathogens and the resulting illness/symptoms as your body flushes them from your system. Remember: Always listen to your gut and follow what feels right for your body.

What Brand Should I Get?

It's very important to use the correct species of oregano; as different species contain different levels of Carvacrol and Thymol. Please follow the specifications here to ensure you get the desired results and don't substitute brands unless they can meet the same criteria (confirmed via an independent lab assay). When purchasing Wild Oregano Oil, make sure you get:

Species: *Oreganum vulgare*
Subspecies: Hirtum is one of several that work well

For Wild Oregano Oil to be effective, it must be high in naturally occurring Carvacrol (ideally 75% or more) – not just have extra Carvacrol added in later. If you get a brand with the correct species and subspecies, this will not be a problem. Effective, good quality Wild Oregano Oil should also be low in Thymol. Thymol is a naturally occurring compound in Oregano Oil that must be present as it works synergistically with Carvacrol. But, too much is hard on the liver, so check that levels do not exceed 5% maximum. Currently, there are only two brands of Wild Oregano Oil that I can recommend that meet these standards for efficacy and bioavailability: Oil of Oregano by Joy of the Mountains *(www.LTYGshoppe.com)* and Oreganol by North American Herb & Spice Company. I find Joy of the Mountains to be the better of the two, however, it also has a 'hotter' feel to it, so if you're using it for children then go with the Oreganol brand. The dosage given for Wild Oregano Oil in this Protocol is for Oregano Oil that has already been diluted in a carrier oil (most brands are) like olive oil. 5 drops of diluted Wild Oregano Oil is equivalent to 1 – 2 drops of pure, undiluted Wild Oregano Oil. If you're using a brand other than the ones recommended here, check carefully to see whether it's diluted or undiluted. Remember to *always*

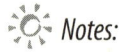 *Notes:*

dilute pure (undiluted) Oregano Oil in a carrier oil before using internally or externally, or it can cause tissue damage. The two brands recommended here have already been diluted with olive oil, so you don't need to dilute them further before using.

Warning: Ideally, for best results, you should wean yourself off all drugs before beginning this Protocol (see your doctor or Chapter Five for weaning instructions). However, if that is not possible, then DO NOT follow this Protocol if you are using three or more prescription drugs. It will not be safe for your liver. Also, Wild Oregano Oil is not recommended for pregnant or breastfeeding women, or for children under age five.

I have not used it whilst pregnant or breastfeeding, but I have used it on my children from four months of age topically and 6 months of age orally. Obviously, I gave it to my kids in very minute doses (congruent with their body weight) and found it caused no harm when used in conjunction with and followed by probiotics. I also gave it in high doses to my breastfeeding cat when she became deathly ill after eating a dead bird, and she and her five kittens showed no ill effects. In fact, when we took the kittens to the pet store three weeks after dosage, the vet said he'd never seen an entire litter of kittens come in with no mouth or ear infections before!

Obviously, this is an area where you'll have to make your own decision since there are no clinical studies on usage with pregnant or breastfeeding women, or with babies and toddlers. My personal opinion is: Avoid it if possible since it is a very strong substance (especially in first trimester pregnancy when your liver is already stressed). But, you have to ask yourself: When faced with antibiotics or steroids as the alternative, do you feel Wild Oregano will do less harm than these potent drugs? Consult your naturopathic physician for more guidance or information and if you decide to take it whilst pregnant or breastfeeding, stay under your physician's care and supervision, and please post your results to my website so that others can benefit from your experience: *www.JiniPatelThompson.com*.

> For Wild Oregano Oil to be effective, it must be high in naturally occurring Carvacrol (ideally 75% or more) – not just have extra Carvacrol added in later. It should also be low in Thymol.

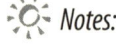
Notes:

Jini's Wild Oregano Oil Protocol

Phase 1 – Until Infection Is Gone

▸ *Wild Oregano Oil* – 10 drops (or 2 capsules of oil), 3 – 5 times per day, on an empty stomach, until infection is resolved. This can take anywhere from two weeks for mild infection, to six months for severe, chronic infection. Use 5 times a day if you have a strong or widespread infection, or, 3 times a day for regular infection. Also apply topically, if needed, 3 times per day till completely healed (see *Usage Instructions* below for detailed instructions).

▸ *Natren Probiotics* – (all three: Megadophilus, Bifido Factor, Digesta-Lac in powder form only) once before bed on an empty stomach until infection is healed; 1 tsp. of each powder mixed together in 6 – 8 ounces of filtered, room temperature water. Do not use the Natren Healthy Trinity capsules at this point since we need the good bacteria to begin colonizing in your mouth (swish around before swallowing if you can) and esophagus, as well as stomach, small intestine and colon. Try to take it at least two hours after your last dose of Wild Oregano Oil.

Phase 2 – Three Months*

▸ *Probiotic Retention Enema* – Perform *Jini's Probiotic Retention Enema* before bed on day one of this Phase (see instructions below in *Probiotic Supplementation* Section). Then, on day three, begin the rest of the procedures for this phase:

▸ *Wild Oregano Oil* – 5 drops (or one capsule of oil), once in the morning, on an empty stomach for three months (see *Usage Instructions* below)

▸ *Natren Probiotics* – (all three: Megadophilus, Bifido Factor, Digesta-Lac) once in the afternoon and once before bed, on an empty stomach, for three months. If you're having loose stools or diarrhea, then take the Natren probiotics in powder form only; 1 tsp. of each mixed in 6 – 8 ounces of filtered, room temperature water. Otherwise you can use either the capsules (Healthy Trinity – 1 capsule only, once before bed on an empty stomach) or the powders, whichever you prefer. But keep in mind the powders will also colonize your mouth and esophagus. For this reason, I prefer the powders if possible. If you don't do *Jini's Probiotic Retention Enema*, then take one more dose of oral probiotics per day (i.e. take the powders 3 times per day and the capsule 2 times per day).

Phase 3 – Three Months
- ***Natren Probiotics*** – (all three: Megadophilus, Bifido Factor, Digesta-Lac) 3 times per day on an empty stomach for three months. If you're having loose stools or diarrhea, then take the Natren probiotics in powder form only; 1 tsp. of each mixed in 6 – 8 ounces of filtered, room temperature water. Otherwise you can use either the capsules (Healthy Trinity – 1 capsule, 1 – 2 times per day on an empty stomach) or the powders, whichever you prefer. Also do *Jini's Probiotic Retention Enema* once per month for 3 months, if you can (highly recommended) – see *Probiotic Supplementation* section below for Enema instructions.

If your infection is only mild, you can probably skip Phase 2 and go directly to Phase 3.

> There are two ways to eliminate infectious microorganisms: Antimicrobial drugs or substances, or high doses of probiotics. This protocol is unique in that it combines the two methods.

Wild Oregano Oil Usage Instructions

Wild Oregano Oil feels 'spicy hot' when you swallow it (or when it touches any mucous membrane). So, the best way to take it is to fill the dropper with 5 – 10 drops, tilt your head back and shoot the contents of the dropper to the back of your throat. Immediately follow with lots of water or juice, and keep drinking water till heat sensation disappears (about 10 seconds). Always shake dropper bottle well before using.

- If you also have mouth ulcers or a gum infection, sip a mouthful of water and hold it in your mouth. Add five drops of Oregano Oil to the mouthful of water and then swish together around your mouth and gums for as long as you can stand it, then swallow. Leave it if you can tolerate the heat, if you can't, then sip water till the heat sensation subsides.

> Inflammation is usually a response to infection, or, the body's attempt to get rid of something undesirable.

- Alternatively, you can simply drop some Oregano Oil onto your finger and rub it directly onto the mouth ulcer(s) or infected gum/tooth. Leave it as long as possible and then drink water if needed. If you can't tolerate the taste or smell of Wild Oregano Oil (some like it, some don't) then you can take it in capsule form. But make sure the capsules contain the oil, not powdered oregano. 1 capsule is equal to 5 drops. Be sure and follow capsules with lots of water to help dilute the oil in your stomach.

- You also MUST apply Wild Oregano Oil directly/topically to any localized infection on skin, nails, mouth, vagina, etc., 2 – 3 times per day. However, when applying to genitalia or anal area you should dilute the Wild Oregano Oil further, or you will be hopping around from the 'burning' sensation! Dilute it with olive oil 10:1 or 15:1 (i.e. 15 drops of olive oil to one drop of oregano oil) before applying to genitalia or anal area.
For babies or toddlers dilute 15:1 or 20:1 for diaper, anal or genital area. Always shake bottle containing dilution well before using. Excellent for treating yeast *(Candida albicans)*, fungal, bacterial infections, herpes, etc. For fistulas, try to drop the diluted Oregano Oil directly into the fistula hole/opening and then massage gently with your finger to rub it in.
A reader who had two fistulas in his anal area chose to use Wild Oregano Oil at full strength because the 'burning' sensation made him feel it was really killing everything and clearing them out. Hey, whatever works! For a vaginal infection, you can either apply the diluted Wild Oregano Oil directly to your labia, vaginal walls and cervix using your finger (really swab it round thoroughly), or you can add about 50 – 60 drops of the dilution to some warm water and douche with it. For more instructions on topical applications, go to: *www.ListenToYourGut.com*

- An added bonus is you probably won't get any flus/colds whilst taking Wild Oregano Oil!

Repeat all three Phases whenever you have a flare, or symptoms begin to return. The Protocol may need to be repeated every 3 – 4 months for 2 – 3 years (the dormant/active cycle of mycobacterium) to completely clear all intestinal infection and restore gut flora. If symptoms start again during Phase 3, return to Phase 1 and begin again.

Natren brand probiotics are VITAL throughout the protocol. Remember that Wild Oregano Oil is a potent antibiotic and just like a pharmaceutical antibiotic, you need to supplement with probiotics to minimize the side of effects of antibiotics *during* treatment and then you need to completely re-populate your gut flora *after* treatment – to prevent recurrent infection. You should use Natren brand probiotics (*www.LTYGshoppe.com* as they are the only brand that currently meets potency and bioavailability standards (at time of consumption, not packaging!) for effective gut reflorastation. See the *Probiotic Supplementation* section following for more details. Remember that the Wild Oregano Oil dosage in Phase 1 is equivalent to a course of Vancomycin, or other potent antibiotic, therefore it MUST be followed with probiotics.

Important: If you abandon this treatment protocol without finishing the third phase, you MUST supplement with Natren brand probiotics to restore good bacterial flora to your gut. Wild Oregano Oil is a very potent antibiotic and MUST be followed with probiotics for at least three months.

> Top quality probiotic supplementation is an integral part of healing the root cause of IBS or IBD and then maintaining ongoing health.

PROBIOTIC (GOOD BACTERIA) SUPPLEMENTATION

Probiotic therapy benefits people with IBD (inflammatory bowel disease) and IBS (irritable bowel syndrome) in many ways. If you get too many 'bad' bacteria in your gut and not enough 'good' bacteria, the bad bacteria (and other pathogenic microorganisms like yeast, fungi, parasites, etc.) will degrade the mucosal lining of your intestine and even penetrate through the intestinal wall. Aside from resulting in an increase of mucous, inflammation, ulceration and bleeding, this will also result in undigested particles of food passing directly into your bloodstream – where they are perceived as allergens and trigger an immune response. Repopulating your bacterial flora to contain predominantly good bacteria (via probiotic supplementation) will result in a drastic reduction – if not elimination – of many harmful pathogens like yeast, fungus, mold, parasites, viruses and bad bacteria from your gut environment. The good bacteria will also form a protective coating of your mucosal cell lining and produce B vitamins and digestive enzymes. As a result, proper digestion and absorption of nutrients will gradually be restored. Top quality probiotic supplementation is an integral part of healing the root cause of IBS or IBD and then maintaining ongoing health. Symptoms that can be automatically resolved as a result of this healing include: heartburn, gas, bloating, constipation, diarrhea, excess mucous, intestinal spasms or cramping, ulceration, inflammation, and bleeding.

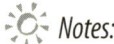
Notes:

Benefits Of Probiotics

Friendly bacteria, such as *Lactobacillus acidophilus, Bifidobacterium bifidum and Lactobacillus bulgaricus*, provide the following benefits to our bodies:

- Produce natural antibiotics (acidophilin, lactocidin and acidolin) to fend off bacterial pathogens such as salmonella, shigella, staphylococcus, and *Helicobacter pylori*.
- Produce lactic acid that discourages the growth of unfavorable organisms
- Inhibit yeast (*Candida albicans*)
- As a result of the above points, they prevent intestinal, bladder and vaginal infections and bowel toxicity
- Synthesize B vitamins and vitamin K
- Synthesize butyric acid (butyrate), which is a primary fuel and healer for cells lining the colon and an important anticancer agent
- Aid in nutrient uptake (especially calcium)
- Synthesize acetic acid, which inhibits cholesterol synthesis in the liver and helps lower serum cholesterol levels
- Improve lactose metabolism
- Help metabolize toxic environmental chemicals
- Calm the liver, thereby resulting in better sleep when taken before bed

(Sources: *Optimal Wellness* by Ralph Golan, MD and *Probiotics: Nature's Internal Healers* by Natasha Trenev)

Sara Horowitz, PhD, wrote an article titled *Promoting Gut Health with Probiotics*, in which she summarized a lot of the recent research concerning probiotics and IBD. Here are some interesting data she highlighted (see her article for original reference sources).

1. Scientists purposely create mice with high levels of bad bacteria in their gut. Then they restore normal levels of good bacteria and show that it prevents colitis.
   "'Knockout' experimental models of IBD, in which genetic engineering methods breed selectively for the lack of a protective element in the immune system, have shown that animals bred in this way experience an increase in aerobic luminal bacteria that invade their intestinal linings aggressively. Mice born without IL-10 have decreased GI levels of beneficial *Lactobacillus* bacteria. When normal Lactobacillus levels were restored in one study, the levels of problematic bacteria were reduced and the development of colitis was prevented." [11]

2. Dr. Lichtenstein (a gastroenterologist), says that probiotics have an anti-inflammatory effect and they also help to tone down hyper-active immune systems in people with IBD:
   "After noting that preliminary results regarding probiotics for management of IBD are promising, Gary R. Lichtenstein, MD, in the department of gastroenterology, University of Pennsylvania School of Medicine, Philadelphia, similarly summarized the probable mechanisms of action of probiotics as basically involving increased immunosuppressive and decreased proinflammatory mediators." [12]

3. Probiotics can help get the immune system out of "attack mode" and improve the intestinal mucosa:
   "It has been hypothesized that probiotics can help to turn off the inappropriate, overreactive immune response in IBD by controlling regulatory signaling between the bacteria and these cells, and influencing mucosal integrity favorably." [13]

> Probiotics can help get the immune system out of "attack mode" and improve the intestinal mucosa.

4. IBS patients treated with *L. acidophilus* showed 50% improvement in eight weeks:

> "In a double-blinded clinical trial of 18 patients with IBS, subjects were treated for six weeks with *L. acidophilus* in capsule form. After a 2-week washout period, the subjects continued to take the supplement for another six weeks. The patients who received the probiotic experienced a 50% improvement compared to placebo" [14]

In Natasha Trenev's book, *Probiotics: Nature's Internal Healers*, she recounts a clinical trial that used probiotics to induce remission in patients with ulcerative colitis and Crohn's Disease. Interesting to note is that the strains of bacteria are actually listed (not just the species) and the *acidophilus* and *bifidum* strains are the same ones that Natren Inc. uses in their probiotic products:

> "In 1994, Dr. Michael L. McCann and colleagues published a paper entitled, "Recolonization Therapy with *Nonadhesive Escherichia coli* for Treatment of inflammatory bowel disease," in the *Journal of the New York Academy of Sciences*. This work reported on a process called "reflorastation" and a three-year study that focused on normalizing the bowel bacteria using *L. acidophilus* (DDS-1 strain), *B. bifidum* (Malyoth strain) and benign *E. coli* bacteria (Nissel 1917 strain). Remember, *E. coli* is a common bowel bacteria that we all carry. With the exception of the lethal H:0157 strain, which contaminates the food chain, most strains of *E. coli* are harmless. Because they are normal bowel residents they can even be considered beneficial.
>
> Dr. McCann's study involved patients who suffered from an inflammatory bowel disease, either Crohn's disease or ulcerative colitis. His reflorastation protocol began with the use of heavy-duty antibiotics and antifungals to completely rid the body of all bacteria – the good as well as the bad. Once the intestines had been thoroughly denuded, the normal bacteria were reintroduced, both orally and via retention enemas. As a result, each patient so treated

went into remission, and those who continued with the bacterial supplementation remain disease-free at the time of this writing [1998].

The paper concludes, "A subset of patients with inflammatory bowel disease who are successfully recolonized with nonadhesive *E. coli* [and the friendly bacteria] achieved complete, sustained, drug-free remissions....Reflorastation is not only a method that has the potential to identify putative etiologic antigens, but is also a clinical method to induce long-term remissions without the use of toxic drugs." [15]

Are Crohn's & Colitis Infectious Diseases?

There is also a growing field of research suggesting that Crohn's and ulcerative colitis are not auto-immune diseases, but rather, infectious diseases as a result of harmful bacteria or other pathogens in the gastrointestinal tract. Doctors who are treating patients from this position, like Dr. McCann above, are using potent cocktails of antibiotics to wipe out the existing flora in the gut. Some then repopulate the gut with good bacteria, and some don't. Personally, I'm convinced the permanence of the cure or remission would be directly related to whether or not the gut was repopulated sufficiently (and perhaps supplementation maintained indefinitely) with beneficial bacteria. Also, keep in mind that *Jini's Wild Oregano Oil Protocol* above is as potent and effective (and in some cases moreso) than pharmaceutical antibiotics, antifungals, antiyeast, antiparasitic, etc. products.

Mycobacterium avium paratuberculosis (MAP) is a bacterium whose RNA has consistently been isolated in 92 – 100% of patients tested with Crohn's Disease (the incidence varies from study to study). MAP is occasionally found in milk – even in milk that has been pasteurized. However, UHT milk (sealed, boxed milk that can sit on the shelf till opened) is subjected to much higher temperatures than pasteurized milk and may be less likely to contain MAP (they're not sure at this point). John Herman-Taylor, a researcher at St. George's Hospital Medical School in London, thinks there is also evidence that MAP is at the root of irritable bowel syndrome, "In animals, MAP inflames the nerves of the gut. Recent work from Sweden

A 1994 clinical trial used antibiotics and antifungals folllowed by high dose probiotic supplementation to induce remission in patients with ulcerative colitis and Crohn's Disease.

shows that people with (IBS) also have inflamed gut nerves." Kelly Karper, PhD, RPh, recently published a paper in a journal for pharmacists titled, *Crohn's: An Infectious Disease?*:

> "Like other mycobacterial strains, MAP reproduces very slowly. For antibiotics to effectively eliminate MAP, a cocktail of antimycobacterial drugs must be used for extended periods of time. And that is just what the doctor orders for patients with Crohn's disease in Sydney, Australia. Thomas Borody, M.D., director of the Centre for Digestive Diseases, utilizes triple antimycobacterial therapy for his Crohn's patients…for at least three years…In his experience, 'cures are achieved in 20 – 25% of his patients and the rest go into total remission.' By cure, he means that when his patients are off all medications, they not only have no symptoms, but, endoscopically, they have no inflammation, no histologic evidence of Crohn's disease, and their blood work is negative for markers of inflammation. In contrast, those patients that 'go into total remission' experience only minor symptoms, and there is still slight evidence of the disease in endoscopic examination." [16]

I can't help wondering what Dr. Borody's cure and remission rates would be like if he also followed his antimycobacterial protocol with one to two years of high quality probiotic supplementation. As Kelly Karpa goes on to say in her article:

> "Some other gastroenterologists who believe an infectious agent may underlie Crohn's disease have taken a different approach to treating the illness. Instead of using antibiotics to wipe out infectious microorganisms, they have instead opted to treat patients with therapeutic doses of 'healthy bacteria', or probiotics. Rather than using antibiotics to kill bacteria, this novel approach lets bacteria kill bacteria." [17]

Probiotic Species & Strains

Regardless of whether IBD and IBS are initially caused by pathogenic microorganisms (like MAP), or not, the fact remains that probiotic supplementation results in many benefits to the gut and overall health of people with IBD and IBS. Adequate probiotic supplementation is an integral part of healing the root causes of your digestive disorder. And when I say 'adequate probiotic supplementation', I mean high-dose supplementation with effective, potent strains. There have been many human studies done with probiotics to monitor the effect of supplementation on things such as candidiasis, diarrhea, cystitis, etc. and the same probiotics taken at lower levels had very little or no effect. However, the same probiotics taken at high doses (typically 7 – 10 billion cfu per day in adults) showed impressive results. So, you can be taking the right probiotics, but if you're not taking them in high enough doses, you won't see the desired results.

It's also important to ingest the right strain of each species. Different strains of *acidophilus* (for example) can produce completely different results. Out of 200 different strains of *acidophilus*, only 13 have potent antibiotic and antiviral capabilities. If you have IBS or IBD, you need to ingest potent strains that are capable of wiping out the bad bacteria in your gut, strong enough to protect against re-infection, and capable of restoring your mucosal lining and help balance your immune system. There have been human trials performed where (for example) probiotic supplementation consisting of strain 'A' of *L. acidophilus* and strain 'B' of *Bifidobacterium* was ingested by subjects with diarrhea, and supplementation significantly reduced the incidence of diarrhea. However, the other half of the 132 member study who consumed strain 'X' of *L. acidophilus* and strain 'Y' of *Bifidobacterium* showed no results of any statistical significance.[18]
Just ingesting high doses of *L acidophilus* or *B. bifidus* is not enough. You need to ingest high doses of the correct strains of *acidophilus* and *bifidus*.

Many probiotic manufacturers have tried to tell me that the strain doesn't matter, or isn't important. All this shows is that they are either lying or ignorant, as there are dozens of human trials that illustrate quite clearly that the strain is extremely important to the potency and efficacy of the probiotic – i.e. can it adhere to walls of the intestine and colonize effectively? Can it produce beneficial enzymes, vitamins, healing agents and

> To see results from probiotic supplementation, you have to ingest the right strain of each species, and you also have to ingest high enough doses.

anti-cancer agents? Can it inhibit or exclude pathogenic microorganisms like bad bacteria, yeast, fungi and parasites? Etc. etc.

The species and strain of bacteria (along with manufacturing process and environment) are also very important when considering safety issues. Here's an example to help you distinguish between the name of the species and the name of the strain:

Lactobacillus acidophilus DDS-1 (often written *L. acidophilus* DDS-1)
Genus – *Lactobacillus*
Species – *acidophilus*
Strain – DDS-1

Some species that are routinely included in commercial probiotic blends simply do not have a long-term record of human safety and not enough is known about their actions/ramification in the gut under varying conditions. For example, a study on immunodeficient mice found that supplementing with a certain strain of *L. reuteri* (used in many probiotic blends) caused some of the mice to die, leading the researchers to recommend "the need to proceed cautiously when using high doses of this strain in neonatal, immunocompromised hosts." [19] Therefore, you only want to purchase a probiotic supplement that contains species and strains with a proven, long-term record of human safety.

The manufacturing of probiotics is another area that can result in a dangerous product if incredibly strict, sterile-environment procedures are not followed. An Australian manufacturer was completely shut down after their product was found to be contaminated with lead and other toxic materials. Again, there is no independent, third-party regulating probiotic manufacture, advertising or distribution, so you're completely at the mercy of the manufacturer to ensure you're consuming a safe, potent, effective probiotic. I have heard from so many people who developed further complications after ingesting unsafe probiotics, or, who had been taking probiotics (usually recommended by a health professional) for one or two years and yet seen no change in symptoms. Once these clients switch to Natren probiotics and scale up to the appropriate dosage, they can't believe the difference. One of my consultation clients even saw a dramatic reduction in mucus and bloating after only four days – but she is an exception, not the norm.

I have communicated directly with several popular, well-known probiotic manufacturers (other than Natren) and they were all very helpful with my initial inquiries. However, once I started asking specific questions about strains used and/or asking to see independent lab assays of the product, most simply stopped responding to my questions and refused to talk to me anymore and one even started yelling at me, accusing me of being ridiculous and unreasonable – I kid you not!

Choosing The Right Probiotics

So, you need to be very careful when choosing a probiotic brand to supplement with as the field of misinformation in this arena is vast. In my opinion, probiotics are so powerful, they should be even more stringently regulated than prescription drugs. Swallowing live microorganisms, which are highly adaptive, intelligent beings, should be undertaken with great caution and safety should always be paramount. Unfortunately, currently probiotics are not regulated at all, and many probiotic manufacturers do not even comply with labeling guidelines. In addition, when I refer to 'probiotics' I'm referring to food-cultured beneficial bacteria only. Bacterial soil organisms, (bacteria that exist in the soil) are a completely different proposition and something I strongly recommend you do *not* ingest – although many manufacturers are now referring to this kind of bacterial organism as a 'probiotic' as well. For more information and my opinion on bacterial soil organisms (also referred to as SO's, SBO's, or HSO's), please see Chapter Eight. *Saccharomyces boulardii* is also referred to a probiotic, but it is not a bacteria, it is a yeast. It has been shown to be beneficial in clinical trials with both Crohn's and ulcerative colitis. I tried it myself many years ago and before I discovered Natren probiotics, but it exacerbated my symptoms. If you feel led to try *Saccharomyces boulardii*, it is probably safe, however, I don't recommend long-term or ongoing supplementation with

> Swallowing live microorganisms, which are highly adaptive, intelligent beings, should be undertaken with great caution and safety should always be paramount.

it. Simply because it doesn't have the track record of human safety that the other probiotics (recommended here) do.

Therefore, to ensure both safety and potency, when choosing a brand of probiotics, you need to make sure the product fulfills *all* of the following criteria:

1. **cGMP Facility and stored in dark, glass bottles only**
   Make sure the probiotic is manufactured in a facility that carries the cGMP (current Good Manufacturing Practices) certification, otherwise you risk consuming a contaminated product. Contaminants could consist of lead, mercury (and other poisonous heavy metals), and undesirable bacteria. A 1990 independent laboratory study found that nine out of ten brands of popular *Lactobacillus acidophilus* probiotics actually contained no acidophilus at all. All nine contained contaminants and other species of lactobacilli instead.[20] Probiotics are also sensitive to (and damaged by) light and moisture. Only a glass bottle will keep out all moisture – all plastic is permeable to varying degrees of moisture. In addition, the glass must be dark (or amber colored) to keep out light, which also damages bacteria.

2. **Different species must not be touching each other**
   Different species of bacteria placed together will compete for space and try to dominate each other, resulting in competitive exclusion by the dominant species. In vitro studies have shown that when you place different species together, the dominant (strongest) species will usually produce bacteriocins that kill closely related species. For example, one study in a prestigious microbiology journal showed that a certain strain of *L. acidophilus* produced bacteriocins (antibiotics that work against same, or closely related species by adsorption to receptors on the target cells) that inhibited *L. delbrueckii, L. bulgaricus, L. fermentum, Lactococcus lactis,* and *Enterococcus fecalis*.[21] Look at the list of ingredients, and you'll see that many probiotic companies package these same species together all in one bottle or capsule. If *L.acidophilus* can

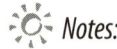
Notes:

inhibit or competitively exclude all these other species, how much of each species is going to be left by the time you ingest it?

Therefore, each species (eg. *acidophilus, bifidum, bulgaricus*) must be kept in its own bottle or in separate capsules to prevent the dominant species from inhibiting or killing off the other species. Refrigeration does not prevent this from happening either, since certain bacteriocins have proved stable at temperatures as low as −20 degrees Celcius. Currently, Natren Inc. is the only company I know of that has worked out a patented system for keeping the species of bacteria separate, yet within the same capsule. The bacteria are added one species at a time to the capsule, over the course of a week, and each species is encapsulated within its own oil bubble, so although you just swallow one capsule, within that capsule, the different bacteria are completely isolated and not touching each other (hence the high price of the product). I know most probiotic manufacturers sell regular capsules or powders with anywhere from 3 to 14 different species packaged together in one jar, or one capsule. Again, I'm absolutely mystified as to why they do this. However, check the bottle and you'll see that none of these manufacturers guarantees the number of live, viable bacteria in their product at the time of opening, or consumption. Nor do they guarantee how many of each species and strain remains alive and viable for effective colonization in the gut at *time of consumption*. One can only conclude that they know that different species inhibit and compete with each other, but yet they continue to package them this way. Perhaps they're relying on the ignorance of the consumer, supported by poorly researched magazine articles that tell people to consume a full spectrum of probiotics, but don't give enough guidelines to ensure safety and potency of the probiotic products. Or, amazing at it may seem, the more probiotic manufacturers I talk to, the more it becomes clear that they themselves are actually ignorant of the problems of packaging different species together! Again, as I've stated before, this is a rapidly-expanding segment of alternative medicine with the potential for huge, quick profits due to the ignorance of both health professionals and the consumer.

> Different species of bacteria placed together will compete for space and try to dominate each other, resulting in competitive exclusion by the dominant species.

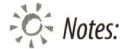 Notes:

3. Must be kept refrigerated at all times

The bacteria need to be stored in a fridge at the store and they must also be shipped in refrigerated trucks to the store. Heat quickly kills bacteria and even at room temperature they will become active and soon live out their life cycle – think of what happens if you leave yoghurt on the counter. The best way to preserve bacterial potency is by keeping it cold at all times, until you're ready to ingest it. Freeze drying is the best method of preserving the bacteria and for this to be maintained, they must be kept very cold at all times until you're ready to ingest them. Of course, keep your probiotics refrigerated at home too. When I travel to third world countries, I pack my probiotics in a cooler, on ice, and make sure the hotel where I'm staying has a bar fridge. Alternatively, you can just keep them in a filled ice bucket in your room, but that's a bit more hassle as you have to keep filling the bucket with fresh ice.

4. Strain and number of bacteria per serving must be listed on the bottle

Only certain strains of bacteria are potent and effective (eg. *L. bulgaricus* DDS-14 is excellent, *L. bulgaricus* DDS-13 is useless – remember, '*bulgaricus*' is the species, 'DDS-14' is the strain). If the manufacturer just lists '*acidophilus*' for example, chances are they've used a cheap and ineffective strain of *L. acidophilus*. There are approximately 200 identified strains of L. acidophilus, of these, only 13 have good antibiotic (against bad bacteria) qualities, thus, the strain is indeed very important. They must also list the number of bacteria guaranteed per serving (and this should be between 2 – 5 billion colony forming units per serving) *at the time of opening*. This guarantee is key: If a manufacturer only guarantees the number of bacteria *at the time of manufacture*, this is meaningless. At manufacture, a bottle may contain 2 billion cfu (colony forming units) per serving – however, by the time that bottle gets to you, the bacteria may be mostly dead. Another trick to watch out for is that manufacturers will list (for example) two different strains of *L. acidophilus*, one of which is a good strain and the other a cheap useless one. Then they will list the total guaranteed bacteria per serving at 2 billion cfu. However, they haven't told you how much of that total count is the effective strain and how much is the ineffective one. To increase profitability, the product probably consists mostly of the cheap, ineffective strain, with a tiny amount of the potent strain sprinkled in. It's also a good idea to use human strains (vs. bovine or porcine strains) for safety's sake. Probiotics are one of the fastest growing segments of the healthcare industry and thereby attracting innumerable get-rich-quick artists – know what to look for and you won't get ripped off.

5. Avoid centrifuged or filter-extracted bacteria
The cheapest way of extracting the bacteria from their growing culture is by centrifuge extraction. In centrifugal extraction, the bacteria (which are embedded/attached to their growth medium) are put in a centrifuge and whirled around with great force at high speed. This greatly damages the bacteria as they're hurled against the walls of the centrifuge and many of them are left ruptured and useless. However, the manufacturer can still put this damaged, ruptured bacteria in a bottle and include it in the guaranteed count per serving. Technically, you'll still be ingesting that amount of bacteria, it just won't do you any good. In ultrafiltration extraction methods, the bacteria are pressed through a filter that removes the larger molecules of their growth medium. However, when bacteria are growing in their culture, they form into chains as they multiply. Ultrafiltration results in the breakup of these chains, separates the bacteria from their beneficial growth medium (supernatant) and can also damage the bacteria themselves. The best method of preserving bacteria (and the most expensive) is to freeze dry it along with its growth medium. Many scientists maintain it's best to consume bacteria along with it's growth medium (also known as the substrate or supernatant) since this protects the bacteria from stomach acid and provides a ready food source for the bacteria to consume as they establish themselves in your gastrointestinal tract. Also, as the bacteria grow in the culture (of milk or vegetable matter), the growth and culturing process produces valuable substances such as vitamins, antioxidants, immune system factors, antimicrobial compounds and digestive enzymes that greatly benefit your body when ingested. Make sure your brand of bacteria states on the

> The manufacturer can still put damaged, ruptured bacteria in a bottle and include it in the guaranteed count per serving. Technically, you'll still be ingesting that amount of bacteria, it just won't do you any good.

bottle that it doesn't use ultrafiltration or centrifugal extraction methods (if it doesn't say so, chances are it does use these methods) and ideally, purchase bacteria that's freeze dried along with its growth medium.

6. Avoid prebiotics

Some companies package their probiotics with fructooligosaccharides (FOS) and/or inulin – indigestible substances referred to as prebiotics, which they claim feed the bacteria, thereby improving performance. Keep in mind though, that many bacteria (both good and bad) can feed on these substances. So if you have a predominantly bad bacterial flora (as most, if not all people with IBD do) consuming prebiotics is probably going to exacerbate your symptoms. Also, most FOS is manufactured via chemical synthesis and in many instances has been shown to cause abdominal pain, bloating and gas. I especially don't recommend it for people with IBS or IBD. Also avoid FOS and inulin in vitamin/mineral supplements, whey protein powders, etc. Be sure to read labels as it's become popular to add it to all kinds of products. For perfectly healthy people with an established good bacterial flora, prebiotics are probably okay, especially if they are not able to obtain these substances naturally through a good diet.

Unfortunately, to date, the only brand of probiotics I've found that meets all the requisite criteria (as listed above) is Natren Inc. And let me state here that I receive NO commissions, royalties or other compensation from Natren for recommending their products. Like George's Aloe Vera Juice and Udo's Choice Oil Blend, I'm simply recommending the best product that I've found, in order to save my readers time, hassle and the pain (symptom exacerbation) of unsuccessful experimentation. Natasha Trenev is the passionate founder and owner of Natren Inc. and as long as she owns the company, you can be assured the same level of quality and safety will continue. If the company is ever sold, then check to make sure the products still meet all the above criteria. Now, if any of you manage to find another brand of probiotics that meets all the criteria listed above – please let me know! I would love to have another brand to recommend to people, it's always nice to have choices.

 Notes:

With probiotics being such an expanding field and numerous different companies producing them, I'm really mystified as to why everyone else is producing such inferior products. I can only surmise that it's due to profits and ignorance. It's very expensive to produce and ship bacteria according to the standards required for full potency, safety, and bioavailability (as outlined above). Perhaps these other companies just aren't aware of all the factors involved in successful culturing, extraction and storage of bacteria, or, perhaps they're counting on the fact that the consumer is not aware and therefore will buy their products anyway. Don't be surprised when even your naturopathic physician or gastroenterologist doesn't know the above criteria for ensuring potent, viable bacteria. As I said, there's a lot of money being invested in probiotics by people/manufacturers who know very little about these highly sensitive microorganisms. Unfortunately, they care more about their profits than your health.

When I first began recommending Natren probiotics to my readers, I did so for one reason only; they worked. At that time, I knew a fraction of what I know now about probiotic strain selection, manufacturing, storage, and other factors effecting potency and efficacy. I had experimented with different brands of probiotics off and on for seven years and each time I tried supplementing, my symptoms (gas, bloating, bleeding) worsened. Although the science behind probiotics and why they should benefit me seemed sound, my experience proved contrary. When I was nearly ready to give up on the whole subject, my naturopathic physician Dr. David Wang, convinced me to try Natren brand probiotics. He insisted they were the best brand he knew of and that I would see good results from them. I started with Natren's Bifido Factor powder (*Bifidobacterium bifidum* Malyoth strain) and for the first time, experienced an improvement as a result.

Prior to taking Natren's *B. bifidum*, the only thing that had worked to stem my chronic diarrhea was L-Glutamine (on an empty stomach only). However, within three doses of Natren's bifidobacteria, my stools began to firm up and excess water was reabsorbed. I tried Natren's Megadophilus (*Lactobacillus acidophilus* DDS-1) next but did not tolerate that as well as the *bifidum*. In searching for reasons why, I came across this bit of research

> When purchasing probiotics, make sure the manufacturer guarantees the number of live bacteria, of each strain (not just of each species), at the time of *consumption* – not at the time of packaging.

that showed that in states of inflammation the overall tolerance to bacterial flora is greatly reduced:

> "It is possible that the products of the commensal flora promote inflammation in the presence of an impaired mucosal barrier or injury to the mucosa… These results indicate that, in health, there is tolerance to autologous [your own] but not allogeneic [foreign source] intestinal flora, and tolerance is lost during inflammation. Evidence also exists that animals are tolerant to their own flora in health but not after colitis develops." [22]

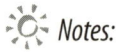

Notes:

Unfortunately, this bit of research doesn't specify which species of bacteria the body loses tolerance for, and which strains of which species – perhaps all of them? Nevertheless, it provided me with a clue by which to proceed, and I stayed on just the *B. bifidum* bacteria for another three months before trying the *L. acidophilus* again and I then tolerated it well. By that time (I surmise) the *B. bifidum* and other supplements I was taking had healed my intestine to the point where it was able to tolerate – and benefit from – additional probiotic supplementation. About a month after that, I added Natren's *L. bulgaricus* and tolerated that successfully as well. I have since continued to recommend the same conservative course of action to my readers.

However, in March 2005, *gastroenterology* journal published results of a human trial on 75 people with IBS, supplementing with 10 billion cfu of *B. infantis*, once per day in a malted milk drink. Now, *Bifidobacterium infantis* is, as the title suggests, a strain typically used for infants. But as Dr. Quigley and his colleagues note in their paper, the symptom relief achieved with *B. infantis* in the trial was comparable to that seen with Zelnorm (tegaserod) and Lotronex (alosetron) – two drugs used in the treatment of irritable bowel syndrome.[23]

B. Infantis is the predominant bacteria found in the bowel of healthy breastfed infants. As the infant begins to eat solid foods, the more 'adult' strains like *B. bifidum* come to dominate. However, what if you never had a healthy bacterial flora as an infant? Then maybe it would be best for you to start with what was missing from the very beginning and work up from there? This approach makes sense to me both logically and intuitively. Interestingly, I had a bottle of Natren's Life Start *(B. infantis)* in my fridge (that I had given to my daughter) and about six months before this research came out I had begun taking it myself (along with the three adult species/strains) just because I intuitively felt like trying it. In light of this research, you may want to consider beginning probiotic supplementation with *B. infantis*, especially if you try *B. bifidum* and can't tolerate it. And just to confuse you even more, I have talked with readers who couldn't tolerate *B. bifidum* at first, but could tolerate *L. acidophilus*. So, essentially, I've provided you with a guideline, but within that you may need to experiment and find what works best for your particular body and gut environment. The only thing I can tell you for sure is: Don't give up! You do need to establish a healthy bacterial flora (consisting of all three species) to enjoy long-term, lasting health.

I know many people have experienced good results from more aggressive supplementation and also from beginning supplementation immediately (with ulceration and bleeding still present). Feedback from hundreds of readers has confirmed the effectiveness of the slower approach (as outlined above), but it certainly does take more time to see results since you're proceeding so slowly. However, if your gut is really toxic, proceeding slowly helps minimize the die-off effect (Herxheimer Reaction), so while it takes longer to see any results, at least you don't have the nausea, bloating, headaches, etc. that can result from a rapid die-off of pathogens in the gut. As in all things, please follow your own gut instinct first. If you feel you should pursue aggressive supplementation, then please do so. I know of a colon clinic in Sydney, Australia that treats people with active, bleeding Crohn's with high doses of Natren brand probiotics orally and also via retention enemas and they have had good success with this approach. I will give you instructions below for doing *Jini's Probiotic Retention Enema* and I certainly recommend this as one of the fastest, most effective ways of changing your gut ecology and seeing quick, positive results (not including the die-off effect!).

> If you try all the adult strains and can't tolerate them, then try the infant strain: *B. infantis* (Life Start by Natren). Maybe you have to start with what you never had as a baby, and gradually move on from there.

How Much Should I Take And When?

If you're a highly reactive, sensitive person, you may want to get your ulceration and bleeding healed (using the therapies recommended in this program) before beginning probiotic supplementation. However, I do recommend you try supplementing with Natren's Bifido Factor (*B. bifidum* Malyoth) right away because if you can tolerate it, it will help speed your healing. If you can't tolerate the *B. bifidum*, then try Natren's Life Start (*B. infantis*). Life Start is available in stores only in a dairy-based formula at this time. If you want the goat milk-based formula, you'll need to order it online, direct from Natren. By the way, when ordering Natren probiotics online, I recommend you ONLY order from www.natren.com or from my store, www.LTYGshoppe.com, as there are a lot of counterfeit operations that have imitated Natren's label, claiming to sell Natren's probiotics, but while the label looks the same, inside the bottle is a completely different product!

Once you've successfully used Natren's *bifidum* bacteria for a month, next try adding Natren's Megadophilus (*L. acidophilus* DDS-1). If you tolerate that well, then finally add their Digesta-Lac product (*L. bulgaricus* LB-51) to your regimen. If you don't tolerate a new species of bacteria well, then stay on just what's working for you for another few weeks or a month before trying again. You ultimately need to ingest the complete spectrum of probiotics as each is particularly active and healing for different parts of your intestine: *Acidophilus* for the esophageal tube, stomach and small intestine, bifidum for the large intestine, and *bulgaricus* is a transient species that travels throughout the intestinal tract and also assists the action of *acidophilus* and *bifidum*. If you suffer from irritable bowel syndrome (IBS) you can start immediately with all three (Megadophilus, Bifido Factor, Digesta-Lac) and/or, with Life Start (*B. infantis*) as discussed above. Whether you tend toward diarrhea or constipation or some mixture of both, probiotics will normalize your bowel function and you should start to see positive results within a month or so.

Natren probiotics are available in both dairy-based, and non-dairy preparations. If you have a dairy intolerance, then use the non-dairy versions. Again, if you're having trouble getting exactly what you want from your health store (most don't carry the full line), then order it direct from Natren *(www.natren.com)* or the LTYG Holistic Health Shoppe *(www.LTYGshoppe.com)*. However, after you've been taking probiotics for a year or so, you may be able to tolerate dairy again – especially since they produce the enzyme lactase, which helps your body digest the lactose in milk products, and *L. bulgaricus* also helps you digest milk proteins. If you don't have a problem with dairy, then test each of them and see which one you get better results from. My body seems to prefer the dairy-based probiotics now, although initially I consumed the non-dairy line. Also, for young children who won't drink the probiotics mixed in water, it's also effective to mix the Natren dairy-based line in with yoghurt (flavored or plain are both ok). Because the probiotics are in a dairy growth medium they blend perfectly with the yoghurt and kids can't even taste that they're there (mix well and don't let them see you putting it in if your kids are finicky!). The probiotics can also be mixed in a non-acidic juice like apple or pear for kids, but again, consume on an empty stomach.

I recommend people with IBD take their probiotics in powder form so that (a) you can reap the benefits in your mouth (mouth ulcers), esophagus and stomach (*L. acidophilus* reduces or eliminates heartburn – even while pregnant) and (b) to ensure effective utilisation as people with IBD often have very fast transit times through their gastrointestinal tract, so capsules are not always broken down/absorbed properly. Also, when you take the powder form, you're also ingesting the valuable supernatant (growth medium) along with the beneficial bacteria. If your system tends to be constipated, then you'll probably be fine with taking the capsules (if you prefer).

When you first begin probiotic supplementation, I recommend proceeding slowly. This is due to a phenomena called The Herxheimer Reaction (first documented by Dr. Karl Herxheimer) where the die-off of pathogens in the gut (caused by the good bacteria) causes various unpleasant symptoms. Bloating, gas, headaches, colds, flu, diarrhea, etc., can result as these toxins die off and your body tries to expel them as quickly as possible. To

> For young children who won't drink the probiotics mixed in water, it's also effective to mix the Natren dairy-based line in with yoghurt (flavored or plain are both ok).

avoid or minimize this temporary reaction, start with only ¼ tsp. of each (Bifido Factor, Megadophilus, Digesta-Lac) 1 – 2 times per day, or, 1 capsule (Healthy Trinity) every second day, on an empty stomach (15 – 20 minutes before food, or 2 hours after food). Some people's guts are so toxic, they are only able to tolerate 1 capsule every four days. So listen to your gut and proceed at the pace that's right for your body. Eventually work your way up to 1 tsp of each powder (Bifido Factor, Megadophilus, Digesta-Lac), 3 times per day, or, 1 capsule (Healthy Trinity) 1 – 2 times per day on an empty stomach (15 – 20 minutes before food, or 2 hours after food).

You can follow dosage instructions on the bottle (but try to work up to 1 tsp. 3 times per day) and you can mix all three powders together in one glass of room temperature, filtered or spring water (no tap water as the chlorine in tap water kills bacteria). If you want to be careful about not contaminating each bottle, you can wipe the spoon off with a piece of tissue in between scooping from each bottle (so you don't transfer *acidophilus* to your *bulgaricus* bottle, for example). Or, even better, you can hold the spoon below the mouth of the bottle and shake the powder into the spoon, so it doesn't even touch the remaining contents of the bottle. Make sure you *always* take probiotics on an empty stomach (15 – 20 minutes before food, or 2 hours after food) as digestive juices destroy the bacteria. I also like to take 1 tsp. of each powder (mixed together in a glass of room temperature filtered or spring water) before bed (on an empty stomach) so the bacteria have all night to colonize undisturbed. You need to work up to a full teaspoon of each powder (Bifido Factor, Megadophilus, Digesta-Lac), three times a day, or, 1 capsule (Healthy Trinity), 1 – 2 times per day, for at least three months to see really good, lasting results. If you have IBD, your gut flora is so compromised that you need consistent, high doses of the full spectrum of probiotics to effect any kind of lasting change.

For ongoing maintenance, once you're completely healed and symptom-free, I recommend taking one dose (1 tsp. of each powder) before bed, on an empty stomach (2 hours after food). Or, if you prefer, you can just take 1 Healthy Trinity capsule before bed, on an empty stomach, for ongoing maintenance.

Things That Kill Good Bacteria

Keep in mind that numerous drugs used in IBS/IBD therapy also kill off the good bacteria in your gut, so if you're on medication, you should also simultaneously be using probiotics (at least 2 – 3 times per day). Prednisone is one of the worst drugs for disrupting bacterial flora in the gut since it produces an alkaline pH, which promotes the growth of yeast *(Candida albicans)*, fungi and bad bacteria. Birth control pills have the same effect. Other substances that also disrupt the growth and balance of beneficial bacteria in your gut include antibiotics, some antidepressants, laxatives, antacids, chlorinated water, anal intercourse, nonsteroidal anti-inflammatory agents (NSAIDS) and steroids (including corticosteroids like Prednisone and Hydrocortisone). See Chapter Nine for alternative methods of birth control to the oral contraceptive pill. If you are using any of these substances, you will have to continue probiotic supplementation indefinitely to counter the effects of these agents. Once you stop using these substances, you will then need to do at least three month's of high dose probiotic supplementation and then continue as needed.

Dosage Summary

Cautious / Sensitive Approach: Skip this section if you favor a more aggressive approach, if you've successfully taken probiotics before, or, if you only have IBS.

- Start with ¼ tsp. of Bifido Factor powder 1 – 2 times per day, mixed in 4 ounces of room temperature, filtered or spring water, on an empty stomach (20 minutes before food, or, 2 hours after food). Gradually work up to 1 tsp. of Bifido Factor powder 3 times per day, mixed in 8 ounces of room temperature, filtered or spring water, on an empty stomach.

- Next, introduce ¼ tsp. of Megadophilus powder 1 – 2 times per day, mixed together with the 1 tsp. of Bifido Factor in 8 ounces of room temperature, filtered or spring water, on an empty stomach (20 minutes before food, or, 2 hours after food). Keep your dosage of the Bifido Factor

> Whether you tend toward diarrhea or constipation or some mixture of both, probiotics will normalize your bowel function and you should see some positive results within a month or so. For faster results, do *Jini's Probiotic Retention Enema.*

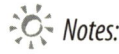 Notes:

the same as above. Gradually work up to 1 tsp. of Megadophilus powder and 1 tsp. of Bifido Factor powder 3 times per day, mixed together in 8 ounces of room temperature, filtered or spring water, on an empty stomach (20 minutes before food, or, 2 hours after food).

- Finally, (keeping existing probiotics at existing dosage) introduce ½ tsp. Digesta-Lac in powder form along with the 1 tsp. of Megadophilus powder and 1 tsp. of Bifido Factor powder 1 – 2 times per day, mixed in 8 ounces of room temperature, filtered or spring water, on an empty stomach. Increase to 1 tsp. Digesta-Lac in powder form along with the 1 tsp. of Megadophilus powder and 1 tsp. of Bifido Factor powder 3 times per day, mixed in 8 ounces of room temperature, filtered or spring water, on an empty stomach (20 minutes before food, or, 2 hours after food). Continue on this dosage for three months. Also perform *Jini's Probiotic Retention Enema* once per month, for three months (see instructions below).

- For the next six months, take 1 tsp. each of Megadophilus, Bifido Factor and Digesta-Lac powder once before bed, mixed in 8 ounces of room temperature, filtered or spring water, on an empty stomach (20 minutes before food, or, 2 hours after food). Monitor your symptoms and if you need it then also take a dose first thing in the morning as well. Or, if you prefer, and you have no diarrhea or heartburn, take 1 Healthy Trinity capsule (instead of the powders) once before bed, on an empty stomach.

- For ongoing maintenance, see *How Long Should I Take Probiotics?* section below.

Moderate Approach: If you have IBS, or, if you've taken probiotics successfully before, you may want to start with this dosage method.

- Start with ¼ tsp. each of Megadophilus, Bifido Factor and Digesta-Lac powder 1 – 2 times per day, mixed in 6 ounces of room temperature, filtered or spring water, on an empty stomach (20 minutes before food, or, 2 hours after food). Based on the study mentioned above, you may also want to add ¼ tsp. Life Start *(B. infantis)*.

SUPPLEMENTS & TREATMENT PROTOCOLS — CHAPTER 2

- Gradually work up to 1 tsp. each of Megadophilus, Bifido Factor and Digesta-Lac powder 3 times per day, mixed in 8 ounces of room temperature, filtered or spring water, on an empty stomach (20 minutes before food, or, 2 hours after food). Ideally, take your last dose right before bed. Continue on this dose for 3 months. Or, if you prefer, and you have no diarrhea or heartburn, take 1 Healthy Trinity capsule (instead of the powders) once in the morning and once before bed. Also perform *Jini's Probiotic Retention Enema* once per month, for three months (see instructions below).

- For the next six months, take 1 tsp. each of Megadophilus, Bifido Factor and Digesta-Lac powder once before bed, mixed in 8 ounces of room temperature, filtered or spring water, on an empty stomach. Monitor your symptoms and if you need it then also take a dose first thing in the morning as well (20 minutes before breakfast). Or, if you prefer, and you have no diarrhea or heartburn, take 1 Healthy Trinity capsule (instead of the powders) once before bed, on an empty stomach.

- For ongoing maintenance, see *How Long Should I Take Probiotics?* section below.

Fast Approach: If you've taken probiotics successfully before, or you feel intuitively this would work well for you, then you may want to follow this dosage method. Remember, you can always cut back if the Herxheimer Reaction (die-off of pathogens) is too severe.

- Start with ½ tsp. each of Megadophilus, Bifido Factor and Digesta-Lac powder 3 times per day, mixed in 8 ounces of room temperature, filtered or spring water, on an empty stomach (20 minutes before food, or, 2 hours after food) for two weeks.

- Perform *Jini's Probiotic Retention Enema* (see instructions below) once.

- Next, increase to 1 tsp. each of Megadophilus, Bifido Factor and Digesta-Lac powder 3 times per day, mixed in 8 ounces of room temperature, filtered or spring water, on an empty stomach (20 minutes before food, or,

> Studies show that you need to ingest 7 – 10 billion c.f.u. of a probiotic species per day in order to see a therapeutic effect. Therefore, you need to take 1 tsp. of each Natren probiotic powder, two to three times per day. Or, 1 capsule twice per day.

 Notes:

2 hours after food). Ideally, take your last dose right before bed. Continue on this dose for 3 months. Or, if you prefer, and you have no diarrhea or heartburn, take 1 Healthy Trinity capsule (instead of the powders) once in the morning and once before bed. Also perform *Jini's Probiotic Retention Enema* once per month, for three months (see instructions below).

- For the next six months, take 1 tsp. each of Megadophilus, Bifido Factor and Digesta-Lac powder once before bed, mixed in 8 ounces of room temperature, filtered or spring water, on an empty stomach. Monitor your symptoms and if you need it then also take a dose first thing in the morning as well (20 minutes before breakfast). Or, if you prefer, and you have no diarrhea or heartburn, take 1 Healthy Trinity capsule (instead of the powders) once before bed, on an empty stomach.

- For ongoing maintenance, see *How Long Should I Take Probiotics?* section below.

Dosage Instructions Following Antibiotics Or Exploratory Tests

If you're taking an antibiotic, you can either wait until the course of treatment is over before beginning probiotic supplementation, or, you can take probiotics during the course of antibiotic treatment. If you take probiotics during antibiotic treatment, the probiotics will help to further encourage the exit of undesirable bacteria from your gut and will also simultaneously inhibit the overgrowth of yeast, fungi and parasites – which can flourish in the absence of good bacteria (which have been killed off by the antibiotic). If you know you have a *Candida albicans* problem, for example, then you definitely want to take probiotics at the same time as the antibiotics to prevent an explosive proliferation of this yeast that will then be difficult to control. If you've supplemented with probiotics prior to antibiotic treatment, then take your probiotics as follows:

- Two hours after you take each prescribed dose of antibiotics, take 1 tsp. of each Natren brand probiotic (Megadophilus, Bifido Factor, Digesta-Lac) mixed in 8 ounces of room temperature, filtered water (not tap water) on an empty stomach (15 – 20 minutes before food, or 2 hours after food), then take an additional dose (1 tsp. of each) before bed. When your course of antibiotics is finished, do *Jini's Probiotic Retention Enema* and take 1 tsp. of each powder on an empty stomach (15 – 20 minutes before food, or 2 hours after food) three times a day for three months and then once or twice a day (always on an empty stomach) for the following three months.

If you haven't supplemented with probiotics prior to antibiotic treatment, then you may want to proceed more slowly to avoid the Herxheimer Reaction :

▶ Two hours after you take each prescribed dose of antibiotics, take ¼ – ½ tsp. of each Natren brand probiotic (Megadophilus, Bifido Factor, Digesta-Lac) mixed in 6-8 ounces of room temperature, filtered water (no tap water) on an empty stomach (15 – 20 minutes before food, or 2 hours after food), then take an additional dose (½ tsp. of each) before bed. When your course of antibiotics is finished, do *Jini's Probiotic Retention Enema* and take 1 tsp. of each three times a day on an empty stomach (15 – 20 minutes before food, or 2 hours after food) for three months. And then take 1 tsp. of each powder once or twice a day (always on an empty stomach) for the next three months as well.

When undergoing a digestive diagnostic or exploratory test (stomach, small or large intestine), immediately follow it with probiotic supplementation. These tests are all very disruptive to bacterial flora and you leave yourself wide open to infection by yeast, bad bacteria, viruses and fungi following these procedures. If you've already been taking probiotics regularly, then follow any of these procedures (gastroscopy, colonoscopy, barium enema, etc.) with 1 tsp. of each Natren brand probiotic (Megadophilus, Bifido Factor, Digesta-Lac) in powder form mixed in 8 ounces of room temperature, filtered water (no tap water) on an empty stomach (15 – 20 minutes before food, or 2 hours after food), three times a day for three months and then 1 tsp. of each powder (or 1 Healthy Trinity capsule) once or twice a day (always on an empty stomach) for the following three months. If you

> ☼ If you take probiotics during antibiotic treatment, the probiotics will help to further encourage the exit of undesirable bacteria from your gut and will also simultaneously inhibit the overgrowth of yeast, fungi and parasites – which can flourish in the absence of good bacteria (which have been killed off by the antibiotic).

haven't been taking probiotics prior to the diagnostic/exploratory tests, then you should proceed more slowly with supplementation to avoid the Herxheimer Reaction. Take ¼ tsp. of each Natren brand probiotic powder (Megadophilus, Bifido Factor, Digesta-Lac) mixed in 6 – 8 ounces of room temperature, filtered water (no tap water) on an empty stomach (15 – 20 minutes before food, or 2 hours after food), two to three times a day for two weeks, then ½ tsp. of each three times a day for two weeks, then 1 tsp. of each powder, three times a day (always on an empty stomach) for the following three to six months. If you don't have loose stools, or tend towards constipation, you can also take one Healthy Trinity capsule before bed, on an empty stomach, if you prefer. Perform *Jini's Probiotic Retention Enema* if the procedure involved your colon.

Dosage Instructions For Babies

For an infant with bowel problems (or skin problems), supplement with Natren's Life Start (*Bifidobacteria infantis* bacteria) only – do not give the other probiotic species directly to an infant (although a nursing mother can and should ingest other species including *B. infantis*). ⅛ – ¼ tsp. 2 – 3 times a day should produce fairly swift results. You can let your baby suck it off your finger (on an empty stomach), or mix it with room temperature filtered or spring water, or mix it with applesauce (wait 20 minutes before following that with any food other than breastmilk – breastmilk they can have fairly soon after probiotics). My daughter developed a bacterial infection diaper rash at three weeks of age. Then at four months of age she developed a yeast infection in the folds of her skin – which started out looking like the normal baby 'skin rot' and within two months became a bloody, weeping mess. This then progressed to include a fungal infection on her skin, all over her body.

I did not give her any drugs whatsoever (and I won't subject you to a list of all the different natural remedies I tried) but completely healed the yeast and fungus using diluted wild oregano oil applied topically and Natren's *B. infantis* bacteria, ⅛ tsp. 2 – 3 times per day. She actually loved sucking/gumming the probiotic off my finger (it tastes like malted milk).

When she began eating solids at six months, she also became constipated, but as a result of the probiotic supplementation (I increased it), her bowel movements normalized within a week. Remember that skin conditions are always a sign of gut problems, so although the Wild Oregano Oil would have eliminated the visible symptoms, the underlying problem still needed to be addressed. Her body has also shown me (via the yeast/fungal skin infections and tendency towards constipation) where her genetic weakness lies (or where she carries stress in her body), so I continue to give her probiotics regularly. If I'd known then, what I know now about probiotics, I also would have taken high dose probiotics throughout my pregnancy. It's interesting that my son's body, in contrast, shows a healthy gut flora. And he was conceived shortly after I completed a seven week course on The IBD Remission Diet (which involves high dose probiotic supplementation for three months after the Diet).

> Life Start *(B. infantis)* tastes like malted milk – quite yummy. I would put the dose in a little dish, dip my finger in it and then let my daughter suck/gum it off my finger – she loved it.

Jini's Probiotic Retention Enema

This retention enema, which delivers very high dose probiotics directly to your colon (and lower part of your ileum) can provide dramatic healing results. As the name suggests, this is not a cleansing or flushing enema, but rather it is an implant or retention enema – where the goal is to hold the mixture in your colon until the liquid is completely absorbed (about 2 hours). If you can't retain it until the liquid is absorbed, don't worry, continue with oral probiotic supplementation and try again in a few weeks. You will still retain some benefits though, no matter how short the retention time, so don't worry, the effort is not wasted.

Many people use *Jini's Probiotic Retention Enema* during severe inflammation and bleeding for quick healing, whilst others prefer to wait until things have calmed down a bit and they're tolerating the probiotics well orally first. You really have to just follow your own body wisdom (intuition) on when would be best for you. Even people who have not seen great results from oral probiotic supplementation (it takes longer and can be more difficult to colonize via oral supplementation) see significant symptom clearing following this retention enema. It's definitely something you should do at least once to provide a solid foundation of good gut flora. You can also perform *Jini's Probiotic Retention Enema* during the IBD Remission Diet.

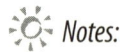 Notes:

1. Ideally, for best results, first clear the colon of fecal matter, until an enema bag of warm water runs clear when expelled from your colon/rectum. You can clear the colon by giving repeated enemas of warm, filtered water. Use an enema bag to put 8 – 16 ounces (1 – 2 cups) of warm, filtered water into your colon, massage around for as long as you can (or up to 10 minutes) and then expel liquid and feces into the toilet. Then, give yourself another enema of 8 – 16 ounces (1 – 2 cups) of warm, filtered water, massage water around the colon, and expel. Continue until the water expelled is clear of fecal matter. If you think that repeated enemas will only aggravate your colon, then just do one.

   If your rectum is sore or sensitive, first coat the tip of the enema tube and your anus/rectum with a clear lubricant (such as KY Jelly). Do not use Vaseline.

   If you're currently on an elemental (liquid) diet, or suffer from constant diarrhea, you may not need to do this step if you'd really prefer not to. If having enemas doesn't bother you though, it would still be best if you could administer at least one warm water enema to flush the colon before proceeding.

2. Once your colon is clear of fecal matter, you can give yourself *Jini's Probiotic Retention Enema*. Unlike the previous enemas, the goal of this one is to NOT expel the contents into the toilet, but rather to retain (hold) it in your colon until all the water has been absorbed and thus the bacteria has a chance to colonize at full capacity.

Jini's Probiotic Retention Enema

2 tablespoons Natren's Bifido Factor powder

2 tablespoons Natren's Digesta-Lac powder
1 tablespoon of Natren's Megadophilus* powder
8 ounces (1 cup) of warm spring or filtered water

Mix together well (no lumps) and then pour into enema bag.

*Although the *L. acidophilus* (contained in the Megadophilus product) is primarily active in the small intestine, in disease states the ileocecal valve (between the large and small intestine) is often malfunctioning and bacteria from the colon washes up into the small intestine. Therefore I like to add some *acidophilus* to the retention enema mixture 'just in case' this may be occurring.

It's preferred if you can use the dairy-based powders for all three probiotics, if tolerated. If you can't tolerate the dairy-based, then use the non-dairy powders. However, Digesta-Lac is only available in capsules in the non-dairy formulation, so you either have to open a lot of capsules, or don't include it.

Elevate your hips using rolled towels or a pillow, lie on your right side and insert the enema tube 1 – 2 inches up your rectum (lubricate tube and anus with your saliva, or saline lubricant if necessary). Slowly release the clamp so the mixture flows slowly into your colon. Stop flow and rest periodically if needed. Continue until enema bag is empty and then slowly withdraw the enema tube. Continue to lie on your right side for the next 10 minutes. Then lie on your back for 10 minutes. Then lie on your left side for 10 minutes. Rotate back through the positions (right side, back, left side) every 10 minutes for the next hour or two. However, if lying on your left side makes you feel you need to expel the mixture, then just lie on your right side and your back. If you can, massage your colon gently in each position to really work the probiotics into all the folds and crevices of your colon. However, take care to massage *away* from the rectum to help prevent expulsion: Massage *from* your left side *towards* the right side of the colon. Having a good book to read can really help keep your mind off the enema

> ☼ There is a colon clinic in Sydney, Australia that successfully uses this retention enema for clients with active, bleeding Crohn's and colitis.

and help you to relax during this time. The best time to do this retention enema, if possible, is last thing before bed – then the bacteria have the whole night (hopefully!) to colonize undisturbed.

How Long Should I Take Probiotics?

Again, this is an area where there are vastly differing opinions:

Opinion 1: You should take probiotics every day for the rest of your life. Thirty years ago, it took about 25,000 colony forming units to cause food poisoning, today it can take only 10 colony forming units. Therefore, you need to daily make sure you have a protective population of beneficial bacteria in your gut to prevent and fight off invading pathogens. As the probiotics discussed also have anti-viral, anti-fungal and anti-bacterial (against 'bad' bacteria) capabilities, taking them daily supports your ongoing health. The other argument for this position is that people who've demonstrated a gut weakness, or, susceptibility (as in the case of someone with IBD) need extra support and protection against pathogenic microorganisms and thus should take the beneficial bacteria daily. If you ever eat at fast food restaurants, or buy non-organic ground meat, you also need to know that:

> "Every day in the United States, roughly 200,000 people are sickened by a foodborne disease, 900 are hospitalized, and fourteen die. … American meat production has never before been so centralized: thirteen large packinghouses now slaughter most of the beef consumed in the United States. The meatpacking system that arose to supply the nation's fast food chains – an industry molded to serve their needs, to provide massive amounts of uniform ground beef so that all of McDonald's hamburgers would taste the same – has proved to be an extremely efficient system for spreading disease. …The medical literature on the causes of food poisoning is full of euphemisms and dry scientific terms: coliform levels, aerobic plate counts, sorbitol, MacConkey agar, and so on. Behind them lies a simple explanation for why eating a hamburger can now make you seriously ill: There is shit in the meat." [24]

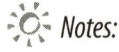 Notes:

SUPPLEMENTS & TREATMENT PROTOCOLS — CHAPTER 2

Natasha Trenev, the founder of Natren Inc., maintains that if you lived on your own farm where you grew your own organic vegetables, raised your own organic meat and eggs and were in control of your own water supply (with appropriate filtration), then you could probably live happily without ongoing probiotic supplementation. For the rest of us, she advises daily supplementation.

Opinion 2: You should only take probiotics when your system shows you it needs them. Gas, bloating, diarrhea, constipation, etc. are all signs that your gut needs more beneficial bacteria. Once the symptoms have subsided, you can stop supplementing with probiotics until your body asks for them again. On a daily basis, for maintenance, be sure to consume foods that contain probiotics such as miso, tamari-shoyu, organic or homemade yoghurt (Natren sells a Yoghurt Starter for making homemade yoghurt that contains good strains of bacteria), sauerkraut, kefir, etc.

Opinion 3: Take the probiotics 2 – 3 times per day until you have completely normal digestive and bowel function. Then continue taking them 1 – 2 times per day for the next six months to two years (depending on the length of time you've had IBS or IBD). Thereafter, take only as needed – when symptoms in your gut arise (gas, bloating, diarrhea, constipation, heartburn, etc.).

I'm not going to tell you which of these three opinions to follow. This is definitely one of those times when the best course of action is to 'listen to your gut'! You know what's right for your body and you'll soon discover what works best for you. For myself, I use a mix of Opinion #2 and #3 and if I ever travel to less developed countries, or travel anywhere for longer than two weeks, I carry probiotics with me and take them prophylactically (daily).

> Thirty years ago, it took about 25,000 colony forming units to cause food poisoning, today it can take only 10 colony forming units.

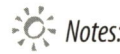 Notes:

VITAMIN AND MINERAL SUPPLEMENTATION

If you've had IBD or IBS for any length of time, you probably have a medium to severe deficiency of the following vitamins and minerals due to decreased nutritional absorption and excess fecal losses (Source: *Encyclopedia of Natural Medicine*, by Michael Murray N.D., and Joseph Pizzorno, N.D.):

Zinc – Zinc picolinate or zinc citrate are much better absorbed than other forms (e.g., zinc sulphate). Also, if you're on the birth control pill then you're going to be extra-low in zinc.

Magnesium – Magnesium chelates (citrate, aspartate, etc.) are much better absorbed than magnesium salts (e.g., magnesium carbonate). However, magnesium can have a laxative effect, so give your body time to adjust by starting with a lower dose and working up. Recent studies have shown an average of 40% of Americans are deficient in magnesium.

Calcium – A vitamin D deficiency (among other things) can result in a calcium deficiency even though you're ingesting sufficient calcium.

Potassium – Another reason to eat bananas and papayas. If you tend to get leg and foot cramps, then you're probably low in calcium and potassium.

Vitamin A* – This vitamin directly affects the intestinal mucosal lining; it increases the production of mucins, increases the secretion of mucus and restores normal barrier function.

Vitamin D – sunshine! Do not always cover up your skin or use sunscreen as you do need to be able to absorb the sun's rays to get enough vitamin D for your body.

Vitamin E* – Inhibits inflammation and reduces free radical damage.

Selenium* – Another excellent antioxidant, best taken with vitamin E (they increase each other's absorption), but take your vitamin C at another time as it interferes with the absorption of some forms of selenium. Liquid selenium is virtually tasteless and odorless.

Vitamin K – Also present in parsley.

Folic Acid – Intestinal mucosal cells need a constant supply of folic acid (or folate), also necessary for iron absorption.

Vitamin B12 – Sublingual pills (dissolve when placed under your tongue) or drops are the most easily absorbed form of B12, especially if you have any inflammation or have had any surgery done on your terminal ileum. Also, I like to take the whole B group of vitamins in addition to the B12.

Vitamin C* – Can cause an increase in diarrhea in ascorbic acid form, so if this is a problem take at night rather than in the morning and adjust the dosage to what works for you, or, avoid the problem altogether by taking it in mineral ascorbate form (e.g., vitamin C as calcium ascorbate), which causes no diarrhea.

Vitamins A, C, E and Selenium are all excellent antioxidants and beneficial for people with inflammatory bowel disease since "IBD mucosa is relatively depleted of antioxidant defenses, rendering it susceptible to oxidative injury..." [25]

You also need to take a look at the drugs you're currently on to determine which vitamins and minerals they leach from your body, or inhibit the absorption of, so you can take extra to make up for it. Look up the drugs in your pharmacist's CPS (drug handbook) or ask your doctor for the pharmaceutical printout on each drug he prescribes you (don't trust your doctor to know about this, he may have little to no idea of the extended ramifications of the drugs he's prescribing). Here's an example of two common drugs used in the treatment of IBD and their effects (Source: *Encyclopedia of Natural Medicine*, by Michael Murray N.D., and Joseph Pizzorno, N.D.):

1. Corticosteroids
    - decrease the absorption of calcium and phosphorous
    - depress protein synthesis
    - decrease bone formation and impair wound healing

> If you've had IBD or IBS for any length of time, you probably have a medium to severe deficiency of numerous vitamins and minerals due to decreased nutritional absorption and excess fecal losses.

- increase urinary excretion of vitamin C, calcium, potassium, and zinc
- increase blood glucose, serum triglycerides, serum cholesterol and blood pressure
- increase requirements for vitamin B6, ascorbic acid, folate and vitamin D
- increase risk of cataracts

2. Sulphasalazine
   - inhibits transport and absorption of folate
   - decreases iron and serum folate
   - increases urinary excretion of ascorbic acid (vitamin C)

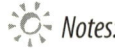
Notes:

You're also going to need information on which glands, organs, etc. are also affected by your drug intake (your naturopathic doctor should be able to figure this out by looking at the pharmaceutical printout on the drug) and then take the necessary herbal therapy or treatment to remedy the effects. For example, steroids suppress adrenal gland functioning and are taxing on the liver. So part of your treatment to heal the effects of this drug may include a herb to stimulate the adrenals, a herb to cleanse the liver and another one to strengthen it, and acupressure or acupuncture to further stimulate and strengthen the adrenals and liver. Make an appointment with a good naturopathic doctor (N.D.) and take in the list of drugs you're on or have been on in the last two years, and he/she will be able to advise you on which herbs to take. But remember, always trial-test new substances one at a time and follow your own intuition above all else. Also, you may want to wait until your digestive tract is reasonably healed – no intestinal bleeding and no more than five bowel movements per day – before starting any additional herbal therapy (i.e. other than those recommended in this chapter). Acupressure or acupuncture can be done at any time.

We've had a lot of media hype and information about the importance of vitamins, but less attention has been given to minerals. However, due to deficient and declining soil and water quality, it's actually harder now to get a sufficient amount of minerals from our diet. Also, many people with IBD tend towards a hyper-acidic bodily state and certain minerals act as alkalizing agents to bring your overall body's pH back into balance. Depending on how overly acidic your body is (i.e. low pH), you may need mega-doses of certain minerals to bring it back into balance. A good naturopathic physician will be able to test you for this using BTA (Biological Terrain Analysis), where the biochemistry of your blood, urine and saliva are all tested and compared. You get a much better picture of what's going on holistically with your body than you do from just regular blood tests. If you have difficulty swallowing pills, you can take your minerals by crushing them up finely (use a pill-crusher, or mortar and pestle) and mixing them with either oatmeal, yogurt, fruit juice or half a mashed banana. You can also get many of them (calcium, magnesium, zinc, selenium, etc.) in liquid or capsule preparations.

I have found with both vitamins and minerals, that liquid or chewable preparations are the most easily absorbed, especially if you've had sections of your intestine removed. I strongly recommend that, wherever possible, you take your supplements (herbal, vitamin, mineral) in liquid form. However, a problem with taking your vitamins/minerals in liquid form is that they are often mixed with other herbs and flavorings (e.g., citrus juices, peppermint), which can be irritating to a sensitized gastro-intestinal tract. Therefore, an excellent and highly recommended way to get your daily vitamins/minerals is to buy them in capsule form and mix them in with an Absorb Plus or protein shake. Simply open the capsule and empty the contents into the blender with the supplement powder. Even if you don't need to gain weight, you may want to replace breakfast with a delicious liquid shake simply because it's such an effective way to absorb and digest your daily nutrients. You can also add other supplements at this time, like extra iron capsules, coenzyme Q10, a tablespoon of Udo's Choice EFA oil, etc. See the section above on *Malnutrition*, and the *Bowel Rest Elemental Diet* section in Chapter Three for more information on Absorb Plus and protein shakes.

> Due to deficient and declining soil and water quality, it's actually harder now to get a sufficient amount of minerals from our diet. Also, many people with IBD tend towards a hyper-acidic bodily state and certain minerals act as alkalizing agents to bring your overall body's pH back into balance.

In some regions you can get vitamins and minerals in a spray form and this also increases absorption – just watch out for any possible irritation to the tissue you're spraying, but unless you're super sensitive it should be fine.

Buy your vitamins and minerals from a reputable health food store or alternative health pharmacy as they carry a much greater selection and better quality than a drugstore. Or, you can buy online from *www.LTYGshoppe.com*. Again, try to get preparations from a certified organic or wild source, plant derivatives are better than animal sources, and make sure the product has no added fillers (starch, sugar, yeast, etc.). After literally years of searching, I have finally found an adult chewable multi-vitamin/mineral supplement that's free of artificial sweeteners or fillers and actually tastes good: Nature's Plus Natural Pineapple Flavor Adult's Chewable Multi-Vitamin & Mineral (ingest 2 – 3 times per day).

See Appendix C for supplier details. Again, take it at mealtimes to ensure absorption.

I've found my body initially tolerates, on average, half the recommended dose for each of the vitamins and minerals that can cause diarrhea (see the list above). If you think this might be a problem then it's best to start slowly and gradually work your way up to the recommended dose or beyond it, if needed. However, if you simultaneously supplement with L-Glutamine, Psyllium Seed, or Bentonite Clay (see outlines above) these will greatly lessen your diarrhea and you may be able to ingest the normal dose right away.

Vitamin and mineral supplementation is a vital part of giving your body the tools and energy it needs to heal itself. To make sure you're getting ideal amounts of all the vitamins and minerals necessary, I recommend the following easy daily supplementation plan:

> **Vitamins associated with lower Colon-Cancer risk**
> A recent study has shown that supplements of multivitamins and vitamin E are associated with a lower risk of colon cancer. American researchers assessed the frequency, duration, and daily dose of individual vitamin supplements and multivitamins, for a ten year interval ending two years before diagnosis of cancer. After controlling for other predictors of colon-cancer risk such as intake of dietary vitamins, alcohol, and fibre, the risk of colon cancer was lower in men and women who took supplements of vitamins A, C, E, folic acid, calcium, and multivitamins. But the association was strongest for vitamin E and multivitamins: people who used multivitamins daily for the entire 10-year interval had half the risk of those who had not taken multivitamins. Those who averaged 200 IU or more of vitamin E per day for the 10 years had a 57% risk reduction compared to non-users.
> Macready, N. *The Lancet* 1997, 350 (9089) 1452

- High quality multi-vitamin/mineral supplement in capsule form, with extra vitamin A and B spectrum.
- 2 capsules of a fairly dissolvable mineral blend for extra mineral supplementation needed for vital bodily functions and to regulate acidity.
- 60 – 100 mg. Coenzyme Q10 and 60 – 100 mg. Pycnogenol or Grape Seed Extract antioxidant supplements.
- One or two 25 mg. capsules of Ferrasorb iron, from Thorne Research Ltd. (only if anemic).
- 1 – 2 tablespoons of Udo's Choice Ultimate Oil Blend, from Flora Manufacturing, containing Omega-3 and 6 essential fatty acids, evening primrose oil and vitamin E. Even the super-sensitive should have no problem tolerating and digesting this oil, but if you do, reduce it to ½ tablespoon per day (or whatever you can tolerate). Also available in capsule form, if you prefer.

Add all of these together (simply open capsules and empty the contents) once or twice a day in an Absorb Plus (for added energy and tissue repair/healing) or protein shake. I add all my supplements to an Absorb Plus shake in the morning for breakfast. See *www.LTYGshoppe.com* or Appendix C for details on suppliers of these products.

> I have found with both vitamins and minerals, that liquid or chewable preparations are the most easily absorbed, especially if you've had sections of your intestine removed.

SUPPLEMENT INTRODUCTION ORDER

Now that you've read about all the different supplements you can take to address your particular symptom profile, let's talk about the best order for introducing supplements. I've had many private consultations with readers who are super-sensitive to any new substance. So, to reduce the risk of adverse reactions, they want to know which supplements are safest to introduce first. Of course, each person's body is going to be different and react to different things, but here's a rough idea of how to proceed based on my experience and feedback from readers. Supplements are listed in the order they're least likely to cause an adverse reaction (i.e. the 'safest' supplement is listed first). However, please keep in mind that ALL of these supplements have now been used and tolerated well by many thousands of my readers, so you only need to follow this order if you're very frightened/nervous:

- Homeopathic iron or other homeopathic remedies
- FissureHeal suppositories
- George's 'Always Active' Aloe Vera Juice
- L-Glutamine and N-Acetyl Glucosamine
- Wild Oregano Oil
- *Jini's Healing Implant Enema*
- Flax Oil
- Fish Oil
- Natren probiotics (but take in the order suggested in *Probiotic Supplementation* section)
- Grape Seed Extract or Pycnogenol
- CoEnzyme Q10
- Astragalus
- Maitake
- Deglycyrrhizinated licorice (DGL) tablets
- Multi-Vitamin/Mineral
- Ferrasorb iron
- Absorb Plus
- MucosaHeal
- Vitamin C in mineral ascorbate form
- Liquid Chlorophyll
- Auxima Fera or Flouradix iron
- Iron Transfusion

Notes:

Remember, you can order all of the products recommended in this chapter from *www.HolisticHealthShoppe.com* or call 1-888-866-7745 (toll-free, open 24/7), or see Appendix C for details on ordering directly from the manufacturers. Even if you prefer to buy your supplements at your local health store, you may still want to check out the Holistic Health Shoppe, since I have pre-screened all the supplements available, and my comments are listed beside each – this will give you a better idea of exactly what to look for at your local health store.

Now turn to the *Healing Journey Workbook* on the *Listen To Your Gut CD* and complete the section for this chapter – Chapter Two.

3

Food As Medicine

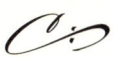

"Virtually every bit of food you eat has been treated with some chemical somewhere along the line. Dyes, bleaches, emulsifiers, preservatives, flavors, buffers, noxious sprays, acidifiers, alkalizers, deodorants, moisteners, drying agents, gases, extenders, thickeners, disinfectancts, fungicides, neutralizers, anticaking and antifoaming agents, conditioners, curers, hydrolizers, hydrogenerators, and many others.

These are the tools of the food technician... His alchemy can make stale food appear fresh, permit unsanitary practices, mask inferior quality, substitute nutritionally inferior or worthless chemicals for more costly ingredients."

William Longgood

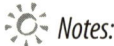 *Notes:*

This chapter contains specific dietary guidelines that I've established through extensive testing, trial and error, and some research or clinical data. Many of the 'do's' and 'don'ts' are likely to be things you've already noticed affect your body positively or negatively. Like most people with an illness, you're going to have to resign yourself to giving up the junk food, chemical-laden, processed food, fast food diet you may be on. A "normal" western diet places tremendous stress on the digestive system and pollutes your body with all kinds of substances that irritate your gastrointestinal tract.

ORGANIC FOOD AND BEVERAGES

It is very important that you consider switching to certified organic food and beverages as much as possible. This includes meat, dairy products, vegetables, fruit, juices, bread, rice and all other grains – basically, anything you put in your mouth. Yes, this is a lot more expensive and will probably involve more hassle as you'll have to go to a special grocer. But again, is your health and wellbeing your number one priority, or not? Keep in mind that you don't have to put yourself in a prison about this. If you go out to eat with family or friends, just enjoy the food available and relax. Having a good time and relaxing is just as integral to wellness as the physical food you ingest.

Meat & Dairy Products

Non-organic meat is a major source of pollutants for your body because the animals are fed chemically grown and treated feed, they're given a steady diet of antibiotics to combat the unhealthy environment they're raised in and they're also given hormones to make them grow and mature faster for slaughter. All of these toxins are then ingested by you when you eat the meat. Certified organic meat, on the other hand, is fed natural, organic feed, and not injected with antibiotics or hormones. Needless to say, this also means the animals have a better life prior to slaughter and are allowed to mature normally in a natural, free-range environment. You can see why organic farmers need to charge more for their meat, but also why it is well worth it.

Certified organic milk, cheese and other dairy products are also far superior to non-organic because the non-organic cows are continually given hormones to unnaturally increase and prolong their milk production (in addition to pesticide and antibiotic consumption). This means that non-organic (i.e. regular) milk and dairy products have very high levels of hormones in them. The harmful effects of secondary hormone consumption (via animal products) are not currently understood properly. However, there is increasing research available showing the negative effects of estrogen-mimicking compounds (xenoestrogens) in plastics, and increased breast cancer rates have been shown, among other harmful effects.

Fruits & Vegetables

As for certified organic fruit and vegetables, let me give you a little example to show you the difference. Let's take a look at the typical growing and storage cycle of a non-organic potato. First the soil is mixed with a chemical fertilizer so that the seed potatoes from the beginning of their growth cycle are absorbing toxic chemicals. During the above-ground growth cycle of the potato plants, they will probably be sprayed with chemical pesticides at least twice. These pesticides are directly absorbed by the plant and also leach into the soil in which it's growing. After harvest, some of the potatoes are shipped directly to grocery stores, the rest of them are sealed in an airtight storage container. These stored potatoes are then blasted with a toxic gas designed to kill anything it comes into contact with (to prevent decay).

The potatoes sit, surrounded by and absorbing this poisonous gas in the sealed, airtight container, until they're shipped to the stores and sold for your consumption.

Certified organic potatoes, by comparison, are grown in naturally fertilized soil, no pesticides or chemicals of any sort are used during the growing cycle of the plant and after harvest they remain untreated and natural. When you buy a certified organic potato at the grocery store you get a

> A "normal" western diet places tremendous stress on the digestive system and pollutes your body with all kinds of substances that irritate your gastrointestinal tract.

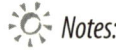 Notes:

plain, natural potato with no added chemicals, toxins or poisons. I think you may be beginning to comprehend why it makes sense to pay extra for certified organic food. Remember, you need to create a healthy, supportive environment that helps your body to heal itself – not one that makes it harder and poisons your body with even more toxins to process.

Make Sure It's Certified

You may notice that several times I've used the term 'certified organic' instead of just 'organic'. This is because, unfortunately, some states and provinces have no regulations governing organic food and there's nothing to prevent an unscrupulous grocer or supplier from just slapping the label "organic" on a product that's actually full of chemicals. However, if you buy food and produce that's labeled "certified organic" (and the regulatory board will also probably be listed) you can be pretty certain you're getting what you're paying for. Typically, "certified organic" produce means that the soil has been free of prohibited pesticides and chemical fertilizers for at least three years; with regard to meat it means the animals have been fed certified organic feed and not given hormones or antibiotics.

Organic Food = Healthier Rats

A 2005 study done by the Danish Institute of Agricultural Sciences and the School of Agriculture at the University of Newcastle, compared the results between rats fed a diet of organic food since weaning and rats fed conventional food. Scientists found that, compared to rats that ate conventional diets, organically fed rats experienced various health benefits:

- Improved immune system status
- Better sleeping habits
- Less adipose tissue (fat)
- Higher vitamin E content in their blood

Of course, rats are not human, but the results are certainly meaningful.

I hope I've impressed upon you the importance of eating organic food and beverages. However, as with anything we "should" do, when it comes time to actually implement it in our lives, several other factors can come into play. If you have a choice between eating lunch at work or taking an organic packed lunch from home, then pack your own lunch – as long as it doesn't stress you out. It's better to eat one organic meal a day in a happy and relaxed state, than to eat three organic meals a day simultaneously feeling stressed out and unhappy over the amount of time you've spent preparing food. Our goal is to reduce toxins ingested, so whatever amount of organic food you can consume is better than none.

Shopping For Organic Food

As consumer awareness increases, we are seeing more foods in regular grocery stores with labels like, "No artificial preservatives or additives", or "No sugar added". This is a good trend as it's also bringing down the price of pure foods. Remember that every little bit helps, so if you absolutely cannot afford organic food or you can't get it where you live, then start at your local supermarket and buy the purest of what they're stocking. Here are some guidelines:

▶ Hothouse tomatoes and other vegetables tend to be grown with less chemicals than outdoor varieties.

▶ You can get a natural vegetable/fruit wash product that will remove some of the pesticide residues from the skin of fruits and vegetables.

▶ Whenever possible, peel your non-organic produce before cooking or eating.

▶ In my opinion, it's more important to eat organic meat, eggs, and dairy, than organic vegetables and fruit.

Also, you may want to look at scaling back your meat consumption and eating less meat and more vegetables – not only is this good for your health, but it will considerably bring down your food bills. For years when I would eat at my parents' house I couldn't believe the portions of meat they ate at

☼ Remember, you need to create a healthy, supportive environment that helps your body to heal itself – not one that makes it harder and poisons your body with even more toxins to process.

one sitting – I used to say to my mum, "you know, the amount of chicken on your plate alone would feed three of us at my house." Unsurprisingly, my mum and dad both developed very high blood pressure. In the last year, my mum has cut way back on their meat consumption and sometimes serves entirely vegetarian meals and now her blood pressure is normal. My dad still smokes and drinks quite a bit however, so his blood pressure hasn't seen such marked results! However, if reducing your meat intake is going to cause you to increase your bread, pasta, potatoes, and other starchy carbohydrates intake – then don't do it. Of the two scenarios, for someone with IBS or IBD, it's better to eat more meat and less starchy carbohydrates. If you can reduce your meat consumption and increase your non-starchy vegetable consumption, then that's ideal.

RESTRICTIONS & GUIDELINES

Here are some issues that may or may not be applicable to your situation. Keep in mind that all of *The Healing Diets* following assume you have read and incorporated these suggestions into your dietary practice.

Preserving The Nutritive Value Of Food

In order to get the highest level of nutrition from your food, in the most easily digestible form, it's best to eat fresh meats and vegetables and cook them in a conventional oven or stovetop. Eating raw foods is definitely beneficial and usually contains the highest amount of live enzymes. However, until your system is quite healed you may find it difficult, if not impossible, to tolerate raw foods. The best way to cook vegetables for maximum nutrient retention is to steam them. You can do this using a steaming basket suspended in a pot with water on the stove, or you can buy a steamer that you just fill with water and plug it in – both ways are equally easy. Otherwise, if you boil vegetables in water, make sure you use the least amount of water (filtered, not tap) possible as this will help reduce nutrient loss. Most of us put far too much water in the pot – usually you only need the water to come about half way up the vegetables and then cover the pot with a lid to produce a 'steaming' effect (turn the heat down low). If you can

---

☼ Pesticides are directly absorbed by plants and also leach into the soil in which they're growing. Water run-off from the soil then carries these pesticides into our rivers, lake and oceans, where they further damage our wildlife and environment.

either drink this cooking water, or use it in a soup, sauce or stew, that's ideal. See Chapter Four for detailed instructions on what kind of pots and pans to use, and why you should never use a microwave.

Eliminating Sugar

White sugar (and brown sugar) also interfere with your healing process. Numerous clinical studies have shown that the immune system stays markedly depressed for 4 – 8 hours following the consumption of even a small amount of sugar. Therefore, it's best to reduce or eliminate as much refined, unnecessary sugar from your diet as possible. This means:

 *Notes:*

- Drink only fresh, natural juices with no added sugar and even then, dilute with ½ water to reduce sugar intake.
- Switch to all-fruit sugarless jams and jellies (sweetened with grape juice or fructose – the naturally occurring sugar in fruit).
- Reduce or stop putting sugar in your tea.
- Use honey, stevia or pure maple syrup instead of sugar wherever possible, especially in baking.
- Where you must have sugar, use brown Rapadura sugar. Rapadura (sometimes called turbinado sugar) is the most natural-state form of sugar available. Most other brown sugars are first bleached and then dyed brown again – using molasses or an artificial coloring agent.
- Always check labels (especially on canned foods) to ensure there's no added sugar, or artifical sweeteners.
- Switch to natural cereals flavored with honey, rice syrup, molasses, fruit juice, or fructose (the naturally occurring sugar in fruits). When you're cooking oatmeal or any other hot cereal, add raisins and/or chopped apples towards the end of cooking, and they'll automatically sweeten it for you so you won't have to add much (if any) additional sweetener.

Fructose (a natural fruit sugar) has been getting some negative media coverage lately. However, the media reports do not distinguish between regular fructose and high fructose corn syrup. Regular fructose is often extracted from corn (since it's a sweet vegetable), but, high fructose corn syrup is fructose that's been extracted from corn, and then combined with glucose to produce a completely different substance. Research shows that consuming high fructose corn syrup causes great spikes in blood sugar and disrupts normal insulin production and response. Therefore, I don't recommend you consume it. Be sure and check labels as it's often added to drinks, cereals and other packaged foods.

However, regular fructose does not impair insulin function and in fact, actually improves insulin response. Fructose is not transported directly into the bloodstream after digestion and absorption, but is converted into glycogen in the liver, where it is stored and used for energy at a later time. A recent trial demonstrated that no increase is seen in blood glucose after ingestion of fructose at 15 grams or less. This lowered glycemic response with fructose ingestion appeared to be most effective in those individuals who had the poorest glucose tolerance profiles. In non-diabetic individuals, fructose consumption results in little to no discernable rise in blood insulin levels.[1] Because fructose must be changed to glucose in the liver in order to be utilized by the body, blood glucose levels do not rise as rapidly after fructose consumption compared to other simple sugars or even complex carbohydrates. For example, the glycemic load calculation for 10 grams of fructose is only 2. In comparison, the glycemic load for a slice of bread is 10, an apple is 7, and a cup of white rice is 26.

My philosophy is to save your sugar for when it really counts. If you eliminate most of the unnecessary sugars from your diet, then you can enjoy that occasional chocolate bar or sugar-packed piece of cake without feeling guilty.

The good news about all of these restrictions is that when you switch to doing your grocery shopping at a natural/ whole foods/ organic grocery store, most of the products they carry will already conform to these guidelines; no added sugar, no preservatives, chemicals, MSG, nitrates, nitrites, etc. Still, you should check the labels just to make sure.

> High fructose corn syrup causes great spikes in blood sugar and disrupts normal insulin production and response. Regular fructose does not impair insulin function and in fact, actually improves insulin response.

Reduce Grains/Carbohydrates

If you have IBS or IBD, there's a good chance you also have an overgrowth of yeast (*Candida albicans*) in your body. Yeast loves to feed on sugars, and all carbohydrates – when broken down via digestion – are sugars. Therefore, it's almost always a good idea for people with IBS or IBD to reduce their grain and starchy carbohydrate intake and increase their intake of protein, non-starchy vegetables, and good fats. Grains include wheat, rice, corn, amaranth, quinoa, cous-cous, millet, oats, rye, barley, kamut, spelt, etc. Other carbohydrates to reduce or avoid include potatoes, sweet potatoes, yams, beans, legumes, and fruit. If you suspect a *Candida* overgrowth, you also need to avoid fermented foods such as soy sauce, tempeh, natto, miso, cheese, alcohol, vinegar, sauerkraut, pickles etc. as well as mushrooms and sugar alcohols (sweeteners like xylitol, sorbitol, etc.). Once you have no more symptoms of bowel dysfunction and you have restored a healthy bacterial flora to your gut, you can begin to eat these foods again.

When you do eat grains, try to eat other varieties like millet, spelt, rye, amaranth, quinoa, and kamut, instead of just eating wheat all the time. Health stores now carry many different varieties of bread and pasta made from spelt, kamut and rye. For myself, I still continue to minimize grains and starchy vegetables like potatoes, just because my gut tells me to. Sometimes I won't eat bread at all – other times I'll minimize intake by having an open-face sandwich (for example), thereby consuming one slice of bread, rather than two. Likewise, I continue to minimize sugar consumption and use Stevia (a natural herb that is 200 – 300 times sweeter than sugar) as much as possible.

> **Refined Carbs Increase Colon Cancer**
> Researchers in Italy conducted a multi-centre case-control study including 1,953 cases and 4,154 hospitalised controls. Subjects from 6 Italian regions were interviewed, using a food frequency questionnaire, over a period of 4 years. Results showed that individuals with the highest consumption of refined bread had a 28% higher risk of colorectal cancer than those with the lowest. For refined sugar, an increase of one serving (4 teaspoons) per day showed an 11% increase in colorectal cancer risk. Both results remained statistically significant after adjustment for confounders. Eating either raw or cooked vegetables showed a protective effect. An increase of one serving of vegetables per day resulted in a 13% reduction in risk.
> Franceschi, S .et al, *Eur. J. of Cancer Prevention* 7 (Suppl 2) S19-S23.

Sufficient Water Intake

People with IBD and IBS tend to need more water due to increased bowel movements and/or the need to flush toxins and drug residues. Make sure you're getting at least 8 – 10 glasses of water per day. Spring water is ideal since it contains natural minerals that help alkalize your body, but filtered is okay. Do not drink tap water as it is often contaminated with pathogenic microorganisms and/or chlorine, which will kill off the good bacteria in your gut. Also do not drink carbonated, or 'fizzy' water as it will likely bloat your gut and the carbonation leaches minerals from your bones. A great book on the importance of drinking water is Dr. F Batmanghelidj's book, *Your Body's Many Cries for Water*.

Mealtimes

Remember that the way and manner in which you consume your food can be almost as important as what you're eating. Always take the time and peace necessary to sit down and relax while you're enjoying your food. Don't discuss sensitive or emotional issues right before, during, or right after a meal. Ask your friend, family, or spouse to please wait until later, when you'll be more than happy to discuss the issue. Remember that digestion begins with the enzymes in your saliva, so take the time to eat slowly and thoroughly chew each mouthful before swallowing. If these guidelines seem tedious to you, just give it a chance and you'll soon be enjoying your food and mealtimes as a wonderful time to relax and savor.

Vegetarianism

If you're a vegetarian, you're going to have to make sure you're getting an adequate intake of nutrients, particularly since beans, lentils and the entire cabbage family (onions, Brussels sprouts, broccoli, cauliflower, etc.) are not allowed on most of *The Healing Diets*. To make up for the prohibited beans, vegetables and cheese, you'll need to make sure you're eating plenty of couscous, brown rice and more nutritious grains and pastas like kamut (has 40% more protein than wheat), amaranth and quinoa. Vegetarians also need an alternative source of protein since dairy products (except certain types of whey protein) are not allowed, or restricted on most of the Diets. Therefore, if you're vegetarian, you'll also need to supplement daily with whey protein or hemp protein shakes. People in disease states need a lot of extra protein and without it, your body can't heal properly. I even recommend that meat eaters ingest one whey protein isolate shake per day since the protein is alkaline and highly absorbable. If you don't want to eat these other sources of protein and iron, then you may want to consider eating meat until

---

☼ People in disease states need a lot of extra protein and without it, your body can't heal properly. Therefore, if you're vegetarian, you'll also need to supplement daily with whey protein or hemp protein shakes.

your body is healed to the point where you're completely off drugs, have acceptable hemoglobin levels, no more than three formed bowel movements per day, and no cramping or bleeding. At that point, you'll be able to eat beans, lentils and whatever other vegetables you want and so can probably become a vegetarian again, if you wish.

High Fibre & Raw Foods

I know there are many dieticians and naturopaths who recommend a high fibre diet as the best therapy for people with IBS and IBD. I'm sorry, but I must disagree with them. When your intestines are in an inflamed, aggravated state, they simply cannot digest and absorb the nutrients from high fibre foods (whole grains, legumes, dark green leafy vegetables, celery, etc.). In fact, if you eat these foods you'll probably find the result is flatulence (gas), bloating, diarrhea and sometimes a trigger or increase in intestinal bleeding. However, after you've used *The Healing Diets* to heal yourself, you can most certainly start consuming high fibre and cabbage family (cruciferous) foods again. In terms of preserving and maintaining intestinal health I highly recommend these whole, unrefined foods. But, your intestines need to be fairly healthy before you'll be able to digest these foods properly. For myself, after following *The Healing Diets* for two years (keep in mind I was testing and developing them simultaneously) I was able to start eating onions, broccoli, beans, wild rice and all kinds of high fibre and raw foods again with absolutely no bloating or gas as a result. Yes, dietary freedom is possible! But first you need to heal your system and bring your digestive and absorptive abilities up to normal – or at least close to it.

Likewise, once you're healed, you want to eat as many raw foods as you can. When you consume raw vegetables and fruits (preferably naturally ripened before picking) you will receive the maximum amount of live enzymes, phytonutrients, vitamins and minerals possible. However, until your digestive system is fairly healed (especially if your stomach and small intestine are compromised) it is difficult to digest raw foods; they can be irritating and cause gas, bloating and diarrhea. Therefore, until you reach

> Your intestines need to be fairly healthy before you'll be able to digest high fibre or raw foods properly. Even raw vegetable juices can trigger diarrhea.

the *Maintenance Diet*, I recommend you cook all vegetables, and on some of the diets you'll need to cook fruit as well. If you want to try juicing raw vegetables, then start with really small amounts, otherwise you may find they trigger diarrhea.

Soy Products

I recommend that all people (from infants to adults) avoid or greatly minimize unfermented soy product consumption – this includes tofu, soybeans, soybean oil, soy milk, soy protein, etc. You especially need to read the labels on vegetarian processed foods as many are composed predominantly of some form of soy or soy protein. Here's why I recommend you avoid consuming unfermented soy products:

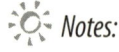
Notes:

- Soy contains very high amounts of phyto-estrogens (plant based chemicals that mimic estrogen). The daily exposure of infants who consume soy formulas is 6 – 11 times higher than adults consuming soy foods, and the concentration of these phyto-estrogen hormones in the blood is 13,000 to 22,000 times higher than normal estrogen.[2] This is detrimental both from a hormonal/glandular balance point of view and also from an 'increased propensity to breast, uterine and cervical cancer' point of view.

- The phytic acid naturally contained in soy inhibits mineral absorption and depresses thyroid function. These are both very harmful factors for normal people, but especially so for people with IBS and IBD.

- Soybeans contain enzyme inhibitors that block the action of trypsin and other enzymes needed for protein digestion. These enzyme inhibitors can produce gastric distress, reduce protein digestion and result in chronic deficiencies in amino acid uptake. In test animals, diets high in trypsin inhibitors caused enlargement and pathological conditions of the pancreas, including cancer.[3]

Fermented soy products, like natto, miso, tempeh and soy sauce, are fine to consume and actually beneficial, since the fermentation process greatly reduces the phytic acid, and deactivates the enzyme inhibitors. As well, your phyto-estrogen intake, in the amounts you'd normally eat of these foods, would be fairly low. For many more excellent articles on why you should not consume unfermented soy (or only a minimal amount) see *www.mercola. com* – in particular, read the article by Sally Fallon and Mary G. Enig, PhD.

If you've been using soy as a dairy substitute, try switching to rice milk or goat's milk instead. Almond milk is also good but you may have to make your own as I've been thus far unable to find a commercial product that doesn't have added carrageenan. If you've been using soy as a protein source, then good alternatives include cold-extracted, whey protein isolate, cheddar cheese made from raw milk, and hemp protein.

Wild vs. Farmed Salmon

Before you buy salmon or order it in a restaurant, confirm that the salmon is wild, not farmed. Farmed salmon is an unhealthy food choice and the salmon farms are causing serious damage to the ocean environment and wild salmon populations. Farmers need to feed the farmed salmon food pellets that have been chemically dyed orange, otherwise the farmed salmon would be grey in color – what does that tell you about the health and abnormal condition of these fish? The waste products from these fish then fall to the ocean floor in such quantity that all natural life on the ocean floor below them is smothered and poisoned. Farmed salmon, like many commercially farmed animals, are unhealthy (due to confinement and overcrowding) and often covered in sea lice. To get rid of the lice, veterinary substances designed to be used on land animals are released into the pens and then flow out into the ocean – with unknown consequences. Every so often, these lice-infested fish break out of their pens and infect wild salmon (particularly the young fish), who then die. Farmed salmon also have much lower levels of beneficial Omega-3 fatty acids – one of the principle reasons why eating salmon is so good for people. Obviously, an unhealthy fish is not going to deliver the same health benefits to the person who eats it, as a healthy fish will. Farmed salmon also have higher levels of contaminants (like PCB's, mercury, etc.) than wild salmon, probably because they're

> The farmed salmon are fed food pellets that have been chemically dyed orange, otherwise the farmed salmon would be grey in color – what does that tell you about the health and abnormal conditions of these fish? Farmed salmon are often covered in sea lice, have lower levels of Omega-3 and higher levels of PCB's and other contaminants.

penned close to shore where toxin levels are higher. So, at all times, check that the salmon is wild (not farmed) before consuming.

If you're going to eat salmon sashimi or other raw fish, make sure the fish has been frozen for 3 – 7 days prior to consumption. Freezing the fish for that length of time causes the worms (anisakiasis, diphyllobothrium) that may be in the fish to die. There is also a simple 'candle test' you can do to check for worms in the sashimi. Simply hold the fish up to a candle and any worms will appear as round, coiled occlusions in the flesh. Also check to make sure the restaurant uses wild salmon, not farmed.

Mercury In Fish

Some fish are now also contaminated with unacceptably high levels of mercury. Mercury is an extremely damaging substance, especially since it is able to cross the blood/brain barrier. The Environmental Protection Agency has released these guidelines to minimize human mercury contamination through seafood:

1. Do not eat Shark, Swordfish, King Mackerel, or Tilefish because they contain high levels of mercury.

2. Only eat up to 12 ounces (2 average meals) a week of a variety of fish and shellfish that are lower in mercury, i.e. don't eat seafood more than twice a week.

3. Five of the most commonly eaten fish that are low in mercury are shrimp, canned light tuna, wild salmon, pollock, and catfish.

4. Another commonly eaten fish, albacore ("white") tuna has more mercury than canned light tuna. So, when choosing your two meals of fish and shellfish, you may eat up to 6 ounces (one average meal) of albacore tuna per week.*

5. Check local advisories about the safety of fish caught by family and friends in your local lakes, rivers, and coastal areas. If no advice is available, eat up to 6 ounces (one average meal) per week of fish you

catch from local waters, but don't consume any other fish during that week.

6. Follow these same recommendations when feeding fish and shellfish to your young child, but serve smaller portions.

*Many other environmental groups now feel that albacore tuna has moved into the 'high mercury' category as well. So if you're going to eat canned tuna, make sure it's the 'light' tuna variety. Since pollution is increasing rapidly in our world, it's a good idea to periodically check with the Environmental Protection Agency (EPA) or Environmental Working Group (EWG) to find out which fish are still okay, and which have now moved into the 'high risk' category.

> Mercury is an extremely damaging substance, especially since it is able to cross the blood/brain barrier.

THE HEALING DIETS

The Healing Diets are one of your most effective tools for healing yourself. They are meant to be used in conjunction with the healing protocols outlined in Chapter Two. The Diets progress through increasing levels of strictness, depending on the severity of your symptoms:

▶ *Maintenance Diet* – this is the diet to be used for ongoing maintenance by anyone who has ever had IBS or IBD, and their children as well (as a preventive). It could also be called 'The Common Sense Diet' and this should be your ongoing, normal diet for the rest of your life.

▶ *Minimize Gas & Bloating Diet* – if you have no diarrhea, but experience bloating, gas, flatulence, constipation, indigestion and/or belching, then follow this diet till your symptoms resolve.

▶ *Reduce Diarrhea Diet* – use this diet if you're having gas and bloating symptoms along with five or more bowel movements per day. Or, if you're just experiencing diarrhea. You can also follow this diet if you're bleeding from your rectum only.

▶ *Stop Intestinal Bleeding Diet* – this is a very strict, bland diet to be used in conjunction with the appropriate supplements (outlined in Chapter Two) to stop bleeding from your stomach, small intestine or large intestine. It is not necessary to follow this diet if your bleeding is from your rectum only (in that case just follow the *Reduce Diarrhea Diet*).

- **Bowel Rest Elemental Diet** – this is a completely liquid, pre-digested diet and usually used when you're so ill that you're facing surgery, or you're facing, or already on TPN (total parenteral nutrition), or you're currently receiving elemental food through a shunt (tube that goes directly into your stomach). Alternatively, it can be used as a fast way to clear symptoms, gain weight, induce disease remission and test for food sensitivities/allergies.

Use whichever diet corresponds to where you're at in your healing process. You may need to switch back and forth between diets depending on how you're doing each month and the stress levels in your life. Let your symptoms be your guide and choose the diet according to your most severe symptom. For example, if you're experiencing excessive gas, bloating and diarrhea, then follow the *Reduce Diarrhea Diet*. Once you have the diarrhea under control, switch to the more lenient *Minimize Gas & Bloating Diet*. When you're no longer experiencing any flatulence or bloating, switch to the *Maintenance Diet*.

If you switch diets and experience a recurrence of symptoms, it means that you've switched too soon. Go back to the stricter diet for another few months and then try the more lenient diet again. As well, as you become more in tune with your body, you'll be able to sense if your system's getting run down or aggravated due to stress and then you can switch right away to one of the stricter diets. This will help you to prevent flare-ups before they manifest full-blown in your body. There are Quick Reference Guides for each Diet listed at the end of this chapter. These Quick Reference Guides summarize each of the diet guidelines on one page, making them easy to refer to at a glance. I've also made these one-page Quick Reference Guides available to you on the *Listen To Your Gut CD*, so you can print them out and tack them up on your fridge. You can also take a copy with you when you go grocery shopping, or out to restaurants to aid you in your food selection.

> If you switch diets and experience a recurrence of symptoms, it means that you've switched too soon.

All of *The Healing Diets* have the following guidelines or principles in common:

- **No processed foods containing nitrates/nitrites, preservatives, MSG, carrageenan, artificial flavors or colors.** There is a new class of chemicals that have just been released which are 'flavor blockers or enhancers' and these work by blocking or stimulating receptors on your brain associated with certain tastes and flavors. This means that a food company could release 'reduced salt' potato chips (for example) that taste just as salty as regular potato chips – because they're using a 'salt enhancer' chemical that tells your brain there's more salt in the chips then there actually is. Obviously, as these chemicals are new, there's no feedback yet on safety, however, keep in mind that MSG works in a similar manner and many scientists now classify MSG as a "neurotoxin". The really awful thing about this new class of flavor blockers/enhancers is that the FDA does not require manufacturers to list them specifically on the label, they will just automatically be included under the 'artificial flavor' category. This makes it even more important to avoid anything with 'artificial flavor' listed on the label.

- **Reducing or eliminating milk products (depending on your sensitivity).** Raw milk is much better tolerated and digested than pasteurized milk. Many health professionals classify pasteurized (and homogenized) milk as a toxic product since it has been denatured to the point where the body cannot digest it properly or extract many nutrients from it. In fact, homogenized milk has been shown to destroy plasmalogen (which makes up 30% of the membrane system in human heart cells) resulting in atherosclerosis.[4] Raw milk (milk that has not been heated or homogenized) however, has not been denatured and still contains the beneficial enzymes and bacteria that help your body to digest and absorb it properly. Cheddar made from raw milk (available in many natural food stores) is a good place to start testing, as it is tolerated by many

> **Processed Food and IBD**
> Sulphate-reducing bacteria can proliferate in the colon as a result of large amounts of animal protein and processed food, especially those which contain sulphur-based preservatives.
> One of the end products, hydrogen sulphide, is as toxic as cyanide, and can turn into sulphuric acid. A study showed that as meat consumption rises from 60 to 600 grams per day sulphates in the urine double, and sulphites in faeces increase tenfold. In people with ulcerative colitis the epithelial cells that line the colon lack the ability to oxidise butyrate, a vital fatty acid, and this abnormality could be the first step in the development of the disease, as exposure to sulphides selectively inhibits the ability of colon cells to use butyrate.
> *New Scientist*, 8th Aug. 1998, 26-30.

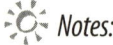
Notes:

people who cannot tolerate pasteurized milk products. To find a raw milk supplier in your area, go to **www.realmilk.com**. You can also read more about this issue on the website and the site will point you to other relevant resources. I eat raw milk cheddar all the time with no problems and it is an excellent source of calcium and protein. I can't get raw milk where I live, so haven't been able to test that, but I suspect I would be fine with it. Pasteurized milk, however, will often cause me to have a bowel movement within an hour of consumption. The odd time my kids insist on drinking cow's milk (because they've had it at friends' houses and realize it tastes pretty darn good!), I mix in a ¼ tsp. of Natren's dairy-based Megadophilus or Bifido Factor probiotics. They can't taste any difference (because it's dairy-based) and the probiotics help them digest the milk better and avoid bloating.

▶ **Reducing or eliminating acidic foods;** tomatoes, citrus fruits and juices, tomato-based sauces and condiments, vinegar-based sauces and condiments, etc. (dependant upon your sensitivity and until your system can handle them). People whose mucosal lining is inflamed or ulcerated are very sensitive to anything acidic, so best to avoid acidic foods and beverages until inflammation and ulceration is healed.

▶ **No caffeine.** Caffeine inhibits the absorption of vitamin C and leaches calcium, magnesium, potassium, iron and trace minerals from the body, and it stimulates bowel movements. Coffee is the worst thing you could drink; it really aggravates the colon in particular. A fantastic herbal coffee substitute is Bambu by Bioforce Inc. (available in many health stores, or online), but you'll still need to test it to make sure it doesn't aggravate your colon or cause heartburn. Even de-caffeinated coffee is not tolerated well and can result in cramping or increased bowel movements. Pure hot chocolate may be okay (test it and see), but make it with ¾ water and only ¼ milk.

▶ **No alcohol.** Alcohol is also extremely acidic and therefore very irritating to the mucosal lining of the stomach and intestines. Once you're healed and on the *Maintenance Diet* you may want to test small amounts – but try to stick to wine or beer and avoid all hard liquor. If you've adjusted fine to getting along without alcohol, then why drink at all? There are no health benefits to consuming alcohol, only negatives. If you need the 'drug' aspect of it, then personally, I feel marijuana (in small and infrequent amounts) does less damage to your health than alcohol. Personally, I consume neither.

▶ **No carbonated drinks (e.g., soda pop).** Carbonated drinks are packed with sugar, artificial flavors and colors. Even if you buy natural carbonated beverages, or plain soda water, the carbonation still leaches minerals from your bones (especially calcium) and produces gas and bloating in your abdomen. Emergen-C vitamin C drink packets are an excellent alternative to carbonated drinks since the mineral ascorbates go a bit fizzy when you add water and they taste as good, if not better, than a soda.

▶ **No hydrogenated oils/fats.** During the processing of commercial vegetable oils, they are heated to the point where their molecular structure is altered (similar to margarine) resulting in trans-fatty acids that damage cell walls and DNA. Margarine (and some other butter substitutes) is treated with chemical solvents and bleaches resulting in deformed, highly toxic, trans-fatty acids. These trans-fatty acids are also suspected carcinogens.

▶ **No artificial sweeteners.** Aspartame has the largest list of complaints and adverse reactions of any substance listed with the FDA. Aspartame has been proven to cause memory loss, can also be highly addictive and cause seizures and hyperactivity in some people. There is also a large body of mounting evidence against sucralose (Splenda), saccharine and acesulfame-K. An Internet search using the keywords "dangers of [name of sweetener]" can bring up lots of research on any one of them, pointing out the dangers and adverse reactions reported to date.

The best sugar alternative that has virtually no calories and is actually beneficial to your body is a plant extract called Stevia. Stevia is 100% natural and is 200-300 times sweeter than sugar. Xylitol is also another

---

People whose mucosal lining is inflamed or ulcerated are very sensitive to anything acidic, so best to avoid acidic foods and beverages until inflammation and ulceration is healed.

natural sweetener that works well, however Xylitol also flushes bacteria and prevents them from adhering to mucous membranes. This is a benefit if you're using Xylitol as a nasal spray (for example) during a cold, however, for ongoing use it's not a good idea as it will interfere with the necessary good bacteria colonizing your body. In small amounts, occasionally, Xylitol is okay. Stevia can be used any time and in any amounts you wish and it is now available in many forms in health stores and grocery stores.

▶ **Reducing roughage and cabbage family vegetables, until your system can handle them.** Roughage includes any type of bran, husk, or insoluble fibre (raw fruit, raw vegetables, sprouts, seeds, celery, green leafy vegetables). Certain other vegetables and fruit like grapes, blueberries, cherries, celery, corn, bell peppers also have a tough 'skin' that is very hard to digest and should be avoided, or removed before cooking and eating. Cabbage (or cruciferous) family vegetables should also be avoided and these include garlic, onions, leeks, cauliflower, broccoli, Brussels sprouts and cabbage. These foods will cause lots of gas and bloating until your mucosal lining is healed and your bacterial flora normalized. You also won't be able to digest them properly or absorb the nutrients from them until your digestive system is fairly healed, and will see lots of undigested particles floating in your stools, so there's no point in consuming them until you're healed enough to switch to the *Maintenance Diet*.

Therefore, you'll notice that each of the diets has numerous 'Do's' and 'Don'ts' in common. The *Stop Intestinal Bleeding Diet* has the greatest number of 'Don'ts' and the list gets progressively shorter (or less strict) as you move to the *Reduce Diarrhea Diet*, then the *Minimize Gas & Bloating Diet*. Finally, the *Maintenance Diet* has the smallest number of 'Don'ts' and is the most lenient of all *The Healing Diets*. The *Bowel Rest Elemental Diet* is in a class by itself as it doesn't involve ingesting normal food at all.

Notes:

Food Combining

If you have severe or widespread Crohn's (particularly if inflammation is present in your stomach and/or small intestine), you may have a higher degree of success with these diets if you also practice proper food combining at the same time (fully outlined in the book, *Fit For Life*, by Harvey and Marilyn Diamond). The basic tenet that should be followed is simply to not mix your proteins with your starch, or, complex carbohydrates (polysaccharides). The premise for this practice is that the digestive process for protein is very different, requiring different enzymes and fermentation times, from that of starch. Therefore, eating the two together at the same time results in neither being digested or absorbed with maximum efficiency. It's okay to eat protein with simple carbohydrates as the sugars in their mono and disaccharide molecular chains are easily broken down and absorbed directly into the bloodstream. To practice proper food combining, you're going to need some knowledge of which foods classify as complex carbohydrates and which are simple carbohydrates. Following are a few examples to get you started. For a complete list and recipe/meal ideas, pick up the *Fit For Life* book:

Complex Carbohydrates

- Bread, cereals, pasta, cakes, cookies, biscuits, crackers, etc.
- Any grains; wheat, rye, corn, bran, oats, barley, rice, cous-cous, amaranth, millet, quinoa, etc.
- Potatoes, yams, parsnips
- Peas, beans, chick peas, sprouted beans, lentils

* *All of the above should not be eaten with proteins/meats.*

Simple Carbohydrates

- Carrots, zucchini, asparagus
- Acorn, butternut or spaghetti squash
- Lettuce, leafy green vegetables (spinach, bok choy, etc.)

> If you have severe or widespread Crohn's (particularly if inflammation is present in your stomach and/or small intestine), you may have a higher degree of success with these diets if you also practice proper food combining at the same time.

- Tomatoes, cucumber, mushrooms
- Red, green, yellow, orange peppers

All of the above may be eaten with proteins/meats.

Elaine Gottschall's book, initially called *Food And The Gut Reaction* and later renamed *Breaking the Vicious Cycle*, also follows proper food combining principles. So if you have her book you can use it as a food category guide and for recipe ideas as well. All the allowable carbohydrates in her book are simple carbohydrates. Not mixing your proteins and starches (complex carbohydrates) will probably feel really weird at first since we come from such a "meat and potatoes" culture. Eventually, I found myself enjoying just a piece of steak or chicken with gravy (the gravy – just water added to drippings in the pan – is also classified as a protein) for one meal and at the next meal having some vegetables on their own with a bit of butter and salt. I also started learning to cook squash and to think of squash (mashed, cubed, fried, etc.) instead of potatoes. It's a hassle when you eat out, but like anything, you'll adjust to the point where your food choices are automatic. Some people have found that it's okay to eat rice with protein, so after you've been food combining for a month or two, you may want to give it a try and see if it's okay for you.

You may want to follow just *The Healing Diet* guidelines to begin with, and once you're comfortable and have adjusted to that change, then implement the food combining rules, if you still need to. As I've said, if you have Crohn's in the stomach and/or small intestine, you may benefit from practicing proper food combining whilst on *The Healing Diets*. However, if that's too much hassle for you, rest assured that you will still experience substantial relief just from following *The Healing Diets* alone (in conjunction with the therapies in Chapter Two).

Implementation

If you're the parent of a child with IBD, please take the time necessary to explain to your child why you're changing his/her diet and why that's a good idea. Again, your child needs to feel positive and has to want to

---

☼ Your child needs to feel positive and has to want to follow these diets, or there's no point in pursuing them. If someone feels they're being forced to eat a certain way and feels anger and resentment at mealtimes, then the food is not going to benefit their body very much.

follow these diets, or there's no point in pursuing them. If someone feels they're being forced to eat a certain way and feels anger and resentment at mealtimes, then the food is not going to benefit their body very much. Remember that the emotions can affect intestinal health just as much as anything we eat or drink. Also, due to the strong evidence for genetic predisposition to IBD, other family members (particularly children) should follow the *Maintenance Diet* as a preventive measure.

Please keep in mind that everyone's body is different and there may be things that I advise you not to eat that you can actually tolerate quite well. Likewise, there may be foods that I say are okay that don't feel good to you at all. For example, I allow potatoes and bread in *The Healing Diets* because I don't find them harmful. However, my personal intuitive sense is to keep these foods to a minimum and often I'll take a break and not eat them for a few weeks or months at a time. Our bodies are unique, finely tuned composites embodying all the complexity and variety of who we are. No one else's body is going to be or function exactly like yours. So, at all times, keep your own body as your final authority or decision maker in what's right, or not right for you.

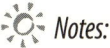 *Notes:*

The Healing Diets are also for you to use while you're simultaneously weaning yourself off prescription drugs. See Chapter Five for more information about the weaning process. For this reason, you'll probably need to switch back and forth between the diets because as you wean yourself off drugs, your symptoms will temporarily worsen as your body adjusts to the change. Here's what the cycle looks like: You reduce your drug intake and your symptoms worsen, so you switch to a stricter diet to get those symptoms in hand. Then you level out for a while, so you switch back to the more lenient diet, then you reduce your drug intake again and your symptoms temporarily worsen again, so you switch back to the stricter diet. And this cycle continues until you're completely drug-free and then the natural, deep healing of your body can begin.

Dependent upon a myriad of factors (length of time you've had IBD, length and intensity of drug use, amount of toxins in your environment and diet, exercise or lack thereof, use of companion healing therapies, mental/emotional state, etc.) you may only need to use these diets for six months or less and be healed enough to switch to the *Maintenance Diet*, or you may need to stay with them for two years or more. Everything in our body/mind/spirit is interconnected. All of the parts affect the whole. If you follow these diets, but implement none of the other changes recommended in this book, you may need to follow these diets for the next five years. The point I'm trying to make is that since we are all different beings, have different rates of change, and respond differently to the same stimulus, there is no cut and dried timetable for the healing of your IBD or IBS. This is your unique process, your healing journey, and it's going to be specific to you and be a little or a lot different from anyone else's. This is why I keep encouraging you to listen to your body, let your own body be your guide and follow your own intuition above anything else.

Maintenance Diet

When you're healed to the point where you're feeling quite good, are not taking any drugs and having fairly normal bowel movements (formed stool that stays in the bottom of the toilet, not more than 2 – 3 bowel movements per day, minimal or no cramping and certainly no intestinal bleeding), this does not mean you should go back to eating and living however you want.

Your body has demonstrated to you that your digestive system is your genetic weak link, or stress outlet. You will probably always need to take special care of your digestive system. If you have fairly mild IBS, this diet alone may be sufficient to keep your symptoms in check. I also recommend that children of people with IBD/IBS follow this diet as a preventive measure due to the strong evidence of a genetic (hereditary) component with these diseases.

Therefore, make it part of your lifestyle, or second-nature, to avoid the following as much as possible:

- Alcohol – very acidic. If you must have alcohol, then have non-pasteurized beer (available from many micro-breweries).

- Caffeine – blocks absorption of vitamin C, leaches minerals and stimulates bowel movements. Even de-caffeinated coffee is not tolerated well. Pure hot chocolate may be okay, but make it with ¾ water and only ¼ milk.

- Carbonated drinks – you certainly don't need more gas, sugar or caffeine in your system.

- Anything containing MSG (interferes with neural functioning) or carrageenan (used in large quantities to induce ulcerative colitis in guinea pigs and primates in clinical trials).

- Margarine or butter substitutes – these are treated with chemical solvents and bleaches resulting in deformed, highly toxic, trans-fatty acids.

- Hot, spicy foods.

- Artificial colors or flavors – especially since the introduction of neural flavor blockers and enhancers.

- Cigarette/cigar/pipe smoke (first or secondhand).

- Artificial sweeteners of any kind – toxic and proven to cause memory loss, can also be highly addictive and cause seizures and hyperactivity in some people.

- Don't consume hydrogenated oils in cooking or in packaged foods. Use a cold-pressed light, extra-virgin, or virgin olive oil wherever oil is called for in cooking, salads, etc. Cold-pressed oils are superior in retaining nutritional value and don't result in toxic trans-fatty acids. Sesame, almond, sunflower, hemp seed and flax seed oil are also okay – basically anything other than mass-market (hydrogenated) vegetable oils.

- Don't eat fruit with other foods, or after a meal. Try to eat fruit in isolation (20 minutes before other food, or 2 hours after) until you've been healed for a year or so and then experiment with mixing it with other foods.

> The standard North American diet is absolutely appalling – it is filled with toxins and damaging substances, and the quality of nutrients is dismal. No wonder cancer rates are one in three. This *Maintenance Diet* should be the standard diet for all westerners.

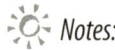 Notes:

- Reduce milk/milk products. If possible, consume raw rather than pasteurized dairy products. Try to use low-fat Lactaid, rice or goat milk, and skim-milk yogurt. Again, after you've been healed for about a year or so, you'll probably be able to drink regular, pasteurized milk in small quantities or from time to time, if you wish. Raw cheddar cheese and raw milk may be tolerated well, test it and see.

- Reduce sugar intake – avoid as much as possible.

- Don't drink milk or juice with meals. If you must have something to drink with your meal, limit yourself to a packet of Emergen-C vitamin C dissolved in four ounces of water, or, ½ glass of warm or room temperature water, sipped slowly and then no liquids for an hour after you've eaten. Liquids will interfere with your digestive juices and cause bloating.

- Keep processed foods, or foods containing preservatives, nitrates, etc. to an absolute minimum, ideally, avoid them completely.

- Eat organic food and beverages as much as possible.

Minimize Gas & Bloating Diet

If your bowel movements are not too frequent (no more than four bowel movements per day) but you're getting a lot of discomfort and cramping from gas, bloating, indigestion or belching, follow the guidelines listed below. After your bowel movements have lessened to no more than three per day, continue on this diet for an additional 2 – 3 months, then switch to the *Maintenance Diet* – but only if you're also drug-free, and have no bloating, cramping or bleeding.

However, if you're currently on Imodium (or a similar anti-diarrhea drug), while it stops/reduces diarrhea it can also cause tremendous, embarrassing amounts of flatulence and bloating. My recommendation would be to go off the Imodium (as with all drugs, never quit "cold turkey" but slowly reduce the dosage one pill at a time every 2 – 3 days, and then half a pill for 2 – 3 days and then quit) and combine the diet listed below with the *Reduce Diarrhea Diet*, depending on the severity of your diarrhea. If you're having over five bowel movements a day, follow just the *Reduce Diarrhea Diet* (it's stricter).

This is the only one of the diets in which yeast and sugar are completely restricted, because excessive bloating is often due to an overabundance of *Candida albicans* (yeast infection) in the colon. If you have a moderate to severe yeast infection, you will also need to eliminate other foods that feed *Candida* like all grains, starchy or complex carbohydrates, mushrooms, all milk products, and fermented foods. Use your own discretion or consult with your naturopathic doctor as to whether you actually need to follow these restrictions.

Eliminate:

- Alcohol – too acidic
- Caffeine – Inhibits absorption of vitamin C, leaches calcium, magnesium, potassium, iron and trace minerals from the body. Coffee is the worst thing you could drink, really aggravates the colon in particular. Pure hot chocolate may be ok, but make it with ¾ water and only ¼ milk. Even de-caffeinated coffee is not tolerated well.
- Carbonated drinks – you certainly don't need more gas, sugar or caffeine in your system.
- The cabbage family (especially onions, cauliflower, broccoli, cabbage and brussel sprouts).
- Beans and lentils.
- Raw vegetables, eat well-cooked vegetables only.
- Roughage (e.g., bran, cracked wheat, corn) or anything else that's 'scratchy' or has a tough fibre matrix (too hard to digest).
- Hot, spicy foods or condiments.
- Yeast or sugar. Be sure and read the ingredient label as many foods contain added yeast.

 *Notes:*

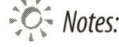 Notes:

- Processed foods, or foods containing preservatives, nitrates, MSG (interferes with neural functioning), carrageenan (used to induce ulcerative colitis in guinea pigs and primates), or anything else that sounds like a manufactured chemical compound.

- Margarine or butter substitutes – treated with chemical solvents and bleaches resulting in deformed, highly toxic, trans-fatty acids.

- Artificial sweeteners of any kind – toxic and proven to cause memory loss, can also be highly addictive and contribute to hyperactivity and seizures in some people.

- Artificial colors or flavors – especially since the introduction of neural flavor blockers and enhancers.

- Deep-fried foods.

- Remove the skin before eating fruits or vegetables.

Reduce:

- Minimize cheese consumption. Use as a garnish rather than a main part of the meal. Hard cheeses made from raw milk, or goat cheeses are preferable.

- Stay away from cream sauces and soft cheeses, minimize milk/milk product consumption and use Lactaid milk when you do drink/eat it. Or, experiment with raw milk, rice or goat's milk.

- Minimize garlic, ginger and cumin consumption.

- When you have a salad, use butter lettuce instead of romaine or iceberg.

- North Americans, on the whole, consume far too many sour, acidic, vinegary foods/condiments (pickles, ketchup, mustard, salad dressings with vinegar, etc.) try to reduce these as much as possible.

- Eat as few tomatoes or tomato-based products as possible.

- When eating fruit or drinking juice, consume in isolation (i.e. minimum of ½ hour before or 1 – 2 hours after any other food or meal). Do not eat/drink citrus fruits in the morning.

- Don't drink anything with your meals. If you must have something to drink with your meal, limit yourself to ½ glass of warm or room temperature water, sipped slowly and then no liquids for an hour after you've eaten. Liquids will interfere with your digestive juices and cause bloating.

Do Eat:

- Six to eight glasses of room temperature or warm mountain spring water per day.

- Japanese green tea, very weak Chinese tea, decaffeinated English tea (never squeeze or re-use the bag as both will release tannins which inhibit iron absorption and irritate the gut.)

- When drinking juice, dilute it with ¼ juice and ¾ water. Juices must be fresh, not from concentrate, with no artificial flavor/color, or added sugar. Avoid citrus juices – apple, pear, mango, papaya and litchi are the best. Remember to always consume in isolation: A minimum of ½ hour before or 1 – 2 hours after any other food or meal.

- Well-ripened bananas, watermelon, apples, pears, mango, papaya, cantaloupe.

- Carrots (peeled and well cooked), zucchini, mushrooms, peas are sometimes okay if well cooked, asparagus, artichokes (natural, not pickled or marinated), pumpkin, plantain, potatoes (no skin), yams. Cook all vegetables well – makes them easier to digest.

- Acorn, butternut or spaghetti squash.

- Avocados, cucumber, regular and shiitake mushrooms.

- Cooked seaweed.

- Eggs, maximum two per day (hard-boiled eggs help stop diarrhea).

Notes:

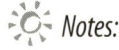 Notes:

- Medium to non-oily fish; sole, cod, wild sea bass, monkfish, wild salmon, tuna. Shrimp, scallops, chicken, extra-lean beef, lamb and pork.

- Sushi, Japanese grilled fish. However, make sure the restaurant is Japanese owned and run (not Chinese, Korean, Caucasian, etc. unless the chef has trained in Japan). A Japanese sushi chef trains meticulously in the healthy cleaning, storing and serving of raw fish. Also check that they don't use MSG in the cooked dishes, as the MSG is likely to make you ill.

- Pasta (spinach or vegetable pastas are good). Make a sauce from pureeing baked squash and water, adding basil and salt for seasoning.

- Brown rice, cous-cous, millet, spelt, amaranth, quinoa, kamut.

- Dry curd cheese (this is cottage cheese without the surrounding milk, it's lactose-free and good for stopping diarrhea).

- 60% whole wheat bread – yeast-free (containing no more than 60% whole wheat flour).

- Use cold-pressed light, extra-virgin, or virgin olive oil wherever oil is called for in cooking, salads, etc. Cold-pressed oils are superior in retaining nutritional value. Sesame, almond, sunflower, hempseed and flax oil are also good – basically anything other than 'normal' hydrogenated vegetable oils (regular sunflower, safflower, canola, etc.). During the processing of commercial vegetable oils, they are heated to the point where the molecular structure is altered resulting in trans-fatty acids that damage cell walls and DNA, and are suspected carcinogens.

- Basil, oregano, cilantro or coriander, thyme, tarragon, fennel, rosemary, Hungarian paprika (non-spicy) and turmeric are good spices to use. Salt is ok unless you have mouth ulcers, then go easy on it.

- Soy Sauce, but make sure there's no added preservatives, alcohol, wheat or sugar.

- Eat only organic foods; meat, vegetables, fruit, grains , milk, cheese, etc.

Reduce Diarrhea Diet

If you're having more than five bowel movements per day, use this diet until you've got it down to three or less bowel movements per day. Then switch to the *Minimize Gas & Bloating Diet* for as long as necessary. If your bowel movements increase after switching to the *Minimize Gas & Bloating Diet*, then switch back to this diet for another three months. Also, check out the information on L-Glutamine in Chapter Two – it's excellent for healing diarrhea and will allow you to move onto the more lenient diet much faster. The *Colonic Massage* technique for *Cramping/Diarrhea* in Chapter Six will also help you spend less time on the toilet.

 *Notes:*

Sore Bum Remedy

If your anus is sore from having so many bowel movements per day, here's a quick remedy that's very effective. After you finish your bowel movement, wipe your bum as usual with soft, dry toilet paper. Then wipe yourself one extra time, but instead of using dry toilet paper, use two, 2-ply tissues (e.g., Kleenex) and quickly flash the tissues under warm tap water to moisten them first. Wipe yourself very gently with the wetted tissues and if you have hemorrhoids or skin tags be sure to clean gently in between and around them. Use a second wad of moistened tissues if necessary. You'll probably be surprised by how much stool shows up on the damp tissues – when you thought your bum was actually clean. Make sure you wipe or dab gently though, otherwise you'll just wind up with little rolls of soggy tissue caught in the surrounding hair (the British actually have a name for these soggy bits: Winnets!) and this will irritate your bum almost as much as leftover stool. If you do this after every bowel movement, your soreness will probably disappear in a few days. Tissues (or Kleenex) work much better than toilet paper since they don't shred so easily and they are softer. Make sure all toilet paper and tissues are not dyed – just plain white – and unscented. Also, make sure you wear 100% cotton underwear during the day and then sleep bare-bum at night on 100% cotton sheets. If the soreness persists, then try Wild Oregano Oil applied topically and just inside your anus – see Chapter Two for detailed dilution and application instructions (you must not use full-strength Wild Oregano Oil on your anus or genitals). Do not use commercial pre-moistened wipes (e.g., Wet Ones) as these will tend to irritate your bum rather than soothe it.

Eliminate:

 Notes:

- Alcohol (alcohol is VERY acidic; drinking it is akin to pouring acid on an open wound).

- Caffeine – Inhibits absorption of vitamin C, leaches calcium, magnesium, potassium, iron and trace minerals from the body. Coffee is the worst thing you could drink, really aggravates the colon in particular. Even de-caffeinated coffee is not tolerated well.

- Carbonated drinks – you certainly don't need more gas, sugar or caffeine in your system. English or Chinese black teas (e.g., Earl Grey, orange pekoe, or any other tea that contains caffeine) or Tangy/citrusy herb teas (e.g., Orange Zinger, tart raspberry, etc.).

- Citrus fruits or juices (e.g., oranges, lemons, grapefruit). Pineapple, cherries, grapes, raspberries.

- Don't drink anything with your meals. If you must have something to drink with your meal, limit yourself to ½ glass of warm water, sipped slowly and then no liquids for an hour after you've eaten. Liquids will interfere with your digestive juices and cause bloating.

- Milk products; milk, yogurt, cheese, ice cream, etc.

- Anything sour, fermented, acidic, or containing vinegar (e.g., all condiments – mustard, ketchup, pickles, Worcestershire sauce, chutneys, etc.).

- Tomatoes.

- Leafy green vegetables (e.g., spinach, lettuce).

- Raw vegetables.

- Beans, lentils.
- Cabbage family vegetables (e.g., onions, broccoli, cauliflower, Brussels sprouts, etc.).
- Garlic, ginger, mustard seed, cumin.
- Spicy or black peppers, chilies, etc.
- Any processed, pre-packaged foods.
- No foods containing preservatives, nitrates, MSG (it interferes with neural functioning), carrageenan (large quantities have been used to induce ulcerative colitis in guinea pigs and primates), or anything else that sounds like a manufactured chemical compound.
- Margarine or butter substitutes – treated with chemical solvents and bleaches, resulting in deformed, highly toxic, trans-fatty acids.
- Artificial sweeteners of any kind – toxic and proven to cause memory loss, can also be highly addictive and contribute to hyperactivity and seizures in some people.
- Artificial colors or flavors – especially since the introduction of neural flavor blockers and enhancers.
- No nuts, seeds, roughage (e.g., bran, cracked wheat, corn,) or anything else that's 'scratchy' or has a tough fibre matrix (difficult to digest).
- Nothing fried or deep-fried, keep butter and oil to a minimum. When you do use oil, make sure it's a light olive oil. Cold-pressed oils are superior in retaining nutritional value. Cold-pressed sesame, almond, hempseed, sunflower and flax oil are also ok – basically anything other than commercial, hydrogenated vegetable oils (regular sunflower, safflower, canola, etc.). During the processing of commercial vegetable oils, they are heated to the point where the molecular structure is altered so that they can no longer be properly digested or eliminated.

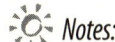 *Notes:*

Do Eat:

- At least eight to ten glasses of room-temperature or warm spring water per day. You lose a lot of fluids with diarrhea, so it's important to stay hydrated.

- Very weak Japanese green tea, weak rooibos or honeybush tea, decaffeinated English tea (never squeeze or re-use the bag as both will release tannins which inhibit iron absorption and irritate the gut.)

- If you really want to drink juice then dilute it with ¼ juice and ¾ water. Juices must be fresh, not from concentrate, with no artificial flavor/color, or added sugar. No citrus juices; apple, mango, pear, papaya and litchi are the best.

- Well-ripened bananas, watermelon, mango, papaya, cantaloupe, pears. Remember to consume fruit in isolation, either ½ hour before or 1 – 2 hours after any other food.

- Carrots (peeled and well cooked), zucchini, mushrooms, asparagus, artichokes (natural, not pickled or marinated), pumpkin, potatoes (no skin), yams. Cook all vegetables well – makes them easier to digest.

- Acorn, butternut or spaghetti squash.

- Avocados, cucumber, shiitake, portobello, oyster mushrooms.

- Cooked seaweed.

- Eggs, maximum two per day (a hard-boiled egg helps stop diarrhea).

- Medium to non-oily fish; sole, cod, wild sea bass, monkfish, wild salmon, tuna. Shrimp, scallops, chicken, extra-lean beef, lamb and pork.

- Sushi, Japanese grilled fish. However, make sure the restaurant is Japanese owned and run (not Chinese, Korean, Caucasian, etc. unless the chef has trained in Japan). A Japanese sushi chef trains meticulously in the healthy cleaning, storing and serving of raw fish.

Also check that they don't use MSG in the cooked dishes, as the MSG is likely to make you ill.

- Pasta (spinach or vegetable pastas are good). Try it with a sauce made from pureeing baked squash and a little water or broth, and adding basil and salt for seasoning. Otherwise, just toss with a bit of olive oil and allowable spices and vegetables.

- Brown rice, cous-cous, millet, amaranth, quinoa, kamut.

- Dry curd (this is cottage cheese without the surrounding milk, lactose-free and especially excellent for stopping diarrhea).

- 60% whole wheat bread.

- Eat only organic foods; meat, vegetables, fruit, grains (wheat, rice, etc.).

- Basil, oregano, thyme, fennel, tarragon, rosemary and cilantro or coriander are good spices to use. A little Hungarian paprika (non-spicy) and turmeric should also be fine. Salt is good (helps you retain fluid and electrolytes) unless you have mouth ulcers, then just eat as much as you can tolerate.

- Soy sauce, but make sure there's no added preservatives or alcohol.

- Keep butter and oil to a minimum, use as little as possible. When you do use oil, make sure it's a cold-pressed, light, extra-virgin or virgin olive oil. Cold-pressed oils are superior in retaining nutritional value. Cold-pressed sesame, almond, hempseed, sunflower and flax oil are also okay – basically anything other than hydrogenated vegetable oils (regular sunflower, safflower, canola, etc.). During the processing of commercial vegetable oils, they are heated to the point where the molecular structure is altered resulting in trans-fatty acids that damage cell walls and DNA, and are suspected carcinogens.

 Notes:

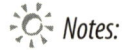 Notes:

Stop Intestinal Bleeding Diet

This diet is for you to use if you're experiencing intermittent intestinal bleeding, or a type and volume of bleeding that you've had before several times and that you know is no cause for immediate or undue alarm. If, however, you're experiencing bleeding that would classify as hemorrhaging or your weight and hemoglobin are dropping rapidly, then you need to follow the steps outlined in the *Bowel Rest Elemental Diet*, listed immediately after this one.

Strictly following this *Stop Intestinal Bleeding Diet* usually stopped my intestinal bleeding within 1 – 3 days. I found if you chill right out, don't go to work or school but just get lots of rest and sleep and strictly follow this diet, within 2 – 3 days you should have the bleeding stopped. However, continue to follow this diet for two more weeks to give yourself time to heal properly, gradually combining it with the guidelines listed under the *Reduce Diarrhea Diet*. See also the herbal therapies in Chapter Two, to help speed healing and stop the bleeding even faster, often within a day or two.

The main difficulty people experience with following this diet is that the food is quite bland, since you're only allowed tiny amounts of butter or oil, and you're not allowed any sauces, condiments, etc. The easiest way around this is to cook with water rather than oil – I know this sounds and will feel really odd, but it actually works very well. Just substitute the water for oil and cook as normal. The other quick way to add a flavor boost to the food is to give it an oriental flavor by adding 1 tsp. of soy sauce and ½ tsp. of cold-pressed sesame oil to 1 – 2 tbsp. of water and then using that, after cooking, to flavor your noodles, rice, vegetables, fish, meat, etc. You will also, by the end of the first week, be able to taste and really appreciate all the natural flavors present in organic meat and vegetables.

If you're having only small amounts of blood in your stool and/or on the toilet paper when you wipe your bum, it's probably just due to an anal or rectal fissure, or internal hemorrhoids and you don't need to follow this diet. See *Rectal Fissures* and *Hemorrhoids* in Chapter Two for a full outline of applicable healing treatments.

Eliminate:

- Cow's milk products; milk, yogurt, cheese, ice cream, etc. (the only exceptions are dry curd and whey protein isolate)

- Rice milk, goat's milk, almond milk, etc.

- Alcohol (alcohol is VERY acidic, drinking it is akin to pouring acid on an open wound).

- Caffeine – Inhibits absorption of vitamin C, leaches calcium, magnesium, potassium, iron and trace minerals from the body. Coffee is the worst thing you could drink, it really aggravates the colon in particular. No de-caffeinated coffee or coffee substitutes either.

- Carbonated drinks – you certainly don't need more gas, sugar or caffeine in your system.

- English or Chinese black teas (e.g., Earl Grey, orange pekoe, or any other tea that contains caffeine) or Tangy/citrusy herb teas (e.g., Orange Zinger, wildberry, etc).

- Citrus fruits or juices (e.g., oranges, lemons, grapefruit). Pineapple, cherries, raspberries, grapes.

- Don't drink anything with your meals. If you must have something to drink with your meal, limit yourself to ½ glass of warm water, sipped slowly and then no liquids for an hour after you've eaten. Liquids will interfere with your digestive juices and cause bloating.

- Anything sour, fermented, acidic, or containing vinegar (e.g., all condiments – mustard, ketchup, pickles, Worcestershire sauce, chutneys, etc.).

- Tomatoes or anything containing tomatoes.

- Leafy green vegetables (e.g., spinach, lettuce, chard, bok choy, etc.).

- Raw vegetables.

- Coconut.

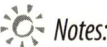 Notes:

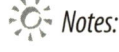 Notes:

- Red meat.
- Beans, lentils.
- Cabbage family vegetables (e.g., onions, broccoli, cauliflower, Brussels sprouts, etc.).
- Garlic, ginger, cumin, mustard seed, paprika, turmeric.
- Spicy or black peppers, chilies, etc.
- Any processed, canned, pre-packaged foods.
- Processed foods, or foods containing preservatives, nitrates, MSG (interferes with neural functioning), carrageenan (shown to cause ulcerative colitis in guinea pigs and primates), or anything else that sounds like a manufactured chemical compound.
- Margarine or butter substitutes – treated with chemical solvents and bleaches resulting in deformed, highly toxic, trans-fatty acids.
- Artificial sweeteners of any kind – toxic and proven to cause memory loss, can also be highly addictive and contribute to hyperactivity in some people.
- Artificial colors or flavors – especially since the introduction of neural flavor blockers and enhancers.
- Nuts, seeds, roughage, whole grains (e.g., bran, cracked wheat, corn, brown rice) or anything else that's 'scratchy' or has a tough fibre matrix (difficult to digest).
- Eat as little butter and oil as possible. Try to keep it to ½ teaspoon or less total per meal. When you use oil, make sure it's a cold-pressed, extra-light olive oil. DO NOT consume hydrogenated vegetable oils (regular sunflower, safflower, canola, etc.). During the processing of commercial vegetable oils, they are heated to the point where the molecular structure is altered so that they can no longer be properly digested or eliminated.

Do Eat:

- Eight to ten glasses of room-temperature or warm spring water per day. You're probably losing a lot of fluid and it's important to stay hydrated.

- Very weak Japanese green tea (if you MUST have decaffeinated English tea, dip the tea bag only twice, never squeeze or re-use the bag as both will release tannins which inhibit iron absorption and irritate the gut).

- Basil, oregano and thyme are good spices to use, but don't use too much – fresh or dried is fine. Dried cilantro (coriander) is okay. Salt is good unless you have mouth ulcers, in which case use only as much as you can tolerate.

- Soy Sauce, but make sure there are no added preservatives or alcohol.

- Well-ripened bananas, watermelon, papaya, cantaloupe, pears, maximum of 1 apple/day (peeled and preferably cooked). Remember to consume fruit in isolation, either ½ hour before or two hours after any other food.

- Carrots (peeled and well cooked), zucchini.

- Acorn, butternut, spaghetti squash (well cooked).

- Avocados, cucumber (peeled).

- Well-cooked potatoes (no skin) but no butter or oil allowed (if you MUST have butter with your vegetables, eat a maximum of ½ tsp. per meal), yams, sweet potatoes, pumpkin. Cook all vegetables really well – makes them easier to digest.

- White rice (jasmine or basmati are good ones).

- Unbleached white or 60% whole wheat bread (containing no more than 60% whole wheat flour).

- Eggs, maximum 2/day.

- Small amounts of chicken or turkey, if tolerated

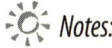 Notes:

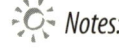 Notes:

- Non-oily fish baked, broiled or steamed; sole, cod, sea bass, monkfish. Shrimp, scallops, broiled or steamed.

- Dry curd (this is cottage cheese without the surrounding milk, lactose-free and especially excellent for stopping diarrhea).

- Whey protein isolate (make sure it's 100% natural and cold-extracted), mixed with water and ½ tsp. Udo's Oil or flax oil only. Alternately, you can use Absorb Plus (tastes much better than plain whey protein) with the same amount of Udo's or flax oil, available at *www.absorbplus.com* (see *Bowel Rest Elemental Diet* below for more details).

- Banana muffins (homemade with no preservatives, 60% whole wheat flour is best, use skim-milk yogurt instead of the butter or oil called for in the recipe).

- Egg noodles or rice noodles, in broth or with a few drops of sesame oil and a teaspoon of soy sauce.

- Pasta (no fillings), tossed with a few drops of extra-light olive oil and fresh basil.

- Beef, chicken, or vegetable broths (homemade is best, but if store bought then make sure they're organic). Homemade broths are a wonderful way to obtain nutrients whilst allowing your digestive system (and bowel) to rest. You may want to drink only water and broths for the first day or two on this diet.

- Eat only organic foods; meat, wild fish, vegetables, fruit, grains (wheat, rice, amaranth, quinoa, etc.).

- Eat as little butter and oil as possible. Try to keep it to ½ teaspoon or less per meal. When you use oil, make sure it's a cold-pressed, organic, virgin or extra-virgin olive oil. Do not consume regular, hydrogenated vegetable oils (regular sunflower, safflower, canola, etc.). During the processing of commercial vegetable oils, they are heated to the point where the molecular structure is altered resulting in trans-fatty acids that damage cell walls and DNA, and are suspected carcinogens.

Here's a sample day's menu on the *Stop Intestinal Bleeding Diet*. Since you'll be resting at home, it's best to eat numerous small meals throughout the day:

Meal #1: 1 poached egg sprinkled with salt

Meal #2: 1 – 2 banana muffins

Meal #3: Linguine with a few drops of extra-light olive oil and fresh basil, chopped finely and added just before serving.

Meal #4: Bowl of beef broth

Meal #5: Filet of sole sprinkled with cilantro, acorn squash (cubed or mashed), steamed zucchini with a sprinkle of oregano.

Now this sample menu may contain more food than you feel comfortable eating, or, you may just want to sip beef broth and aloe vera juice all day for a couple of days. Again, do whatever feels right to you. Listen to your body and give it what it's asking for.

Bowel Rest Elemental Diet

An elemental diet is one in which all the nutrients (protein, carbohydrates) have been pre-digested. The oils (fat) in an elemental diet are all non-hydrogenated, cold-pressed oils, which are essential to your body's functioning and easily absorbed. Elemental diets were originally developed by NASA for astronauts to consume in space so they would only produce a minimal amount of fecal matter. They were later appropriated for use by the medical community. Because they're completely liquid with all the nutrients pre-digested, they also give your digestive system a rest. Colonic wounds are given a chance to heal, as there is a much smaller amount of only liquid or mushy stool being passed. An elemental diet is beneficial when you're recovering from surgery, having severe intestinal bleeding, or when you're malnourished and need to consume as many nutritious calories per day as possible. It is also very effective as a screening tool to determine your particular food allergies or intolerances, and in longer periods to induce disease remission.

 Notes:

Using The Diet To Induce Remission

My gastroenterologist (who has around 700 patients) tells me that in his experience an elemental diet alone (for a duration of about six weeks) produces remission as often as steroids. Recent clinical trials involving children with active Crohn's disease in England and Italy have demonstrated that "elemental diet therapy is as effective as steroids in inducing remission, whilst avoiding steroid side effects" [5]. In the English study, 44 children with Crohn's were put on an elemental diet and 40 of them (90%) achieved clinical remission in an average of six weeks (individual times on the elemental diet ranged from 2 – 12 weeks). In the Italian study, 37 children were assigned to an elemental diet and 10 children were assigned methylprednisone (steroids). 32 (86%) of the children on the elemental diet achieved clinical remission in an average of 2.5 weeks and 9 of the children on steroids achieved clinical remission in an average of 3.7 weeks. However, 7 of the children on the elemental diet showed complete healing of the mucosal lining of the intestine, while none of the children on steroids showed healing of the mucosal lining. As Dr. Robert Canani summarized: "In children with active Crohn's disease, exclusive nutritional therapy shows a more rapid effect than steroids in inducing clinical remission and is markedly more effective than steroids in producing healing of mucosal inflammation." [6]

Many gastroenterologists prefer using an elemental diet because it doesn't result in the "side effects" of steroids or immunosuppressants. However, other gastroenterologists say they don't even bother recommending an elemental diet to their patients because the adherence rate is so low. And they do have a point; an elemental, completely liquid, pre-digested diet is very difficult to stick to for any length of time and requires a lot of discipline. Personally, the first time I went on an elemental diet, I found it extremely difficult. However, I have since heard from numerous readers who actually say they preferred it to eating real food – because they felt so good on it and didn't have to worry about meal planning, grocery shopping, cooking, or cleaning up the kitchen!

The first time I went on an elemental diet was due to intestinal hemorrhaging that left me at 99 lbs (I'm 5'7") and required a transfusion of 6 pints of blood. I had two objectives; to stop the bleeding and to gain weight. Continuing to eat regular food simply re-opened the wounds and started the bleeding again. Therefore, my nutrition needed to come from a completely pre-digested (elemental) liquid source, which my gastroenterologist told me resulted in disease remission as often as Prednisone (steroids). I sampled each of the elemental (pre-digested) products provided by the hospital, but found the taste and ingredient list unacceptable. All of the products contained artificial flavors and sweeteners, large amounts of sugar (in relation to maltodextrin – which results in a 'sugar high', or spike in blood sugar levels) and high levels of low quality oils – which resulted in painful intestinal spasming. Rather than drinking these, or, undergoing a surgical procedure to have a tube inserted in my stomach and the commercial elemental products pumped in, I set out to find a natural, healthy alternative.

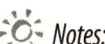 *Notes:*

After an extensive search of health stores and the Internet, I devised my own elemental formula by mixing together six different products. I did this 8 – 9 times a day to give my body the nutrients it needed in elemental (pre-digested for maximum absorption) form. Because all the food I ate (or more accurately, drank) was pre-digested, the elemental diet also gave my bowel a complete rest, which allowed my wounds time and space to heal. In addition, I added numerous supplements to each shake to further facilitate my healing and recovery. Using this formula, I gained 36 pounds of solid weight (not fat) in six weeks and my albumin (blood protein) levels were restored to normal. I went from being so weak I could barely move around my apartment, to cycling and lifting weights at the gym at a solid weight of 135 lbs. One month later I got pregnant, had an excellent pregnancy and gave birth to a healthy baby boy named Oscar.

I had written about this process in the first edition of *Listen To Your Gut* and had given my readers detailed instructions on how to source the same list of products and mix them together to make a good quality, non-toxic elemental shake. After a while, I was approached by one of the directors

> A key benefit of following the IBD Remission Diet is that it provides an ideal vehicle with which to consume large amounts of healing supplements in easily absorbable, liquid form. If you stay on the Diet for longer than two weeks, you'll also experience a gentle detox effect.

of a health company called Imix Naturals Inc. and he asked me if I would be interested in formulating my ideal elemental shake product for their company to manufacture. Of course, I was thrilled to do so and the result is called Absorb Plus. All you have to add to it is cold-pressed flax oil (or Udo's oil), and water. Because Imix gave me the freedom to create my ideal product, Absorb Plus also contains a targeted free-form amino acid blend (that specifically assists the healing of various IBD related conditions) and a carefully selected range of vitamins and minerals (including trace minerals). So you get a lot of benefits automatically, without having to pay for additional supplements. I also spent six months getting the flavoring (all natural of course) as good as it can possibly be with an elemental product – I don't think the lab guys had ever experienced someone as picky as me! However, when you're formulating a product that you know you're going to be using yourself, you have a whole different set of standards than someone who's formulating from a bottom line/profit margin perspective! I could go on and on about exactly why I chose each specific ingredient and the benefits conferred, but it would be better if you just go to their website (*www.absorbplus.com*) as they have extensive information about each of the ingredients in Absorb Plus listed there.

The other thing that happened, following the first outline of an elemental diet in the first edition of *Listen To Your Gut*, is that readers kept contacting me asking for more detailed, specific information on exactly how to implement the diet, for how long, for what conditions, etc. So, in response to that, I wrote a second book called *The IBD Remission Diet* that provides all the information one could possibly need to implement an elemental diet with the highest possibility of success. The IBD Remission Diet is not the same as a doctor-prescribed elemental diet, because it also contains a detailed and targeted supplementation plan specifically chosen to heal the mucosal lining of the intestine, reduce inflammation, repair tissue damage, support enzyme production and hormonal pathways, facilitate optimal cellular function, balance the immune system, and restore a beneficial bacterial flora throughout your gastrointestinal tract. This provides your body with an extended healing regimen where all aspects of digestive healing are supported simultaneously; and as the whole body is inter-linked, you may find that other health issues are also resolved during this time.

Another key benefit of following the IBD Remission Diet is that it provides an ideal vehicle with which to consume large amounts of healing supplements in easily absorbable, liquid form. Swallowing 15 gelcaps, tablets, and capsules (for example) throughout the day for an extended period can be quite difficult and the absorption of these shellacked and capsulated products is not ideal. Emptying all those supplements into several good-tasting shakes and drinking them down is much easier, absorption is improved, and you're more likely to stick with it for the duration. If you stay on the IBD Remission Diet for two weeks or longer, you'll also experience the benefits of a natural, gradual and gentle detoxification. Your cells, organs and digestive system will release and flush toxins, old waste and any impacted fecal matter. If you get pregnant following the IBD Remission Diet, you're likely to experience less nausea, or, 'morning sickness' due to the detoxification of your liver and cells. This detoxification is facilitated not only by the liquid, pre-digested diet, but also by the specific supplements in the Diet that support liver, digestive, and cellular health.

Using The Diet To Gain Healthy Weight

Many people with IBD (inflammatory bowel disease) and IBS (irritable bowel syndrome) also suffer from malnutrition due to inadequate digestion, low absorption of nutrients, and lack of appetite – when everything you eat makes you feel sick or results in pain you quickly lose your appetite! The IBD Remission Diet is a fantastic way to resolve malnutrition and gain some solid weight (muscle, not fat) quickly. Because everything you consume is pre-digested, there is very little digestion required and the nutrients are absorbed rapidly. And because everything is in liquid form, it's easy to consume a large number of calories per day, so you can gain weight more quickly than if you were eating normal food. To eat 3000 – 4000 calories per day of regular food can be quite difficult, but drinking the same number of calories – and being able to actually absorb and utilise all of them – is considerably easier. Also, even though your food is all in liquid form, you will not feel hungry on the elemental diet (as long as you're consuming an

> The IBD Remission Diet is a fantastic way to resolve malnutrition and gain some solid weight – because everything you consume is pre-digested, there is very little digestion required and the nutrients are absorbed rapidly.

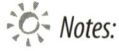
Notes:

adequate number of calories for your body). In fact, some people who've followed the IBD Remission Diet have even been reluctant to go back to eating regular food – they loved the taste of the shakes, felt really energetic, not hungry at all, and very much enjoyed the break from shopping, meal planning, cooking and cleaning the kitchen! If you use the Diet for weight gain or to address malnutrition, I also strongly advise that you start an exercise program – ideally weight-training/body building – at the appropriate time to further encourage muscle growth and development. Later, you can continue to use the shakes in conjunction with your regular diet, for as long as you wish, to further increase your calorie intake (and maintain good quality nutrition) and continue to gain weight. See the section on *Malnutrition/Weight Gain* in Chapter Two for more information on using Absorb Plus along with your regular diet, and for details of a weight-training/bodybuilding program.

For myself, I have a demanding schedule with two young children, so it's hard to get the chance for peaceful, unhurried meals every day. I'm a slow eater and I'm rarely able to eat until I'm full at mealtimes. Therefore, I often drink an Absorb Plus shake for breakfast to make up any calorie/nutrient deficit and simply to maintain my existing weight.

Using The Diet To Lose Weight

Some people have gained excessive weight due to steroid use, lack of physical exercise, unbalanced hormonal system/thyroid function, etc. The IBD Remission Diet is also a good vehicle to lose that extra fat. Many readers have found this an easy way to lose weight because:

a. It's very easy to monitor and control calorie intake when you're on a completely liquid diet. It's actually easier not to eat at all, than to have a wide variety of choices and constantly have to monitor yourself.

b. All the food you consume is of very high quality, with quickly absorbed nutrients, so your body maintains a high level of health and nutrition throughout your weight loss. Another point people are often not aware of is that obese people are often suffering from malnutrition. Fat does not equal nutrition. Indeed the reason some obese people feel so hungry all the time is because their bodies are actually starving! Your body cannot use junk food, hydrogenated fats, and other unhealthy foods to nourish itself or maintain health. So if you're simultaneously obese and malnourished, the IBD Remission Diet is an ideal way to shed some of your fat, whilst addressing your malnutrition.

c. There's absolutely no possibility of eating junk food or typical 'diet-breaker' binge foods on an elemental diet, so that whole avenue of failure/sabotage is closed.

It's important to keep in mind, though, that if you lose weight too quickly it throws your body into 'famine mode' and this can really mess up your metabolism. Then, when you start eating regular food again, you'll gain weight back quickly since your metabolism has slowed down so much to compensate for the 'famine conditions'. Obviously, this is counter-productive and not advised. Since most people don't want or need to be on the IBD Remission Diet for longer than six weeks, you don't really want to lose more than 15 pounds during that time. However, you can continue to use the shakes in conjunction with your regular diet, for as long as you wish, to further control your calorie intake (whilst maintaining good quality nutrition) and encourage ongoing weight loss.

Using The Diet To Test For Food Allergies

The most thorough and reliable method of testing for food allergies or intolerances is to use an elemental diet for 10 – 14 days to completely clear the body of any food allergens. Following the clearance period, you then reintroduce foods, one by one, and test to see if the new food results in any undesirable reaction. Reacting in these ways to consuming a food shows that your body has either an allergy or intolerance to that food.
These reactions can lessen or even disappear as your health improves over time, but it's good to keep them in mind, as during times of stress they'll likely resurface and you'll want to avoid or restrict consumption of these foods again. Undesirable reactions to watch out for include:

▶ increased mucus production

> Obese people are often suffering from malnutrition. Fat does not equal nutrition. Indeed the reason some obese people feel so hungry all the time is because their bodies are actually starving!

- nausea, itchy tongue or skin, swelling, redness, bumps, rash
- bloating/gas, cramps
- heartburn, indigestion
- shortness of breath, fuzzy head or a drugged feeling, sleepiness, etc.
- headache, joint/muscle pain
- any blood mixed in with or accompanying stool. Blood from the colon or rectum will be red. Blood from the small intestine will turn the stool dark green or black (as can iron therapy/supplements, so don't confuse the two). If you only have a bit of blood on the toilet paper when you wipe your bum, it's probably from a minor anal or rectal fissure/wound so don't worry about it.

Once you've been eating completely solid food for a minimum of two weeks, you can also check for these undesirable reactions:

- undigested particles of the test food in the stool or toilet bowl
- watery, slimy, or acidic stool
- increased diarrhea

When you're testing for your own personal food intolerances or allergies, you may want to keep in mind the results of the following study. Thirty-three Crohn's patients were first put on TPN (Total Parenteral Nutrition – liquid nutrients given intravenously) to clear their symptoms. The researchers then gradually reintroduced one food per day to determine which foods were tolerated and which triggered a return of symptoms. Wheat was the highest offender (69%), then dairy products (48%), followed by yeast (31%), corn (24%) and potato (17%).[7]

At the end of this chapter is a *Food Reintroduction Chart* that you can use to screen for allergies or intolerances. When reintroducing foods after the clearance period, test foods from Phase One, column A first. Then gradually move through columns B, C, D and E. Next you would test foods from

Phase Two, column A, and so on throughout the chart. If you know you're allergic or intolerant to a certain food, then wait until you've completed all the foods on the chart (or all the ones you wish to test for), and then test the problem food. If you have a severe allergy, you may want to just leave it alone altogether. Again, use this chart as a guide, but follow your own gut/intuition at all times.

You can use the IBD Remission Diet specifically to test for food allergies, or, you can use it for any of the other purposes listed here and then automatically test for food allergies when you begin introducing solid foods again. Detailed instructions on how to do this are in *The IBD Remission Diet* book (available at: www.IBDremissiondiet.com).

Using The Diet To Prevent Flares
Once you've been on the IBD Remission Diet for an extended period, weaned off all your drugs, and used it as a tool for building solid, foundational health, you may still find you need to use it occasionally, for short periods. If your life is very demanding, or circumstances change resulting in a sudden onslaught of stress or exhaustion, you may find it useful to use the IBD Remission Diet as a relatively quick (usually two weeks is sufficient) recuperation tool.

As with most illness, it was a confluence of events and stressors that led to my second time on an elemental diet. Until I weaned him from night nursing at 18 months, my first baby, Oscar, did not sleep more than three hours in a row, so neither did I. We also went to Singapore when Oscar was eight weeks old, for six months. However, when we came back to Vancouver, the new condo we had bought was far behind its construction schedule. So we then spent the next five and a half months travelling around England, Hawaii and Arizona, living out of suitcases. In addition, Oscar has a voracious appetite (and high metabolism) so he breastfed full feeds about ten times a day. Combined together, the stress of transatlantic flights, no home, no routines for the baby, all the varied adjustments involved for new parents, and the severe extended sleep deprivation eventually became too much for me.

> If your life is very demanding, or you experience a sudden onslaught of stress or exhaustion, the IBD Remission Diet is a relatively quick (usually two weeks is sufficient) and effective recuperation tool.

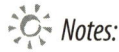 Notes:

I gradually lost weight until I was only 115 lbs and then I took a new calcium/magnesium supplement I'd bought that also contained something called Betaine HCL (Hydrochloride). About eight hours later, my colon started bleeding. After wracking my brain to try and figure out what could have triggered the bleeding, I finally remembered the mystery ingredient and looked it up in one of my encyclopaedias. There I discovered that Betaine HCL is something that stimulates the production of stomach acid. It should never be used by someone with ulcers, and even people with normal digestive systems should start at a very low dose and stop if they experience any discomfort. Obviously, in a digestive system as sensitive as mine, that's all it took to trigger the bleeding and as I was so run down I knew the situation could deteriorate quite quickly.

I've found that you can use all kinds of herbal supplements to prop yourself up and keep going, but when your body becomes too run down and malnourished it loses the ability to heal itself. So even though you give it the tools, your body has no energy or resources left to utilize those tools. Although the bleeding wasn't anywhere near the hemorrhaging I experienced prior to the first time I went on an elemental diet, I didn't want to risk it escalating to that point, so I immediately went on an elemental diet after three days of passing blood, ranging from about 3 tbsp. – ¼ cup per bowel movement, with small blood clots the second and third day.

The good news is that I was also nowhere near as ill and run down as I was the first time round, so although my bleeding had completely stopped by day four, I remained on the diet exclusively for two weeks. I then continued drinking a few shakes a day for an additional ten days as I gradually re-introduced normal food. I also didn't feel the need to gain weight as quickly as I did the first time, so I only consumed six shakes per day. At the end of two weeks I'd gained seven pounds and by the time I was fully back on regular food, I'd gained a total of 14 pounds. During my pregnancy with Oscar, I'd had a shake every morning with all the supplements and flax oil added as it's a wonderful way to ensure excellent health for both myself and the baby.

The third (and hopefully last!) time I had to go on the IBD Remission Diet was following the birth of my second child. Unfortunately, the IBD Remission Diet is such a great rejuvenator of health, that I got pregnant only a few months after my second time on it (described above). Well, my daughter Zara also breastfed all night long, but I now had an energetic toddler (Oscar) to look after during the days as well. The same spiral downward of extended sleep deprivation, inability to eat properly, exhaustion, etc. occurred again and by the time Zara was six months old, I was down to 110 pounds, and chose to go on the IBD Remission Diet again for two weeks. Both kids then slept with Daddy in a separate room and I got uninterrupted sleep for the first time in over three years! You see, even though I'm pretty much healed, with no serious symptoms, and I've been drug and surgery-free for over 16 years, my digestive system is my sensitive area. Load enough stress, exhaustion, lack of nutrients, etc. on me, and my distress will be evidenced in my gut.

> The IBD Remission Diet is such a great rejuvenator of health, that I got pregnant only a few months after my second time on it.

Ordering *The IBD Remission Diet* Book

If you think the IBD Remission Diet may be a useful tool for you and you'd like to order the book, please contact Caramal Publishing first as they will give you a special link to use to order so that you can get a discount on the price (since you've already bought *Listen To Your Gut*). Email Caramal at: service@listentoyourgut.com and tell them that you've already purchased the *Listen To Your Gut* program and now you'd like to purchase *The IBD Remission Diet*. They'll check their database to confirm your information and then they'll give you instructions on how to order via Internet or telephone and receive the price discount. You can read all about *The IBD Remission Diet* at: www.IBDremissionDiet.com

Keep A Food Diary

The point of this program, and *The Healing Diets* in this chapter, is to give you the tools you need to heal yourself – without resorting to drugs or surgery – through all the circumstances of your life. One reader I heard from is a film producer, who always takes Absorb Plus along on location to ensure he doesn't get sick due to the added stress of travel, long shoot days, and the usually unhealthy food on offer. Likewise, one of my phone

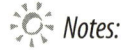 *Notes:*

consultation clients often has to have business dinners in restaurants, so she worked out some ordering guidelines based on *The Healing Diets* to ensure she can maintain her health and not stress her digestive system when she eats out.

It's also helpful to keep a *Food Diary*. Write down exactly what you eat and drink, when, how much, and how you felt at the time. At the end of the day, critique what you ate and how you feel. Describe the type, consistency, and number of bowel movements. Write down any other observations regarding gas, pain, bloating, bleeding, cramping, etc. Also, very important is to note your emotional state and any unpleasant or stressful situations, thoughts, or feelings that occurred. Remember that mind/body/spirit is one, and food is not the only factor that influences your digestive system. *The Healing Diets* give you a pretty good guideline, but keeping a *Food Diary* will help you to really pinpoint what foods are good, or not so good, for your unique body. It will also help you identify, for example, whether it's okay to eat a food once per week, but not three times per week. Our bodies have tolerance thresholds for certain foods or substances and a *Food Diary* can help you map yours out. I've provided a *Food Diary* chart for you on the *Listen To Your Gut CD*, so you can just print out as many sheets as you need.

Turn now to the *Healing Journey Workbook* on the *Listen To Your Gut CD* and complete the exercises for this chapter (Chapter Three).

Following are the Quick Reference Guides for each of *The Healing Diets*, and the *Food Reintroduction Chart* (remember you can also print these out from the *Listen To Your Gut CD*).

Maintenance Diet

Eliminate:
- Alcohol, caffeine, carbonated drinks. When you must have alcohol, then unpasteurized beer (available from micro-breweries) is probably best.
- Anything containing MSG, carrageenan, artificial flavors, artificial colors, artificial sweeteners, preservatives, conditioners, emulsifiers and other chemical additives.
- Processed foods and processed meats (luncheon/deli meat) containing preservatives, nitrates, nitrites, etc.
- Margarine or butter substitutes, or hydrogenated oils (trans-fatty acids) in vegetable oils or packaged foods.
- Fruit with other foods, or after a meal. Try to eat fruit in isolation (20 minutes before other food, or two hours after) until you've been healed for a year or so and then experiment with mixing it with other foods.
- Milk or juice with meals.
- Hot, spicy foods – test very mild chilies after one year and see how your body responds.
- Cigarette/cigar/pipe smoke (first or secondhand).

Reduce:
- Milk/milk products. Consume raw rather than pasteurized dairy products.
- Sugar intake – avoid as much as possible.

Do Eat:
- Organic cold-pressed light, extra-virgin, or virgin olive oil wherever oil is called for in cooking, salads, etc. Organic cold-pressed sesame, almond, sunflower, hemp seed and flax seed oil are also fine.
- Stevia, and small amounts of honey and maple syrup instead of refined sugar.
- Certified organic food and beverages as much as possible. At least, make sure all your meat and dairy is certified organic.
- Unprocessed, fresh food, cooked from scratch (homemade).

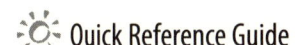 Quick Reference Guide

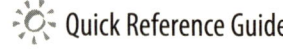
Quick Reference Guide

Minimize Gas & Bloating Diet

Eliminate:
- Alcohol, caffeine, decaffeinated coffee, carbonated drinks.
- Cabbage family vegetables, beans, lentils, raw vegetables, roughage/high fibre foods, hot/spicy foods, deep-fried foods.
- Processed foods; preservatives, MSG, nitrates, artificial flavors, colors, etc.
- Margarine or butter substitutes, artificial sweeteners, carrageenan.
- Yeast, sugar, if necessary.

Reduce:
- Cheese, cream sauces, milk products.
- Sour, vinegary, acidic foods and condiments.
- Tomatoes, tomato-based foods.
- Citrus fruits, consume fruit in isolation.
- Garlic, ginger, cumin.

Do Eat:
- 6 – 8 glasses spring water/day, Japanese green tea, decaffeinated English tea, rooibos or honeybush tea, dilute fruit juices.
- Well-cooked carrots, peas, zucchini, asparagus, natural artichokes, pumpkin, plantain, potatoes, sweet potatoes, yams. Acorn, butternut and spaghetti squash. Avocados, cucumber, button, shiitake, portobello, oyster mushrooms, seaweed.
- 2 eggs/day maximum. Medium to non-oily fish: sole, cod, wild seabass, monkfish, wild salmon, tuna. Shrimp, scallops, chicken, turkey. Extra-lean beef, lamb or pork. Sushi, Japanese grilled fish.
- Pasta, brown rice, cous-cous, millet, amaranth, quinoa, kamut, 60% whole wheat bread, dry curd cheese.
- Well-ripened bananas, watermelon, apples, mango, papaya, pears, cantaloupe.
- Cold-pressed light, extra-virgin or virgin olive oil, cold-pressed sesame, flax, hempseed or sunflower oil.
- Basil, oregano, cilantro, thyme, tarragon, fennel, rosemary, Hungarian paprika (non-spicy), turmeric and soy sauce.

Reduce Diarrhea Diet

Eliminate:
- Alcohol, caffeine, decaffeinated coffee, carbonated drinks.
- Cheese, cream sauces, milk products.
- Cabbage family vegetables, beans, lentils, raw vegetables, roughage/high fibre foods, hot/spicy foods, deep-fried foods.
- Sour, vinegary, acidic foods and condiments.
- Tomatoes, tomato-based foods.
- Citrus fruits, consume fruit in isolation.
- Garlic, ginger, pepper, cumin, mustard seed.
- Processed foods; preservatives, MSG, nitrates, artificial flavors and colors, etc.
- Margarine or butter substitutes, hydrogenated oils, artificial sweeteners, carrageenan.

Reduce:
- Butter and oil consumption, use as little as possible.
- Sugar, yeast.
- Refined carbohydrates – any breads, pastas, cookies etc. made of refined (white) flour.

Do Eat:
- Minimum 8-10 glasses spring water/day, Japanese green tea, decaffeinated English tea, dilute fruit juices.
- Well-cooked carrots, zucchini, asparagus, natural artichokes, pumpkin, plantain, potatoes, sweet potatoes, yams. Acorn, butternut and spaghetti squash. Avocados, cucumber, regular, portobello, oyster and shiitake mushrooms, seaweed.
- 2 eggs/day maximum, medium to non-oily fish; sole, cod, wild seabass, monkfish, wild salmon, tuna. Shrimp, scallops, chicken, turkey. Extra-lean beef, lamb or pork. Sushi, Japanese grilled fish.
- Pasta, brown rice, cous-cous, millet, 60% whole wheat bread, dry curd.
- Well-ripened bananas, watermelon, apples, mango, papaya, cantaloupe, pears.
- Cold-pressed light, extra-virgin or virgin olive oil, cold-pressed sesame, flax, hempseed or sunflower oil.
- Basil, oregano, cilantro, thyme, tarragon, fennel, soy sauce, a little Hungarian paprika, a little turmeric.

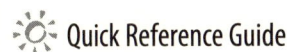 Quick Reference Guide

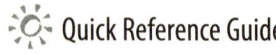
Quick Reference Guide

Stop Intestinal Bleeding Diet

Eliminate:
- Alcohol, caffeine, decaffeinated coffee, carbonated drinks.
- Cow & Goat milk products, rice milk, almond milk, soy milk, etc.
- Sour, vinegary, acidic foods and condiments.
- Tomatoes, tomato-based foods.
- Citrus fruits or juices
- Cabbage family vegetables, beans, lentils, raw vegetables, coconut, roughage/high fibre foods, leafy green vegetables, hot/spicy foods, deep-fried foods, red meat.
- Margarine or butter substitutes, artificial sweeteners, carrageenan.
- Yeast, sugar if necessary.
- Garlic, ginger, cumin, chilies, pepper, paprika, turmeric.
- Processed foods; preservatives, MSG, nitrates, artificial flavors, colors, etc.

Do Eat:
- 8-10 glasses spring water/day, weak Japanese green tea.
- Well-cooked carrots, zucchini, pumpkin, potatoes, sweet potatoes, yams. Acorn, butternut and spaghetti squash. Avocados, peeled cucumber.
- 2 eggs/day maximum, non-oily fish; sole, cod, wild seabass, monkfish, wild salmon, tuna. Shrimp, scallops, small amounts of chicken, turkey. Meat or vegetable broths.
- Pasta, white rice, white or 60% whole wheat bread, dry curd.
- Well-ripened bananas, watermelon, pears, apple, papaya, cantaloupe.
- Cold-pressed, extra-virgin or virgin olive oil, cold-pressed sesame, flax, hempseed or sunflower oil – no more than ½ tsp. or less per meal.
- Basil, oregano, thyme, dried cilantro, and soy sauce (no alcohol added).

Food Reintroduction Chart

PHASE ONE

A	Squash	Zucchini	Mushrooms	Cucumber	
B	White rice	Rice noodles	Rice flour	Rice cereal	Rice milk
C	Sole Tuna	Cod Salmon	Halibut Turkey	Sea bass Trout	Monkfish Chicken
D	Pears Olive oil	Cantaloupe Safflower oil	Apples Hemp oil	Sunflower oil	
E	Vitamins Minerals	Basil Thyme	Oregano Salt	Stevia Fructose	Maple syrup Turbinado sugar

PHASE TWO

A	Peas Amaranth	Snowpeas Bean sprouts	Asparagus Yams	Green beans Sweet potato	Yellow beans Pumpkin Water chestnuts
B	Rice pancakes Quinoa	Sweet rice Spelt	Jasmine rice Brown rice	Millet Basmati rice	Buckwheat Rice bread
C	Plums Peaches	Watermelon Avocado	Mangoes Honeydew	Papaya	Banana
D	Dill Garlic	Sesame oil Cilantro	Soy sauce	Eggs	Rosemary
E	Tapioca	Baking powder	Baking soda	Arrowroot	

PHASE THREE

A	Butter lettuce Spinach	Cauliflower Bok choy	Broccoli Seaweed, Nori	Celery Bamboo	Chives Bamboo shoots
B	Kamut Goose	Beef Sardines	Pork Anchovies	Lamb	Duck
C	Peanuts Cranberries Strawberries	Cashews Apricots	Walnuts Cherries	Raisins Almonds	Blueberries Nectarines
D	Mint Vanilla	Ginger Cinnamon	Paprika Saffron	Turmeric Coconut	Lemon, Limes
E	Daikon Kefir	Bay leaf Goat milk	Mustard Leeks	Olives Butter	Yoghurt Goat cheese

PHASE FOUR

A	Artichokes Lettuce	Turnip Onions	Parsnip Brussel sprouts	Potatoes	Tomatoes
B	Beans Kohlrabi	Lentils Rhubarb	Beets Corn	Cabbage	Chard, Kale
C	Wheat Oranges	Cous-cous Grapefruit	Plantain Raspberries	Currents Blackberries	Figs, Dates
D	Grapes Scallops	Pineapple Lobster	Prunes	Shrimp	Prawns
E	Cornstarch Ketchup	Vinegar Cumin	Lotusroot Cheese	Wasabi Cow's milk	Pickles

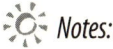 *Notes:*

4
Lifestyle & Environmental Changes

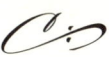

"We now understand our own health as something created through the pattern of our lives; and we are beginning to understand disease, not as something bad or evil that 'comes to get us', but as a symptom of an imbalanced way in which we walk on Mother Earth. With this understanding we can begin the process of healing ourselves through proper nutrition, physical exercise, new belief, and a more healthy environment, as well as through the balancing of energies and the right use of medicines that stimulate the body's innate healing capacities.

In this way our healing becomes an accepting, loving expression of all parts of ourselves. We look at the larger whole and understand that polluting this Earth, from which we receive our physical lives, is the beginning of much disease."

Brooke Medicine Eagle, MA, Native Shaman

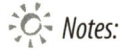 Notes:

Imagine your typical day: You get up in the morning and brush your teeth with toothpaste. Then you have a shower; you use shower gel or soap, shampoo, conditioner and shaving cream. After you've dried yourself off, you apply moisturizer to your skin, makeup to your face and perhaps some hair gel, mousse or hairspray. A final spritz of perfume or cologne, an application of deodorant, and you're ready for breakfast.

You have your usual breakfast of cereal with milk and grab an apple for the road. You're feeling pretty good and refreshed, you're clean, you smell nice and you've just kicked off your metabolism for the day with a nutritious and healthy breakfast. Well, that's one way of looking at it. What you're probably not aware of is the phenomenal amount of toxins you've just absorbed or ingested in your body within your first hour of waking.

The skin is the body's largest organ and it is very efficient at absorbing and transporting to the blood and cells whatever it comes into contact with. Barbara Griggs, the author of *Green Pharmacy: The History and Evolution of Western Herbal Medicine* tells this story of healing via poultices applied to the skin:

> "This hot aromatic poultice of stimulating and antiseptic herbs very probably did the trick – and reminds us that until only very recently, poultices and foot-baths were very common ways of applying medicine, not just because of their local heating or counter-irritant value, but because their virtues are absorbed through the skin. Mustard foot-baths – piping hot – have always been a popular remedy for coughs, colds and chestiness in my family – a folk-remedy of hundreds of years' standing which we have always found highly effective. Research by the German firm Madaus has recently revealed a rationale for this treatment: mustard seeds contain a powerful antibiotic, which is absorbed directly through the particularly sensitive skin of the feet." [1]

When you realize how very efficient the skin is at absorbing and integrating into the body anything it comes into contact with, you might also want to take a second look at exactly what elements you're introducing to your body via your skin. Every single product that you've used during your typical morning outlined above probably contains toxic and carcinogenic elements – from your toothpaste to your deodorant. In addition, many of the products available in North America contain chemicals that have been completely banned in numerous other countries. It's beyond the scope of this book to go into exactly what each of these chemicals are and which products they're found in, but rest assured if you didn't buy all your toiletry products from a reputable health pharmacy, you're likely to be absorbing toxic and carcinogenic elements from every single product you use.

Then there's the supposedly healthy breakfast you ate. But what about the secondary hormones, antibiotics, and pesticide residues in the milk? Your cereal packet was likely sprayed with BHA or BHT (phenolic compounds that are often added to foods to preserve fats):

> "Researchers report that BHA in the diet of pregnant mice results in brain enzyme changes in their offspring including a 50 percent decreased activity in brain cholinesterase, which is responsible for the transmission of nerve impulses. BHA and BHT also affect the animal's sleep, levels of aggression and weight." [2]

Maybe you sweetened your cereal with Aspartame, which is banned in numerous countries and has the longest list of complaints the FDA has ever received. Then there are the pesticide residues found in the cereal itself and also on and in your apple. Your supposedly "normal" morning routine is beginning to look like a toxic nightmare.

We have to wonder why childhood cancer rates are up several hundred percent from the 1970's. What exactly is causing all these auto-immune diseases like lupus, fibromyalgia, Crohn's, multiple sclerosis, etc? And why is it that the incidence rate of cancer in America is now 1 in 3? Could it be that between our diet, environmental pollutants, household cleansers, cookware, toiletries, water supply, synthetic fabrics, building materials and other supposedly "normal" elements, we are slowly and synergistically poisoning ourselves?

What you're probably not aware of is the phenomenal amount of toxins you've just absorbed or ingested in your body within your first hour of waking.

> Why is it that the incidence rate of cancer in America is now 1 in 3? Could it be that between our diet, environmental pollutants, household cleansers, cookware, toiletries, water supply, synthetic fabrics, building materials and other supposedly "normal" elements, we are slowly and synergistically poisoning ourselves?

"The EPA does not have a scientifically acceptable method for determining the risk for multiple chemical exposure. Yet when scientists have done studies on multiple chemical exposure, it seems quite clear that the chemicals act synergistically. In one 1976 study, a scientific team used three chemicals on a group of rats. The chemicals were tested one at a time on the rats without ill-effect. When the scientists gave the rats two at a time, a decline in health was noted. When the rats were given all three chemicals at once, they all died within two weeks." [3]

There are currently over four hundred pesticides and two thousand food additives that have been approved for use in America. Over 69 million Americans live in regions that exceed smog standards and most drinking water contains over seven hundred chemicals. As many as ten thousand chemicals enter our bodies in the form of solvents, emulsifiers and preservatives used in food processing and storage. What on earth makes us think our bodies can withstand such a chemically saturated environment without breaking down? And where do we go from here, how do we progress from feeling depressed and overwhelmed by our current toxin load to a healthier, less toxic state of being?

You can start by becoming aware, and simply take notice of the number of chemicals you're ingesting, absorbing or otherwise exposing your body to. Start reading the labels on products you buy, the food you eat, and toiletries you use. Fortunately, there are non-toxic, environmentally-friendly versions available of nearly every product or food you currently use. Start shopping at organic food stores and health stores. You can eliminate a tremendous amount of daily toxins simply by changing your personal hygiene, household cleaning and dietary habits. Yes, it's more expensive, but would you rather pay the price with your health or your pocketbook? Eliminating the avoidable toxins from your lifestyle and diet will relieve a great deal of stress from your body – leaving it free to use its energy to process the unavoidable toxins and pollutants in our environment.

According to Dr. Claudio Fiocchi at the Division of Gastroenterology, Case Western Reserve University School of Medicine in Cleveland, Ohio:

> "Environmental factors are probably as important as the patient's genetic makeup for the risk of IBD. Potentially relevant environmental factors include prenatal events, breastfeeding, childhood infections, microbial agents, smoking, oral contraceptives, diet, hygiene, occupation, education, climate, pollution, stress and miscellaneous components such as toothpaste, appendectomy, tonsillectomy, blood transfusions, contact with animals, and physical activity." 4

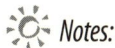 Notes:

You may find this chapter quite overwhelming, and I certainly don't want it to cause you to throw up your hands in despair and give up. This is a difficult chapter and it will cause you to examine ways of living and being that are habitual; things you've done for so long you probably don't even think about them. For this reason, I encourage you to only attempt the changes suggested in this chapter if and when you feel completely ready to. Some of the recommendations in this chapter (for example, having mercury amalgam fillings replaced) have taken me years to get round to implementing, so don't worry if it takes you a long time to work through everything. Just take it nice and slow and don't pressure yourself or stress-out over these recommendations.

Assessing The Toxins In Your Life

Take a look at all the physical factors in your life right now and ask yourself two questions: 1) Am I happy with this? 2) Is this good for my health? Start by taking a look at your living environment:

- ▶ Examine the food you eat and the beverages you drink.

- ▶ What's the air quality like where you live?

- ▶ Are you in a bustling city but would rather be in the peaceful countryside, or vice-versa?

- What's your job like? Does your job build you up or tear you down? Do you look forward to getting up in the morning? Is your level of job-related stress healthy for you, or unhealthy?

- What's your current exercise regimen?

Take the time to go through all of these influencing physical factors in your life and make a list of what should change and a list of what must change (you may want to read this whole chapter first, and then make your list). This will help you to prioritize which changes need to be implemented first. If you want to heal yourself, you must put your body and your needs first. Different people will respond differently to the same stimulus. I'm very affected by air pollution and as a result, I will probably never live in a really polluted city like London or Tokyo again, but you may be only slightly affected by air pollution. Every person is different, with different needs and sensitivities. Listen to your body and to your intuition and you'll know what needs to change for you in your life.

Yes, this is going to be difficult! You may decide you need to change jobs, or take a sabbatical. You may need to change your whole way of eating. You may want to move to a new city, or a new country. You may need to restructure your home life so that you do less of the chores and have more time for relaxation. These are not small changes. But again, just ask yourself the question: Do I want to heal myself? If the answer's "Yes" then you need to make yourself your number one priority and do whatever it takes to put yourself first and get your needs met as much and as often as you can.

You may feel that you can't make the necessary changes or put your needs first because you have a demanding job, or demanding dependents, or not enough money, not enough time, etc. Remember that life is all about choices. You can do anything you choose or decide to do. There's no such thing as "can't". Start taking responsibility for the choices you're making in your life and next time you find yourself saying "can't", change it to "won't". This will actually be a very freeing move, accepting your power and shifting out of victim-mode into driver's seat-mode. Take all the energy that you would normally spend in coming up with reasons why you "can't" do

> There's no such thing as "can't". Start taking responsibility for the choices you're making in your life and next time you find yourself saying "can't", change it to "won't". This will actually be a very freeing move, accepting your power and shifting out of victim-mode into driver's seat-mode.

something and put it into figuring out how you can do that thing. You'll either realize that (a) you actually don't really want to do that thing, or, (b) you'll find a way to do it. Either way, you'll step into your power to make an honest decision about what you want and what's right for you at this time.

It will probably take you a while to implement all of the physical changes that you need to make. No problem! Just take it one step at a time and proceed at the pace of change that's right for you. Don't get discouraged if you feel it's taking you a long time to change your lifestyle, or if some days you feel the task is insurmountable. Look at it this way: Whether it takes you a year to make the changes, or five years, you're still much further ahead than if you'd never made the changes at all. Again, take the time to check-in with yourself regularly and only do what you feel ready for and what you feel is right for you.

ELIMINATING TOXINS

A major part of the healing process involves reducing and eliminating, as much as possible, the toxins in your lifestyle that you sense are detrimental to you. First, let's take a look at environmental toxins. These include:

▶ Cigarette/cigar/pipe smoke, either first or secondhand

▶ Automobile exhaust

▶ Manufacturing or refining byproduct pollutants

▶ Power lines – emit strong electromagnetic energy that is very disturbing to the balance of electromagnetic energy within our bodies. Do not live near power lines, power plants/stations or cell phone towers.

▶ Try not to use cell phones. If you must use one, keep it away from your body and use an ear-pierce *with a ferrite bead attached* to the cord, rather than holding it up to your head to talk. Do not carry a cell phone on your body if it's turned on. See the section below on Cell Phones for more details.

☼ People who are strong and healthy can accept and process a lot of toxins every day without being adversely affected. However, if your body has developed IBD, it is in a hyper-sensitive state and it's up to you to protect it and provide yourself with an environment that supports your healing efforts, not undermines them.

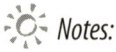 Notes:

- Inhaling any type of air-borne chemical like pesticides from farming or from bug-control in tropical climates, fumes from dry cleaners, auto body repair shops, household cleaning products, perfumes, colognes, or bug sprays, room/car deodorizers, perfumed toilet paper or tissues, formaldehyde in carpets and particle-board furniture, etc.

If you currently have allergies to dust, mold, pollen, animals, etc., chances are you're very sensitive to environmental pollutants and your immune system function is quite imbalanced. If you have medium to severe allergies and you live in a large, polluted city, you may want to give serious thought to relocating somewhere less polluted. People who are strong and healthy can accept and process a lot of toxins every day without being adversely affected. However, if your body has developed IBD, it is in a hyper-sensitive state and it's up to you to protect it and provide yourself with an environment that supports your healing efforts, not undermines them.

Smoking

If you or someone else in your household is a smoker, you may want to consider banning any smoking in the house. Smoking only in a particular room doesn't cut it, because smoke permeates and saturates everything. After your house/apartment has been smoke-free for a week, get all the rugs shampooed, the furniture steam cleaned and all of the drapes and window hangings cleaned. If possible, avoid getting anything dry-cleaned as the chemicals used are very toxic and will then pollute your living environment. If you absolutely cannot avoid dry-cleaning, then hang the fabric or clothing in your garage or outside for a few days to a week to allow the chemicals to disperse as much as possible. Also, wash all of your walls, duvets, pillows and bedding. If you or your partner regularly smoked in the bedroom, you may want to get a new mattress as well. No, I am not going overboard here. After you've been smoke-free for a month or two and you walk into a smoker's house you'll immediately notice a tremendous difference and will probably feel ill from the fumes and smell. Obviously, if you're a smoker, the best gift you could give yourself would be to quit smoking. But again, in your own time and only when/if you feel it's right for you. Although some studies have shown that nicotine can actually have a calming effect on ulcerative colitis (possibly due to increased mucus production in the colon), the negative effects on the body as a whole still far outweigh any short-term benefit that might be derived. Similar studies done with Crohn's patients showed an increase in the number and severity of flare-ups.[5]

Toxins In Food

Most North Americans also consume a phenomenal amount of toxins and chemicals through their food. Part of allowing our bodies to heal themselves involves reducing these toxins to give your immune system as much of a chance as possible. We need to work to create an environment that supports and encourages our healing process. Following are the top polluters of your nutritional environment:

- Processed or packaged foods and beverages.

- Foods/beverages containing preservatives, nitrates/nitrites, MSG (interferes with neural functioning), carrageenan (used in large quantities to induce ulcerative colitis in guinea pigs and primates), chemical dyes, or anything else that sounds like a manufactured chemical compound.

- Non-organic beverages and food; fruit, vegetables, grains, dairy and meat (i.e. The "regular" kind you buy at your local grocer).

- Refined sugar

- Microwaved foods or drinks (alters the molecular composition of food, rendering it toxic)

- Teflon coated (non-stick) cookware. Plastic dishes or containers (chemicals will migrate into the food, even if the food is cold)

If you want to heal your digestive tract, you're probably going to have to eliminate as much of the above from your diet as you can. Go through your diet and your fridge and cupboards. You'll probably be astounded at the amount of food and drinks you normally consume that are packed with

> Avoid getting anything dry-cleaned as the chemicals used are very toxic and will then pollute your living environment.

unnatural additives and chemicals. You're going to have to go back to the beginning and start reading every label on every item you buy. Some foods you're just going to have to give up because they're actually not natural foods and don't exist in a non-toxic form. See Chapter Three and the sections below for detailed information on exactly why all of the above are harmful to your health.

Cell Phones

Cell phone (mobile phone) manufacturers have worked tirelessly to minimize the reporting of adverse effects from cell phone use. However, in November 2000, the prestigious UK medical journal *The Lancet* published two reports on cell phone usage damage, with the author of one report, Dr. Gerald Hyland (a British physicist) stating, "If mobile phones were a type of food, they simply would not be licensed." [6] The two reports point out that cell phone radiation affects a variety of brain functions and this can result in tumors, headaches and disrupted sleep. Cell phone radiation also degrades the immune system. Due to various factors – like head size, a thinner skull, a brain that is still developing and an immune system that is less robust – infants and preadolescents are the most susceptible to the damaging effects of cell phone radiation. A cell phone emits radiation even if it's just turned on (but you're not talking to someone), so make sure you (and your children) don't carry a cell phone anywhere on your body.

If you're at all prone to epilepsy, then the radiation from cell phones can trigger seizures. Here is the actual data from the two reports that explains in technical detail the points I have just communicated:

> "... GSM radiation does seem to affect non-thermally a variety of brain functions (including the neuroendocrine system), and health problems reported anecdotally do tend to be neurological...
> For example:
> ▶ Reports of headache are consistent with the effect of the radiation on the dopamine-opiate system of the brain and the permeability of the blood-brain barrier, both of which have been connected to headache.

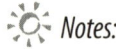 Notes:

- Reports of sleep disruption are consistent with effects of the radiation on melatonin levels and on rapid-eye-movement sleep.

Furthermore, since there is no reason to suppose that the seizure-inducing ability of a flashing visible light does not extend to microwave radiation (which can access the brain through the skull) flashing at a similarly low frequency, together with the fact that exposure to pulsed MWR can induce epileptic activity in rats, reports of epileptic activity in some children exposed to base-station radiation are perhaps not surprising.

Finally, the significant increase (by a factor of between 2 and 3) in the incidence of neuroepithelial tumours (the laterality of which correlates with cell-phone use) found in a nationwide US study is consistent not only with the genotoxicity of GSM radiation, as indicated by increased DNA strand breaks and formation of chromosome aberrations and micronuclei but also with its promotional effect on tumour development.

It is often argued that anecdotal reports of health problems should be dismissed. However, given the paucity of systematic epidemiological studies of this new technology, such reports are an indispensable source of information, a point acknowledged in the 1999 report of the UK parliamentary committee.

Preadolescent children can be expected to be more vulnerable to any adverse health effects than adults because absorption of GSM microwaves is greatest in an object about the size of a child's head, because of the "head resonance" effect and the greater ease with which the radiation can penetrate the thinner skull of an infant.

Also the multiframe repetition frequency of 834 Hz and the 2 Hz pulsing in the DTX mode of cellphones lie in the range of the alpha and delta brain-waves, respectively.

In a child, alpha waves do not replace delta waves as a stable activity until the age of about 12 years. Furthermore, the immune system, whose efficacy is degraded by this kind of radiation, is less robust in children.

> Cell phone radiation affects a variety of brain functions and this can result in tumors, headaches and disrupted sleep, it also degrades the immune system. If you're at all prone to epilepsy, then the radiation from cell phones can trigger seizures.

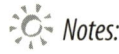 Notes:

> This makes them less able to cope with any adverse health effect that might be provoked by chronic exposure, not only to the pulsed microwave radiation but also to the more penetrating low-frequency magnetic fields associated with the current surges from the handset battery which can reach 40 µT (peak) near the back of the case." [7]

It was originally thought, that since radiation decreases exponentially over the distance between you and your phone, that by using a headset, the phone would be away from your body and thus reduce the radiation intensity. However, a report in the British consumer research magazine *Which?* (www.which.co.uk/) has shown that use of a headset can actually increase your brain's exposure to radiation, depending on the position used.

However, the good news is that you can pretty much neutralize all of the radiation transmitted via the headset by clipping on a ferrite bead device. Professor Lawrie Challis says that clipping a ferrite bead on headsets stops the radio waves from traveling up the wire and into the head, "Using a ferrite bead effectively reduces emissions to the head to zero but as yet manufacturers do not put them on hands-free kits." [8] Dr. Stuart Porter, agrees with Professor Challis' comments:

> "Hands-free kits effectively have two currents, an intentional one that stays within the wires and an unintentional one on the outside. It is the unintentional one the beads stop. They work by blocking the current, a bit like a block in a water pipe." [9]

A ferrite bead is simply a hollow bead or cylinder made of ferrite – a semi-magnetic substance made from iron oxide alloyed with other metals. They work by reducing EMI (electromagnetic interference) and RFI (radio-frequency interference). Jim May, an engineer whose company produces ferrite beads for a variety of industry uses says:

> "Ferrites have a concentrated, homogeneous magnetic structure with high permeability. They are consistently stable over time and over a

wide temperature range, and provide RF suppression without high eddy-current losses." [10]

This may all have been a bit more technical than you'd prefer, but I wanted to present you with the original research, so you can see for yourself that my recommendations are based on hard science. Obviously, it's best if you can avoid using cell phones altogether. But, as that is not always possible, know that you can greatly reduce their harmful radiation by not carrying the cell phone on your body (when it's turned on) and by using a headset (hands-free device) with a ferrite bead clipped to it when speaking on your cell phone. This advice is particularly pertinent for children.

When we lived in Singapore, there was a big media splash about increasing numbers of twenty year olds who were having heart attacks and no one could figure out why. Then, they realized that it was the fashion for these young people to carry their cell phones attached to designer cords worn round their necks. Therefore, their phones hung against their chest – right near their hearts, causing the heart attacks! Knowing this, I cringe when I see mothers tucking their cell phones into baby carriers (right next to the baby's torso) and people putting their cell phones into their pockets.

A good place to get a reasonably priced ferrite bead that is easily attached to your cell phone headset is from *www.mercola.com* – just type in "Ferrite Beads" in mercola.com's search engine. Otherwise, do an Internet search to look for suppliers in your area.

Your Sleeping Environment

Since the normal person spends an average of one third of their life in bed, your bed and sleeping environment can have a significant impact on your health. If your bed, pillow, duvet, etc. are composed of synthetic elements, then they are off-gassing toxins while you sleep, or, you are absorbing toxins through your skin (see the section below on *Absorption Through the Skin* for more details). There are many mattresses now available made from various combinations of the following natural (non-toxic) materials: Natural latex, cotton, coir (coconut fibre), wool, de-magnetized coils, etc. Do an Internet

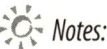 *Notes:*

search using the keywords 'natural mattress' to view a selection of what's available. If you're buying a natural latex mattress, ensure that the mattress is indeed composed of at least 95% pure natural latex. Many manufacturers will mix natural and synthetic latex together and then call it "natural latex". For your bedding, use only natural materials like wool, down, cotton, etc. I prefer to use wool duvets and pillows as I find they're more comfortable than goose or duck down, and wool doesn't shift around or bunch up in places, as down does.

If you can't afford to replace your bed, then at least:

- Get a 100% cotton mattress cover (the padding inside the mattress pad must be cotton as well), or a wool/cotton mattress pad. I had a great deal of trouble finding 100% cotton mattress pads and finally found a great one made by Nautica. Do an Internet (Google) keyword search using "Nautica bedding" to find a supplier near you.

- Use 100% cotton sheets and pillowcases, and replace your pillows and duvet/quilt with ones made from natural materials (wool, down, cotton, etc.).

- Make sure your pajamas are cotton or silk too – no synthetic fabrics.

When you need or want to replace the flooring in your bedroom, choose natural materials like hardwood or cork (durable, warm, and much cheaper than hardwood). Even 100% wool carpeting is not ideal since the glue and underlay are toxic materials. Much better is to get a cork or hardwood floor and then put a cotton or wool rug overtop. If you currently have wall-to-wall carpeting (fitted carpets), when you get it steam cleaned, make sure the cleaners don't use a chemical cleaning solution (specify you want just plain, environmentally-friendly, soap) and do not get it treated afterwards with any kind of stain guard or sealant – these substances are very toxic and off-gas various harmful chemicals including ammonium perfluorooctanoate (C-8).

Make sure the curtains in your bedroom are made from natural materials and if you have blinds, then make sure they're metal or wood, not plastic

Since the normal person spends an average of one third of their life in bed, your bed and sleeping environment can have a significant impact on your health.

(typically PVC). As for bedroom furniture, ensure it's made from solid wood (not particle board, laminates, or melamine), or metal. Lastly, if you have a TV or computer in your bedroom, unplug it before you go to sleep and do not use a clock that plugs in – all give off electromagnetic radiation and interfere with your body's own electromagnetic balance. For this same reason, do not sleep long-term on magnetic sleeping pads, or wear magnets long-term on your body.

Ideally, it's best if you can apply these 'healthy bedroom' guidelines to every room in your house. But that may take some time and quite a bit of money! So, in the meantime, just make sure your bedroom is non-toxic, and when it comes time to buy new floor coverings, window coverings, furniture, etc. for the rest of your house, make sure your new things are 100% natural.

Mercury Poisoning

Toxic poisoning due to the silver-colored, mercury amalgam fillings in your teeth is another issue you may want to look at. Mercury is 80 times more poisonous than arsenic and the mercury in your fillings leaches out into the rest of your body. There are now hundreds of documented cases where people have had their mercury amalgam fillings taken out and replaced with a white resin composite, undergone a mercury detoxification procedure, and all their symptoms of disease have disappeared – this includes people diagnosed with fibromyalgia, nervous disorders, IBS, skin diseases, etc. You can get tested for mercury poisoning by having some of your hair analyzed – your naturopathic physician can advise you on where to go for testing. The technician will then be able to tell you if mercury is present in your system and in what concentration.

However, as with all toxins, different people have differing sensitivity levels and some people do not absorb and store as much mercury in their body as others. Check in with your intuition to see if you feel you should find out more about this issue and whether you should go for testing, or not. At the very least, when you have a new filling done, or one replaced, make sure your dentist uses a rubber dam to prevent the mercury from draining into your throat and some kind of air suction device to suck up the mercury

> There are now hundreds of documented cases where people have had their mercury amalgam fillings taken out and replaced with a white resin composite, undergone a mercury detoxification procedure, and all their symptoms of disease have disappeared.

vapors before you inhale them. Ideally, you should also have a nasal canula with a separate oxygen supply for yourself during the procedure. Also make sure the filling is one of the new white resin composites that are much safer for your body.

Some fish are now also contaminated with unacceptable levels of mercury. See Chapter Three for guidelines released by The Environmental Protection Agency to minimize mercury contamination through seafood.

ABSORPTION THROUGH THE SKIN

As you have read above, the skin is a highly sensitive organ and quickly absorbs any substance applied to it. Reflecting this, many medicines are now available in transdermal formulations like nicotine patches, birth control drugs and hormone creams.

Therefore, we need to have a look at the ingredient list and eliminate the pollutants from everyday products applied to our skin such as:

- Body lotion
- Bubble bath, bath oils, shower gel, etc.
- Soap
- Face cream, face wash, astringent, foundation, other make-up
- Shampoo
- Conditioner
- Sunscreen and self-tanning lotions
- Hair dyes
- Shaving cream
- Toothpaste (fluoride is actually classified as a highly toxic chemical and you're forbidden by law to bury it or put it in a river or ocean – but you can brush your teeth with it!)

> "This may seem like one of the biggest, if not *the* biggest, mistakes the chemical industry has ever made. And how could they [the toxic chemicals emitted] not be in our blood? They're in such a huge range of consumer products. We're talking about *Teflon, Stainmaster, Gore-tex, Silverstone*. So if you buy clothing that's coated with Teflon or something else that protects it from dirt and stains, those chemicals can absorb directly through the skin."
>
> Jane Houlihan, VP, Environmental Working Group

- Perfume, cologne, and perfumed body sprays
- Feminine "hygiene" sprays and powders, tampons or pads bleached with dioxin (unless the package says 'dioxin free' there's a good chance it contains this harmful chemical)
- Dyed and/or perfumed toilet paper or tissues
- Deodorant, anti-perspirant
- Laundry detergent, fabric softeners for the washing machine or dryer, 'fresheners' or other scented products (all these leave chemical residues on your clothes, which touch your skin and are absorbed)
- Dishwashing detergent (leaves chemical residue on dishes, which you then end up eating along with your food/beverages)
- Chlorinated water

Now, obviously, I'm not saying you need to stop using all these products. But you may want to find toxin and chemical-free versions of all these types of products. A good alternative health store or organic grocery will usually carry most if not all of these products in environmentally and health-friendly formulations. An excellent website for all kinds of household and skin products is www.wholefoods.com, and my favorite companies for skin care products are Burt's Bees Inc., Aubrey Organics, Dr. Hauschka, and Lavera. For dishwashing and laundry products I like Seventh Generation. Keep in mind there may be other companies that produce equal or better products to the ones listed here, I'm simply giving you the best I've found from the ones that I've tried.

Chlorine is a very toxic chemical that's added to everyone's water supply in varying degrees. You definitely need to filter your tap water for cooking or boiling in the kettle with either an at-source purification system, or just by using a Brita water filter in your water jug (be sure to change the filter regularly). Become aware of how your body feels after a shower or bath. Remember that chlorine is directly absorbed through your skin. Different people have different sensitivities to chlorine and you may need

> Children who swam regularly in indoor pools had lung damage (from inhaling chlorine vapors) equal to that of an adult smoker.
> The National Post

to add chlorine filters to your bath or shower head as well. I recently read an article in the National Post newspaper outlining how researchers had discovered that children who swam regularly in indoor pools had lung damage (from inhaling chlorine vapors) equal to that of an adult smoker.

THE TOXINS IN YOUR KITCHEN

How you prepare your food and the cooking utensils and methods you use can be just as important as the food itself. Many of you are probably quite unwittingly damaging and adding toxins to your food on a daily basis. This degrades not just your digestive health, but your systemic health as well.

Avoid Teflon And Non-stick Cookware

The chemicals used in making Teflon-coated pots, pans, cookie sheets, bakeware, etc. will also migrate into your food and be released into the air when cooking with them. This includes ammonium perfluorooctanoate (known as C-8), which has been linked to cancer, organ damage and other deleterious health effects in tests on laboratory animals. DuPont (the manufacturer of Teflon) previously asserted that toxins would only be emitted at extremely high temperatures that would not likely be reached in normal cooking. However, in May 2003, a consumer activist organization, the Environmental Working Group (*www.ewg.265org*) conducted their own tests and found that in two to five minutes on a conventional stovetop, cookware coated with Teflon and other non-stick surfaces can exceed temperatures at which the coating breaks apart and emits toxic particles and gases linked to hundreds, perhaps thousands, of pet bird deaths and an unknown number of human illnesses each year. In the cases of 'Teflon toxicosis' as the bird poisonings are called, the lungs of exposed birds (i.e. they're in your house or kitchen while you're cooking/baking with Teflon-coated pans) hemorrhage and fill with fluid, leading to suffocation. The Environmental Working Group also released the following data related to Teflon toxicosis (bird deaths) in people's houses:

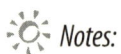 Notes:

"Under ordinary cooking scenarios, Teflon kills birds. A review of the literature and bird owners' accounts of personal experience with Teflon toxicosis shows that Teflon can be lethal at normal cooking temperatures, with no human lapses in judgment or wakefulness.

Bird deaths have been documented during or immediately after the following normal cooking scenarios:
New Teflon-lined Amana oven was used to bake biscuits at 325°F; all the owner's baby parrots died. Four stovetop burners, underlined with Teflon-coated drip pans, were preheated in preparation for Thanksgiving dinner; 14 birds died within 15 minutes. Nonstick cookie sheet was placed under oven broiler to catch the drippings; 107 chicks died. Self-cleaning feature on the oven was used; a $2,000 bird died. Set of Teflon pans, including egg poaching pan, were attributed to seven bird deaths over seven years. Water burned off a hot pan; more than 55 birds died. DuPont claims that its coating remains intact indefinitely at 500°F. Experiences of consumers whose birds have died from fumes generated at lower temperatures show that this is not the case. In one case researchers at the University of Missouri documented the death of about 1,000 broiler chicks exposed to offgas products from coated heat lamps at 396°F." [11]

You simply have to ask yourself: If Teflon and other non-stick cookware are capable of such toxic effects in animals, what are these chemicals doing to us, our children, and our babies? DuPont claims that human illness will be produced only in cases involving gross overheating, or burning the food to an inedible state. Yet DuPont's own scientists have concluded that polymer fume fever in humans is possible at 662°F, a temperature easily exceeded when a pan is preheated on a burner, or placed beneath a broiler, or in a self-cleaning oven. DuPont has also never studied the incidence rates of polymer fume fever among the billions of users of non-stick pots and pans sold around the world. Neither has the company studied the long-term effects from the sickness, or the extent to which Teflon exposures lead to human illnesses believed erroneously to be the common flu.

> The chemicals (like perfluorooctanoate – C8) used in making Teflon-coated pots, pans, cookie sheets, bakeware, etc. will migrate into your food and be released into the air when you cook with them.

Jane Houlihan, vice president for research at the Environmental Working Group said:

> "In retrospect, this may seem like one of the biggest, if not *the* biggest, mistakes the chemical industry has ever made. And how could they [the toxic chemicals emitted] not be in our blood? They're in such a huge range of consumer products. We're talking about *Teflon, Stainmaster, Gore-tex, Silverstone*. So if you buy clothing that's coated with Teflon or something else that protects it from dirt and stains, those chemicals can absorb directly through the skin." [12]

According to the Environmental Protection Agency (EPA), some of the highest C-8 levels were found in children.

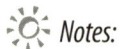 Notes:

You can see why it's really necessary to use stainless steel, cast iron, glass, or ceramic cookware – yes, I know it's more work to clean them, but it's very much worth it for your health. Some health advocates believe the best cookware is ceramic-coated (enameled) metal, as the ceramic is virtually inert and will not transfer any metal ions to the food you cook.
When purchasing stainless steel cookware, make sure the steel content is high enough by seeing if a magnet sticks to it – if the magnet doesn't stick, don't buy it, as it may contain a high nickel content. Nickel is as toxic as mercury to your body and nickel ions will be released into your food during cooking. Also completely avoid aluminum cookware as the aluminum migrates into your food and researchers suspect this is a significant contributor to diseases like Alzheimer's – they found significantly higher levels of aluminum in the brains of people who died with Alzheimer's disease. For baking, I use glass bakeware for cakes, pies, loafs, etc. and ceramic-coated cookie sheets for cookies, squares, etc. If you go to dollar stores you can usually pick up glass bakeware and storage containers very inexpensively. If you can't find ceramic-coated (enameled) cookie sheets, then buy online where there's a fairly good selection (use Google search engine and type in 'ceramic cookie sheets'). Also check other kitchen equipment like kettles, rice cookers, crock pots, etc. to make sure they are not Teflon coated.

Plastic & Xenoestrogens

Plastic bowls, dishes, cups, sandwich bags and storage containers also release chemicals (including organochlorines, bisphenol A, phthalates, xenoestrogens, etc.) into food – even if the food stored in them is cold. Dr. Dan Harper, MD (who specializes in chronic degenerative diseases at the Hamilton Clinic in Montana) writes:

> "The bad news is that xenoestrogens are not only in plastics, but in the hormones the stockmen and farmers use to fatten up their animals for market—beef, chicken, turkey, pork…These little chemicals also do a number on the immune system in general, setting up all kinds of cancers, and a number of autoimmune disorders —fibromyalgias, chronic fatigue, thyroid problems, multiple sclerosis, prostate enlargement, and the list goes on." [13]

Plastic food containers and sandwich bags are certainly difficult to avoid (especially since they're so convenient), but good alternatives do exist. For storing food in the fridge, you can use a glass or ceramic cereal bowl with a small side plate placed on top to cover it – this is a good system because then you can also stack them up. It's a good idea to use glass if you like to see what's in them at a glance. You can also purchase glass storage containers or ceramic casserole dishes with glass lids. Dollar stores are a great place to find cheap glass or ceramic storage containers, or small glass/ceramic bowls. Or, if you have a 'little India' in your town, go there and you can purchase stainless steel containers with airtight stainless steel lids. These Indian containers are very light and very cheap and make the ideal replacement for plastic containers and sandwich bags. They come in a whole range of sizes from those suitable for baby or toddler food, up to cake tin size. For storing food in cupboards, I use large glass 'canning' bottles (also very cheap and ideal for storing soups in the fridge as well) and stainless steel canisters, cake or cookie tins. Also, wrapping or storing food in waxed paper works perfectly well for dry foods or sandwiches. For times when I have to put something in a plastic sandwich bag, I wrap it in wax paper first to shield it from the plastic. You can also freeze soups, stews, and other 'wet' foods in the freezer using glass 'canning' jars. Fill the jars about 1.5 inches

☼ You may also want to avoid wearing plastic clothes (these include polyester, spandex, nylon, elastane, lycra, and other synthetics) as xenoestrogen chemicals are absorbed through the skin from these fabrics.

from the top (you need to leave room for expansion as the contents freeze) and just place the lid lightly on top (but don't screw it on yet). The next day, when the contents are frozen, you can screw the lid on tightly. When you want to eat that soup or stew, either place the jar in the fridge overnight, or place it in a pot or sink of hot water to thaw (not boiling hot though, as you don't want to crack the glass).

It may take a while to clear out all your plastic containers as they are everywhere, but again, it's worth it. Also, be sure and check your kettle as most electric kettles are made of plastic, and switch to stainless steel, if necessary. Check other kitchen items like blenders, mixing bowls, spatulas, kid's dishes, etc. and replace them with acceptable versions. If you have a baby, keep it from sucking or chewing on plastic toys, as much as possible. A lot of research has been done on certain estrogen-mimicking chemicals (xenoestrogens) that migrate into food from plastic containers and these are thought to be a chief contributor to problems with menopause and breast cancer. A great book on this is *What Your Doctor May Not Tell You About Premenopause* by John R. Lee, MD, Jesse Hanley, MD and Virginia Hopkins. You may also want to avoid wearing plastic clothes (these include polyester, spandex, nylon, lycra, elastane and other synthetics) as the estrogen-like chemicals are absorbed through the skin from these fabrics. I wear only natural fabrics next to my skin and though I occasionally wear spandex mixed with cotton, I limit it to a maximum of 5% of the fabric blend. Wearing natural fabrics only will also help you avoid dry-cleaning – which really should be called chemical-cleaning – another source of toxic chemicals absorbed both through the skin and inhaled. If you want more information on which harmful chemicals are involved in dry-cleaning and how they harm the body, do an Internet search using the keywords 'dangers of drycleaning'. Of course, I also apply all these rules to my family's clothing and environment.

The best way to safeguard your health is to use only natural products. If a company offers you an "improved" product, food, clothing, etc. just ask yourself one question: "Is it 100% natural?" If it's not, then don't touch it. You cannot rely on governmental agencies or the manufacturing companies

> You cannot rely on governmental agencies or the manufacturing companies themselves to test for safety and/or advise you of safety issues, because in our current world, money is the primary motivator and determinant of most human behavior.

themselves to test for safety and/or advise you of safety issues, because in our current world, money is the primary motivator and determinant of most human behaviour. According to a study by the National Academy of Sciences, there is adequate information on toxicity for only 2% of the synthetic chemicals released into our environment. If it's not 100% natural, don't touch it, use it, eat it, or have it in your home.

Are you feeling overwhelmed yet?! As I said, take these changes at a pace that's right for you and don't get stressed out or depressed by them. If you start feeling that way, take a break from thinking about these things and just enjoy life for a while. When you feel strong and relaxed again, take another look at this chapter and decide on the next change you'd like to make.

Dangers Of Microwaving

Microwaving food to the "cooked" stage will usually completely destroy its live enzymes. It will also alter the molecular chemistry of foods or beverages, rendering them toxic to the body. When microwave technology was first introduced to the world, Russia (which was under Communist rule at the time) completely banned its use, based on extensive research. If you're interested in this topic, you may want to do an Internet search to pull up some of the original Russian research – it's quite eye-opening.

More recently, a Swiss biologist by the name of Hans U. Hertel researched the effect of microwaved food on participants' blood constituent levels. The changes in blood that were documented include: A decrease in hemoglobin, an increase in negative cholesterol values related to the ratio of HDL (good cholesterol) and LDL (bad cholesterol) values, and white blood cells (lymphocytes) also decreased in the short-term following ingestion of microwaved food. In addition, Dr. Hertel pointed out:

> "Leukocytosis, which cannot be accounted for by normal daily deviations, is taken very seriously by hemotologists. Leukocytes are often signs of pathogenic effects on the living system, such as poisoning and cell damage. The increase of leukocytes with the

"The weakening of cell membranes by microwaves is used in the field of gene altering technology."

Dr Hans Hertel, Swiss Biologist

microwaved foods were more pronounced than with all the other variants. It appears that these marked increases were caused entirely by ingesting the microwaved substances. ... In addition to the violent frictional heat effects, called thermic effects [of microwaving food], there are also athermic effects which have hardly ever been taken into account. These athermic effects are not presently measurable, but they can also deform the structures of molecules and have qualitative consequences. For example the weakening of cell membranes by microwaves is used in the field of gene altering technology. Because of the force involved, the cells are actually broken, thereby neutralizing the electrical potentials, the very life of the cells, between the outer and inner side of the cell membranes. Impaired cells become easy prey for viruses, fungi and other microorganisms. The natural repair mechanisms are suppressed and cells are forced to adapt to a state of energy emergency – they switch from aerobic to anaerobic respiration. Instead of water and carbon dioxide, the cell poisons hydrogen peroxide and carbon monoxide are produced." [14]

> "Leukocytes are often signs of pathogenic effects on the living system, such as poisoning and cell damage. It appears that these marked increases of leukocytes were caused entirely by ingesting the microwaved foods."
>
> Dr. Hans Hertel, Swiss Biologist

In addition, a recent study revealed that microwaving broccoli resulted in up to a 97% loss of antioxidants, as compared to only 11% lost by steaming.[15] Many people I know just use their microwave as a bread box now, and my mum uses hers for storing pies. I don't even have one in the house, because I don't want guests or babysitters using it unwittingly. Like anything, there will be a bit of an adjustment phase, but you'll soon get used to heating things in the oven or on the stovetop, or, you can get a toaster oven for small items (just make sure it's not Teflon-coated!). The good news, health benefits aside, is that food heated conventionally tastes better and stays hot longer!

THE DANGERS OF VACCINATION

Most of you reading this book will likely be vaccinated already. However, knowledge is power and you may still be considering vaccinations for travel, the flu, or your children, so the following information will still be useful. I myself was vaccinated three times as a child – in Kenya, the U.S. and Canada – and I consider this to be one of the key reasons why I developed Crohn's at age 17. I also received a tuberculosis vaccination during my registration for university and three months later developed the first symptoms of Crohn's Disease. After you finish reading this section, you may agree with me that this was not just a coincidence.

▶ An unpublished study by the World Health Organisation (WHO) on a "measles susceptible" (malnourished) group of children showed that the group who hadn't been vaccinated contracted measles at the normal contract rate of 2.4%. Of the group who *had* received the measles vaccine (MMR), 33.5% contracted measles.[16]

▶ In 1975 Japan raised the minimum age for infant vaccinations to two years. As a result, SIDS (Sudden Infant Death Syndrome, or, crib death) and infant convulsions virtually disappeared. In the 80's, Japan lowered the minimum age back down to three months and the rate of SIDS returned to previous levels.[17]

▶ In an Australian study, a group of volunteers were vaccinated for Rubella, and all produced the expected antibodies. When later exposed to the disease, 80% of the recruits contracted it.[18]

▶ According to the U.S. National Childhood Vaccine Injury Act (est.1986): To qualify for compensation, the adverse effects of vaccination must occur within *four hours* of receiving the vaccine. Despite this extremely severe limitation, as of February 28, 1998 compensatory payments totalled $871,800,000.00. This figure is even more alarming when it is revealed that only one in four claimants were awarded compensation.[19]

▶ Some researchers postulate that the use of live viral vaccines introduce foreign genetic material into the human system, which has contributed to the unprecedented escalation of auto-immune disorders (like multiple sclerosis, rheumatoid arthritis, lupus, cancer, Crohn's disease, asthma, etc.) in recent decades.[20]

☼ In Canada, the vaccination schedule for babies begins at two months of age. A baby's body is not even capable of producing antibodies until it is 3-4 months old – so why on earth would you vaccinate a two month old baby?

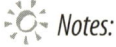 Notes:

The above facts each highlight a different facet of the vaccination question: Effectiveness, adverse effects, and long-term consequences. The unspoken thread running through each of these is a pressing question: Why haven't more people been informed of this evidence, and indeed, why is vaccination presented carte blanche as a positive, imperative requisite for our children's health? When my son Oscar was born, it became important to find out what is really going on with infant and childhood vaccination and whether it is conclusively a beneficial or necessary procedure. Prior to that, I assumed what most of us assume; that vaccination is something that prevents us from getting certain diseases. In short, I had assimilated the carefully disseminated propaganda of the pharmaceutical manufacturers.

Do Vaccines Actually Work?

As I researched the issue, I was amazed to discover that there is a large and growing body of clinical studies, fieldwork (in developing nations) and historical data refuting the safety and efficacy of vaccination. Unfortunately, the propaganda campaign for vaccination has been so successful that most of us automatically believe that vaccines are so effective they are responsible for the virtual eradication of serious childhood illnesses. In reality, this is not so, and if you examine the actual rates of incidence for each disease (from mainstream sources such as *The Lancet*, WHO and UNICEF), the graphs show a clearly different picture.

From the 1800's to the present, *in every case*, each disease had drastically declined decades before the introduction of the relevant vaccine; through improved hygiene, better nutrition, clean drinking water and improved sanitation. Basically, as people's overall health and immune systems improved, they didn't get sick. As the physician W.J. McCormick summarized in 1950 (before vaccines for measles, mumps, scarlet fever and rheumatic fever were introduced):

> "...the decline in diptheria, whooping cough and typhoid fever began fully fifty years prior to the inception of artificial immunization and followed an almost even grade before and after the adoption of these control measures. In the case of scarlet fever, mumps, measles

and rheumatic fever there has been no specific innovation in control measures, yet these also have followed the same general pattern in incidence decline." [21]

Furthermore, research reveals dozens of cases around the world where there was an outbreak of infectious disease (e.g., measles, polio, tetanus, smallpox, etc.) and contract rates were either similar among vaccinated and unvaccinated populations, or higher and more severe among the vaccinated.

For example:

- Massachusetts in 1961 experienced a 'type II' polio outbreak and "there were more paralytic cases in the triple vaccinates than in the unvaccinated." [22]

- In 1976, Dr. G.T. Stewart reported in the *British Medical Journal* that, "of 8,092 cases of whooping cough, 2,940 (36%) were fully immunized, while only 2,424 (30%) were definitely not immunized." [23]

- Professor George Dick, speaking at an environmental conference in Brussels in 1973, admitted that in recent decades, 75% of British people who contracted smallpox had been vaccinated. This, combined with the fact that only 40% of children (and a maximum of 10% of adults) had been vaccinated, clearly shows that vaccinated people have a much higher tendency to contract the disease.[24]

If vaccination is not responsible for the eradication of childhood illnesses, and vaccinated children are actually at a *greater* risk of contracting a disease than unvaccinated children, why is vaccination routinely presented as an effective safeguard for our children's health? When the historical data is referred to by pro-vaccine parties, it is often skewed and presented out of context. For example, in reference to a mass vaccination campaign carried out in Thailand:

> "...the immunization coverage for measles has increased from 6% in 1984 to 63% in 1988, leading to a reduction in measles prevalence from 93.7/100,000 in 1984 to 37.1/100,000 in 1986" [25]

From the 1800's to the present, in *every case*, each disease had been virtually eliminated *decades* before the introduction of the relevant vaccine; through improved hygiene, better nutrition, clean drinking water and improved sanitation.

However, what the report doesn't indicate is that in 1987, the infection rate of measles was 87.1/100,000. And in 1988 it was 59.1/100,000 which is actually *higher* than the rate of infection in 1982 (57.1/100,000) when no one had been vaccinated. These statistics however, are conveniently not included as they don't support the pro-vaccination stance of the report. Aside from establishing that vaccines are not the reason infectious childhood illnesses have virtually disappeared, and that vaccinated children are actually at a *greater* risk of contracting disease, there are also the adverse effects and long-term consequences of vaccination to be considered.

Effects Of Vaccination

Immediate Side Effects

Immediate or short-term effects of vaccination can include the following: encephalopathy (irreversible brain damage), ataxia (incoordination of voluntary muscle movements), mental retardation, aseptic meningitis (inflammation of the membranes of spinal cord or brain), seizure disorders, hemiparesis (half-body paralysis), retinopathy and blindness, hyperactivity, anaphylaxis, high pitched (encephalitic) screaming/prolonged crying, learning disorders, autism, hay fever, asthma, sudden infant death (SIDS), brachial plexus neuropathy (disease affecting nerves which serve the arm, forearm and hand), and abdominal pain. Secondary complications can include juvenile-onset diabetes, Reye's syndrome and multiple sclerosis.

Unfortunately, it's virtually impossible to determine the real incidence of damaging adverse reactions. For example, a British government report claims the rate of permanent neurological damage from the DPT vaccine to be 1 in 300,000.[26] However, other researchers indicate the permanent damage level to be anywhere from 1 in 62,000 to 1 in 300. Research by Coulter and Fisher on the 3.3 million children vaccinated yearly in the U.S. found there to be a total of 33,006 cases of acute neurological reactions (encephalitic screaming, convulsions, collapse) within 48 hours of receiving the DPT shot.

> There is no scientific evidence as to the actual frequency or incidence of vaccine-induced injury, so in fact we have no idea whether reactions are indeed rare, or, statistically significant.

LIFESTYLE & ENVIRONMENTAL FACTORS | **CHAPTER 4**

When the problems with vaccination are addressed in a serious manner by the pro-vaccination side, it usually involves a member of the bio-medical field qualifying that the dangers of vaccination, although real, are very rare, for example:

> "Parents must be informed of the rare possibility of serious adverse effects, including seizure and allergic reaction. Every physician who administers vaccines therefore needs to become familiar with the reactions that may occur with each immunologic agent used. The best safeguard against litigation, when and if a serious reaction follows vaccination, is the indication that these considerations were discussed and that an informed choice was made." [27]

However, there is no scientific evidence as to the actual frequency or incidence of vaccine-induced injury, so in fact we have no idea whether reactions are indeed rare, or, statistically significant. In articles such as the one above, no verifiable statistical evidence, reflecting reliable reporting or monitored studies for this 'rarity' is ever presented. As shown in the official minutes of the *15th session of the US Panel of Review of Bacterial Vaccines and Toxoids with Standards and Potency*:

> "Many physicians are not cognisant of the importance of reporting untoward reactions, or may be unaware of their clinical features. Further, both physicians and manufacturers have been held liable for damage suits by patients who may suffer adverse effects from established vaccines. All of these factors undoubtedly discourage reporting; without some other form of surveillance, definition of the rates and significance of untoward reactions to current and future vaccines cannot be ascertained." [28]

For this reason, it is suspected that the number of adverse reactions and vaccine-damaged children is actually much, much higher than is currently presented by the medical/pharmaceutical community. Instead, there is a growing number of mothers and lay people, whose children have been irrevocably damaged, forming vaccine risk awareness groups.
There continue to be incidents like the one in West Germany in 1967, where

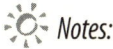 *Notes:*

smallpox vaccination damaged the hearing of 3,296 children, and of these 71 were rendered completely deaf.[29] At the extreme end of the spectrum, we have occurrences like the one in Australia's Northern Territory where malnourished aboriginal children were vaccinated and in some areas 50% of them died.[30] We have to question why autism rates (a common 'side effect' of vaccination) in California have increased 664% since 1997.[31] Whether these adverse reactions are caused by the vaccines themselves or the number of highly toxic additives contained in vaccines (e.g., formaldehyde, mercury, acetone, etc.), or a combination of the two, remains to be determined. As yet, no research has been carried out to resolve this question.

Long-Term Consequences

While these short-term consequences are alarming (especially if it happens to your child) the possible long-term consequences of vaccination are, in my opinion, even more of a worry. When you contract a disease naturally, the virus or bacteria normally enters via the body's natural filtration system – by being inhaled or swallowed and passing through the liver. With measles, for example, the airborne virus is carried first to the tonsils, then the lymph nodes and then into the spleen, blood and other organs. This succession produces a variety of reactions; sneezing, coughing or the secretion of a local antibody within the respiratory tract, all designed to expel or weaken the virus at its port of entry. With vaccines, foreign antigens are usually injected directly into the body's tissues and carried throughout the circulatory system, giving them direct access to all of the body's vital organs and systems. To bypass the body's natural defence system, and at such a young age, is simply asking for trouble. In addition, because the vaccine contains an attenuated (or weakened) form of the virus, the body doesn't activate its major inflammatory response, nor its non-specific immune defences.

Another long-term complication of vaccination involves the 'one cell-one antibody' rule. This means that once a B cell is committed to an antigen (disease-causing virus or bacteria), it becomes inert and incapable of responding to other antigens or attacks on the immune system. If a child contracts childhood diseases naturally, it is estimated that up to a total of

---

☼ Other researchers argue that these attenuated forms of the viruses remain in the body causing continual antigenic stimulation of the immune system – meaning the immune system is always in 'attack' mode – which also weakens it and leads to auto-immune diseases. This immunosuppressive effect is of particular interest to those of us diagnosed with IBD, especially Crohn's disease.

7% of their immune system is taken up with responding to these diseases. However, a child who undergoes the routine course of vaccinations, risks having up to 70% of his/her immune system committed to these antigens and no longer available for other immune challenges. Current research suggests this reduced immune-response capacity is responsible for increased susceptibility to other infections, allergies, and auto-immune diseases. Other researchers argue that these attenuated forms of the viruses remain in the body causing continual antigenic stimulation of the immune system – meaning the immune system is always in 'attack' mode – which also weakens it and leads to auto-immune diseases. This immunosuppressive effect is of particular interest to those of us diagnosed with IBD, especially Crohn's disease.

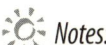
Notes:

A placebo-controlled trial of acellular pertussis vaccines in Sweden, compared vaccinated children with un-vaccinated children of the same birth grouping. During the trial, an invasive bacterial infection occurred among the vaccinated group resulting in numerous deaths. A review of the trial data led researchers to conclude that "The hypothesis of an immunosuppressive effect of the vaccines, which would explain the deaths…could not be refuted by the data." [32] As further evidence, one of the few double-blind trials that have ever been conducted on a vaccine shows the same immunosuppressive effect. In the trial, of the group who were vaccinated with the Salk polio vaccine, over 200 people went on to contract polio. Among the control group (unvaccinated), not one of them developed polio.[33]

Citing references from numerous valid sources, including four recognized textbooks on paediatrics and immunology, Harold Buttram, MD and John Hoffman, PhD, conclude that childhood vaccination "cannot help but have adverse effects on the immunologic system of the child, possibly leaving this system crippled in its ability to protect the child throughout life…opening the way for other diseases as a result of immunologic dysfunction." [34]

The other worrying aspect of live viral vaccines is that they introduce foreign genetic material into the human body. Dr. R. Moskowitz, MD and

> If a child contracts childhood diseases naturally, it is estimated that up to a total of 7% of their immune system is taken up with responding to these diseases. However, a child who undergoes the routine course of vaccinations, risks having up to 70% of his/her immune system committed to these antigens and no longer available for other immune challenges.

Harvard graduate, explains how this can lead to auto-immune disease susceptibility:

> "Vaccinal attenuated viruses attach their own genetic 'episome' to the genome (half set of chromosomes and their genes) of the host cell, and are thus capable of surviving or remaining latent within the host cells for years. The presence of foreign antigenic material within the host cell sets the stage for their unpredictable provocation of various auto-immune phenomena such as herpes, shingles, warts, tumors – both benign and malignant – and diseases of the central nervous system, such as varied forms of paralysis and inflammation of the brain." [35]

Dr. Markowitz states that in addition, vaccines do not just produce mild versions of the original disease, but all of them commonly produce a variety of their own symptoms. In some cases, "these illnesses may be considerably more serious than the original disease, involving deeper structures, more vital organs, and less of a tendency to resolve spontaneously. Even more worrisome is the fact that they are almost always more difficult to recognize." [36]

In addressing scientists at a conference sponsored by the American Cancer Society, Rutgers University professor R. Simpson warned:

> "Immunization Programs against flu, measles, mumps, polio and so forth may actually be seeding humans with RNA to form latent proviruses in cells throughout the body. These latent proviruses could be molecules in search of diseases, including rheumatoid arthritis, multiple sclerosis, systemic lupus erythematosus, Parkinson's disease and perhaps cancer." [37]

The bulk of the evidence gathered from numerous countries points out that not only is vaccination ineffective at preventing the spread of infectious disease, but vaccinated children are actually at a *higher* risk of contracting these illnesses. In addition, the adverse reactions to vaccination are much higher than presently documented in the medico-pharmaceutical literature and the long-term damaging effect of suppressing the immune system is rarely addressed.

In light of all the evidence to the contrary, why have vaccines been pressed upon the public as a necessary, beneficial way of preventing our children from getting sick? In the words of Dr. Raymond Obomsawin (who's held senior positions in UNICEF and CUSO), referring to mass vaccination, "It is reprehensible that such actions continue to be enforced by authorities, while parents and local health workers are not accorded any practical knowledge of the known dangers involved, and the extent to which there prevails a general ignorance of the longer term consequences." [38]

Combine this ignorance with the millions of dollars in profit generated by vaccination that goes straight into the pockets of manufacturing companies, governments and medical doctors, and it becomes clear that vaccination is more of a political and economic issue, than a health issue. Barbara Fisher, who served for ten years on the U.S. National Vaccine Advisory Committee states:

> "We have bad science and bad medicine translated into law to ensure that vaccine manufacturers make big profits, that career bureaucrats at the Public Health Service meet the mass vaccination goals promised to politicians funding their budgets, and pediatricians have a steady flow of patients...As the drug companies have often stated in meetings I have attended, if a vaccine they produce is not mandated to be used on a mass basis, they do not recoup their R&D costs and do not make the profit they want. In the medical literature official studies of vaccine risk are published purportedly proving there is no cause and effect. What the reader does not know is that often the studies have been designed and conducted by physicians who sit on vaccine policy-making committees at the Centers for Disease Control...some of whom receive money from vaccine manufacturers for their universities and for testifying as expert witnesses in vaccine-injury cases. And others are federal employees with an eye on career advancement within HHS and a future job with a vaccine manufacturer after

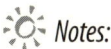
Notes:

retirement from public service. Many of these same physicians sit on the peer review boards of the major medical journals such as *Pediatrics* and *JAMA*, where they refuse space for studies or letters from the few brave physicians who dare to challenge their assertions that there is no cause and effect." [39]

When you take into account the billions of dollars at stake in vaccination campaigns, it is not surprising that vaccination propaganda is foisted upon the public with almost religious fervour. The intense psychological pressure and fear that parents feel about vaccinating their children is no accident, but the result of well-planned, well-funded marketing campaigns.

Needless to say, having completed my research, Oscar and his sister Zara remain completely un-vaccinated. As to whether you should vaccinate your child or not, only you can and should make that decision. It is very difficult to stand strong and resolute against the ubiquitous pressure to vaccinate. It's like having to keep insisting the earth is round when authorities, your community, intellectuals, and the majority of scientists etc. all insist it's flat. As with all matters of health, each of us has to go with what our gut tells us is right, or the best possible option for us at that time.

There are very effective alternatives to vaccination, but it's beyond the scope of this book to address that here (see www.alternativemedicine.com and do a keyword search on vaccination for more info). Also, any good naturopathic physician will be able to advise you of the alternatives and prescribe immune support measures for your child. For those of you who are wary of the dangers of vaccination but not quite strong enough – or convinced enough – to decline vaccination, there are a few options you might wish to explore:

▶ Only give your child the vaccines you feel are most necessary and omit the most dangerous ones, or the ones that have been banned in other countries. For example, opt for diphtheria and tetanus but omit the pertussis component of the DPT shot, skip the hepatitis B vaccine – especially in infants (200 doctors in France have banded together to try to get their government to ban it). The MMR (measles, mumps, rubella) shot has also been banned in several countries. Make sure your doctor uses only single-dose vaccines and shows you the package insert confirming there is no thimerosol (mercury) in it.

▶ If you do vaccinate, assist your child/baby's immune system before, during and after vaccination to reduce the risk of adverse effects. Dr. Lendon Smith (an Oregon pediatrician) administers the following to his patients: 1000 mg. vitamin C, 500 mg. calcium, 50 mg. vitamin B6 the day before, the day of vaccination, and the day after. Consult with your doctor (medical or naturopathic) as to the best amounts and delivery method of these immune support substances for your child. Continue to supplement with a full range of vitamins and minerals daily thereafter (use 100% natural preparations specially formulated for infants or children) along with the full spectrum of Natren brand probiotics. See the section on *Probiotic Supplementation* in Chapter Two for more instructions.

▶ Continue to educate yourself by reading other sources and conduct your own research on vaccination. Consider delaying vaccination until your child is at least two years old to minimize the risk of SIDS (Sudden Infant Death Syndrome).

If your child has already been vaccinated then begin immediately with Natren brand probiotics and daily vitamin C (500 – 1000 mg per day in mineral ascorbate form – Emergen-C is a very easy way to get kids to take their vitamin C) to help your child's immune system cope with and begin to repair the damage. In Canada, the vaccination schedule for babies begins at two months of age. If the whole basis for conferring immunity is the development of antibodies, then this point alone reveals that vaccination is primarily driven by profit, not health concerns: A baby's body is not even *capable* of producing antibodies until it is 3 – 4 months old – so why on earth would you vaccinate a two month old baby?

Obviously, as the mother of two children, this whole issue of vaccination and what's being done to our children's health is very distressing for me. Vaccination (among other factors) has so degraded our children's health in

☼ We have lost perspective on what a 'normal' healthy child looks like. Until we have a majority of people refusing vaccination, and pursuing natural, healthy lifestyles, there won't be a visible control group of what normal, healthy children can look and be like.

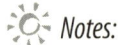 Notes:

the western world that people now think it's 'normal' for kids to be sick all the time. My five year old son Oscar (who has not been vaccinated, takes regular vitamin C and sporadic probiotics with a healthy organic diet) usually goes 6 – 9 months between colds. He's travelled to Malaysia, Hong Kong, Singapore, London, Barbados, Antigua, Mexico, Florida, Arizona, Michigan, California and Washington and the most serious illness he's had was croup. His cousin caught croup at the same time and endured two nights in the hospital, adrenalin drugs, and took five weeks to completely recover. Oscar recovered completely in six days – using only Eucalyptus steams, and receiving vitamin C and Astragalus through my breastmilk. My point in relating this is simply to illustrate that we have lost perspective on what a 'normal' healthy child looks like. Vaccination begins at such a young age now that our children don't stand a chance, and their immune systems are being damaged in a particularly insidious manner. Until we have a majority of people refusing vaccination, and pursuing natural, healthy lifestyles, there won't be a visible control group of what normal, healthy children can look and be like. I really encourage you to take a discriminating look at this issue, there is *much* more information available and I've been able to present only a very small selection of it here. Please educate yourself further until you feel you can make an informed decision. There are many more books, articles, and research papers available where scientists are beginning to speak out against vaccination – an Internet search using the keywords: 'dangers of vaccination' will pull these up for you.

IMPLEMENTING CHANGE

You may be feeling rather overwhelmed at this point by the number of changes you need to make in your diet and lifestyle – that's normal. It's very difficult to change lifelong tastes and habits overnight, so be patient with yourself. Proceed at your own pace of change. Some of you may be able to implement these changes in two weeks and stick to them. Others may require a slow evolution over the course of a year, gradually changing and adjusting to one thing at a time. Some people may take five or six years to complete all the changes they require. We're all different and have different ways of doing things, so do whatever works best for you, keeps you feeling positive and doesn't overwhelm and discourage you.

Your emotions affect your intestinal health just as much as the food you eat and the environment you live in. So if you're a slow-change kind of person and you implement all these changes right away, you're going to be stressed out and miserable, nothing will taste right or good to you and you'll begin to dread food shopping and preparation. These distressing emotions will then very nearly negate all the lifestyle and dietary benefits you're reaping, so what's the point? Slow down and do things at the pace of change that feels comfortable and positive for you. Any changes to promote and encourage your health, no matter how slowly implemented, are better than none. A great website for ongoing information about health, food, environment, etc. is *www.mercola.com*, be sure and sign up for Dr. Mercola's free newsletter as it's an excellent source of well-researched health information. I've been receiving his newsletter for a few years and the only issue to date that I've disagreed with him on is probiotics – he has promoted the use of bacterial soil organisms, which I am strongly opposed to (see Chapter Eight for more on this issue).

Also, be sure to always check in with yourself prior to making any of these changes and only do what feels necessary and right for you. Maybe your body is only nominally affected by toxins and so you only need to change a couple of things. Or maybe your system is very sensitive and you need to eliminate all the toxins listed and a few more besides. Again, only you know what's best for your body, so only change what you feel you need to.

Here in order of importance, are the top ten dietary and lifestyle changes you may want to make, at a pace that suits you:

1. Do not eat/drink foods containing preservatives, nitrites/nitrates, MSG, carrageenan, or any other man-made chemical compound. No processed foods. For specific dietary guidelines, see the *Maintenance Diet* in Chapter Three.

> Your emotions affect your intestinal health just as much as the food you eat and the environment you live in. So slow down and do things at a pace of change that feels comfortable and positive for you.

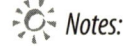 Notes:

2. Consume only organic food and beverages, or as much as possible.

3. Change to natural products for all substances and materials that come into contact with your skin.

4. Buy your food fresh, cook it in the oven or on the stovetop, and don't use a microwave.

5. Examine your job and relationships – do they support you and your health or tear it down? Make changes accordingly.

6. Switch to non-toxic materials for both cooking and storing food (e.g., stainless steel, glass, ceramic, porcelain).

7. Make sure the air pollution in your city is at acceptable levels for you, or else seriously consider moving.

8. Read up on the mercury amalgam filling toxicity issue and go for testing. At least have new fillings or replacement work done with the less toxic, white resin amalgam.

9. Try not to use cell phones. If you must, then don't carry them on your body and use an ear-piece with a ferrite bead attached, rather than holding the phone to your head.

10. Create a non-toxic sleeping environment in your bedroom. Gradually expand these guidelines to the rest of your house.

11. Research vaccination issues and refuse all vaccines for childhood, travel, flu, etc.

Now turn to the *Healing Journey Workbook* on the *Listen To Your Gut CD* and go through the Workbook questions and exercises for this chapter (Chapter Four).

5

Allopathic Medicine

> *"Healing in the deepest sense is a mystery. Even modern medicine with its pretext of being scientific rests upon observations that, at their heart, are unexplained.*
>
> *One of the definitive texts of pharmacology begins by reminding the reader that ultimately no one knows how any drug works. Of course, the average physician conveniently chooses to forget this and actually comes to believe that he knows what he's doing. There is no question that many of these formulations 'work' predictably. Yet when we expect a certain response from a particular treatment, we are more in the business of shuffling symptoms than in the business of healing."*
>
> Dr. Richard Moss, MD

In our society, we have grown up surrounded by an incredibly strong belief in allopathic (Western/modern) medicine and an equally strong belief in the power and authority of medical doctors. This can actually be a positive thing from a 'faith healing' perspective – in that whatever you believe will heal you, is most likely to. However, it can also produce negative results as the treatment protocols in allopathic medicine are often quite invasive and traumatic for the body. The other glaring shortcoming of allopathic (modern) medicine is that it views and treats the body primarily as a rational, logical machine. Drugs and treatments are often prescribed that are designed to affect one part of the body whilst disregarding their effects on other parts of the body. The short-term alleviation of symptoms is usually placed before consequent long-term damage and degeneration.

Fortunately, with the growing awareness of alternative treatment methods, people are also realizing that there are much kinder, gentler ways to effect healing in a manner that supports the whole body. These treatment protocols may take longer and require a bit more effort to implement, but they are worthwhile in that the healing effected is holistic and long-term.

We must take responsibility for the health and treatment of our bodies and determine what is acceptable and what is not. Allopathic (Western/modern) medicine and its beliefs and attitudes did not just spring forth from a void. They came from our culture and our society and were formed by our beliefs and desires. Julie Motz is an energy healer with a master's degree in public health from Colombia University, who has some interesting thoughts on this topic. She accompanies various surgeons in the operating room and administers energy healing whilst the surgery (open heart, neurosurgery, breast cancer, etc.) is in progress. In her book *Hands of Life* she writes:

> "It became more and more apparent to me that we have violent medicine because we have a violent society, and that the root of this violence is the cruelty and humiliation inflicted upon children by their parents. Disease is facilitated by the violence of childhood, and we can think of healing only in terms of matching this violence. That is why

we have a 'war' on cancer, and why surgeons see themselves as heroes on a bloody battlefield, dashing in to save lives. It is probably why we do not practice a great deal more preventive medicine." [1]

In the book, *Women's Bodies, Women's Wisdom*, Dr. Christiane Northrup MD says, "I believe that the modern medical preference for drugs and surgery as treatments is part of the aggressive patriarchal or addictive approach to disease. That which is natural and nontoxic is seen as inferior to the "big guns" of drugs, chemotherapy, and radiation."

Barbara Griggs in her book *Green Pharmacy – The History and Evolution of Western Herbal Medicine* also has an interesting comment to make:

> "It is a curious and depressing truth, demonstrated again and again in medical history, that the desire of the average physician to administer powerful and active drugs is only equalled by the desire of the average patient to have powerful and active drugs administered to him. This seems to have been just as true in the seventeenth century, when the dangers of such drugs were publicly trumpeted, as it is today when their side-effects – except in rare cases – are often merely noted in small type in the medical press." [2]

Take a few moments to examine your own attitudes and beliefs concerning your body and its functioning. Take a look at the type of healthcare and therapies you've chosen and ask yourself why you made those choices. Examine the efficacy of those choices; how and why did they help you or not help you, what are the long-term consequences, what have you learned from your experiences so far? Answering these questions will help you to determine why and how you've chosen your past and current methods of treatment and where you want to go from here. I'm not suggesting that you abandon all forms of allopathic treatment, I'm simply encouraging you to become fully aware of your treatment options and to pursue the methods that work best for you.

My personal belief is that allopathic medicine is very effective and valuable in high trauma, emergency situations – any type of violent accident

☼ In modern medicine, the short-term alleviation of symptoms is usually placed before consequent long-term damage and degeneration.

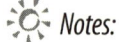 Notes:

situation, extremely premature births, hemorrhaging, intestinal rupture, etc. But for on-going, systemic health, we have other kinds of medicine and treatment protocols that are far more effective in the long-term. It is your responsibility to search out and educate yourself regarding these options and to make the effort required to secure the best treatment for your body. Obviously you're already on this path, or you wouldn't be reading this book. I encourage you to keep going, keep on exploring and experimenting. Hopefully, with all our efforts combined we can leave a much more effective, positive legacy of healthcare knowledge and practice to our children.

DRUGS

When people ingest a drug, the symptom disappears and they assume they're cured. If you want to have any success with natural, holistic healing, you must break out of this paradigm of 'healthcare'. Because, first of all, it's false. Drugs do not heal, they merely suppress symptoms. But, no matter how many times people have it demonstrated to them that drugs do not really heal, they automatically tend to think this way. We live in a short-term, fast food, instant reward society and drugs fit in seamlessly with this mindset. Someone takes a drug for depression and it makes them feel better, but then they become overweight because the drug has damaged their thyroid gland, and they rarely connect the two events. Then they take a drug for their thyroid gland, which then causes problem C, and so on and so on. Drugs do not heal. They merely suppress symptoms for a period of time. Now people with IBD are taking Remicade intravenously to suppress bleeding and ulceration in their intestines and winding up with Hepatitis, or Tuberculosis, or even dead, in exchange.

I'm well aware of the reasons why people take drugs. I grew up not even questioning the allopathic paradigm of healthcare (or, more accurately, disease management). I've been on Prednisone myself because I was ignorant, and I believed what my doctor told me. Don't waste time beating yourself up or lamenting the past. Learn and move forward. If you become aware of your past fears and motivations supporting your drug use, you'll be able to recognize them when they come around again. Knowledge is power. The more you become aware of what motivates you, the better you'll be able to address your shortcomings and change your course of action.

Suppression vs. Healing

It was my opinion that I could not be or feel completely healthy until I got myself off all long-term prescription drugs. As long as I was regularly ingesting such strong substances into my body, how could I expect my body to find its own state of balance and heal itself? Asking my body to heal itself whilst simultaneously overwhelming it with toxic substances (drugs) seemed to be a form of sabotage. The body works and heals holistically, everything works together as a whole.

Drugs do not heal. They merely suppress symptoms.

Unfortunately, when a pharmaceutical company develops a drug, their primary mandate is to develop a product that reliably produces a specific result. All the other results are labeled "side effects" as if they're somehow less important and impact less on the body – which of course they don't. Let's look at steroids as an example: You may take them to suppress inflammation, but at the same time you're sacrificing adrenal gland functioning, inhibiting the absorption of essential vitamins and minerals, stressing the liver and decreasing bone formation. Each of these problems (side effects!) then leads to consequent further (and often synergistic) damage to the body. For example, the adrenal gland produces certain key hormones which then interact with other glands and also play key roles in other hormone production pathways – which in turn interact, balance, and serve your body in hundreds of different ways. I could actually write a small book outlining and tracing the domino-effect damage that steroid medication causes in the body. And if you're a developing child, you're doing even more systemic damage to your body, affecting developing organs and systems:

> "Steroid treatment of asthmatic children has been demonstrated to retard lung maturation and physical growth and to cause a higher incidence of cataracts in children receiving long-term steroid therapy." [3]

When Prednisone was first released, Dr. Mendelsohn relates how it was strictly mandated to be used only in "life threatening conditions".[4] The composition of Prednisone and its effects on the body have not changed. However, it is now used for suppressing a range of symptoms, none of which are classified as 'life threatening'. Why? Is it because doctors have grown familiar and comfortable with prescribing Prednisone? Or is it because they now have drugs that are so much more damaging than Prednisone (like Remicade or Imuran) that they make Prednisone look mild in comparison? Because of the way they're developed and the mindset of the pharmaceutical companies, drugs end up causing a short-term suppression of symptoms, whilst impairing and interfering with long-term healing. Consequently, their use results in damage and malfunction that often takes longer to heal than the original symptom.

It's very difficult to get yourself out of the allopathic paradigm where drugs = cure. In my opinion, drugs do not effect healing. Drugs merely suppress symptoms, for a short period of time. Then your symptoms will recur, or escalate, and become more systemic or more severe. Since pharmaceutical drugs consist of molecularly altered compounds that do not exist in nature, they will also function as poisons, or toxins in your body. So, in addition to the damage they cause your organs, tissues, bones, hormonal and immune system, etc., the drugs you ingest will then also need to be cleansed from your body before true, root-level healing can take place. In his book, *Tales From the Medicine Trail*, Chris Kilham writes:

> "I am committed to the development and promotion of plant-based medicines, because they are far and away safer, gentler, and better for human health than synthetic drugs. This is so because human beings have co-evolved with plants over the past few million years. We eat plants, drink their juices, ferment and distill libations from them, and consume them in a thousand forms. Ingredients in plants, from carbohydrates, fats and protein to vitamins and minerals, are part of our body composition and chemistry. Some compounds perform the same functions in plants that they do in the body. Natural antioxidant phenols in plants, for example, protect plant cells from oxidation, and

☼ When Prednisone was first released, it was strictly mandated – by the manufacturer – to be used only in "life threatening conditions".

they often perform the same function in the human body. Our bodies know the substances that occur in plants, and they possess sophisticated mechanisms for metabolizing plant materials. The same cannot be said about synthetic drugs. These agents are most often alien to the chemistry of the human body, and they're separate and apart from the careful crafting of evolution. Synthetic drugs often act in the body as irritants and toxins, upsetting the balance of whole systems and producing side effects that can be lethal." [5]

You may have initially taken a drug to suppress a distressing symptom – thereby giving yourself temporary relief from pain, worry, fear, difficulty, depression, etc. However, you will then have an even bigger problem on your hands as you are now left with not only the symptom (which will eventually return as you have not addressed or healed the root cause), but also the damage caused by the drug to numerous other parts and systems of your body, plus the burden of detoxifying your body from the poisonous drug. You have sacrificed the long-term health and functioning of your body. Your fear and pain (and often ignorance) has caused you to ingest a damaging substance that provides only short-term relief.

> Drugs merely suppress symptoms, for a short period of time. Then your symptoms will recur, or escalate, and become more systemic, or more severe.

Symptoms Or Messages?

I once heard from a young woman who was following the exclusively elemental diet and supplementation plan from my book, *The IBD Remission Diet,* and she had completely weaned off all prescription drugs and seen real improvement in her health. However, in her fifth week of the diet she developed joint pain and erythema nodosum (swollen, painful nodules on the skin). So she immediately went back on Prednisone! Do joint pain and swollen, painful nodules constitute a life threatening condition? She didn't give her body any time to work through these symptoms, or question what was the root cause of them. Maybe these symptoms were byproducts of the detoxification process – two of the drugs she'd been on for a long time cause joint pain and erythema nodosum as 'side effects'. Maybe they were symptoms of a severely unbalanced hormonal system that required natural hormone supplementation to be brought back into balance.

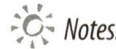 Notes:

Maybe these two symptoms would have automatically resolved when she began probiotic supplementation at the end of the diet. She didn't take the time to find out, or support her body in its healing path. Instead, she quickly ingested a very damaging drug to suppress the symptoms. Whether she did so out of fear or ignorance, I was still saddened that she would sabotage her health and efforts thus far in this manner. Well, who can speak for another person? And she probably had numerous reasons for her actions. But the end result was two steps forward, one step back (or maybe two steps back). Unfortunately, she concluded from this that the elemental diet didn't work very well for her.

But natural healing doesn't work that way. We've been trained by the medical system to expect instant relief (suppression of symptoms) and when we don't get it, we think the natural treatment method isn't working. A pathway of natural healing involves many twists and turns, especially since true healing involves healing the mind, body and spirit. When a symptom comes up (or reappears), instead of just finding out how to get rid of it, you need to first ask yourself, "Why is this symptom here? What's my body trying to tell me? What is the message here for me?" The answer will form part of the treatment to heal that symptom. As your body sends you messages (symptoms) for what needs healing next, try to stick with your body and continue to support it and heal it, rather than just using a drug to suppress the symptom. Replace words like 'flare' and 'symptom' with the word 'message' and see how that alters your feelings and attitude towards your body. Instead of saying, "The erythema nodosum have reappeared again, how do I get rid of them?" Try saying, "My body's developed swollen, painful, nodules…what does that mean…what's my body trying to tell me?" The answer will probably be a mixture of physical and emotional reasons, and only you will be able to decipher the message from your body telling you what it needs you to do next.

Let me give you an example from my own life of how this whole process of 'symptoms as messages' can work: I started bleeding from my colon seven months after the birth of my second child. I passed out from dehydration, so went to the hospital and received four bags of saline. I refused a blood transfusion as my hemoglobin was only 73 and that's not low enough to warrant the risk of a transfusion, in my opinion. I immediately used *Jini's Healing Implant Enema* to stop the bleeding (it took only two applications) and then went on the IBD Remission Diet for two weeks to facilitate thorough healing. When I connected with my body/spirit to find out why this had occurred and what my body was trying to tell me, I realized several things. First of all, my body had been trying for months to get the message to me using lesser signs; mouth ulcers, gas, fatigue, sugar cravings, mild pain after or during eating, etc. Only when I failed to heed any of these messages did it clunk me over the head with the one sign/message I couldn't ignore – intestinal bleeding gets my attention like nothing else!

The message or teaching my body/higher self was trying to give me encompassed several issues in my life – some physical and some emotional. Firstly, I wasn't getting nearly enough sleep at night as my daughter was teething, and waking up to ten times a night in discomfort, wanting to be breastfed back to sleep. I was then getting up after only a few hours sleep and doing a full day's work looking after both children, cooking, housekeeping, and working in my office when I could. My husband and I share parenting and housekeeping duties equally. But to give you an idea of the workload, he's a very healthy, fit/muscular man, getting a full night's sleep and he was still exhausted. Secondly, due to the demands of the kids and my escalating stress levels, I wasn't eating enough at mealtimes, and due to my fatigue I was then using sugary foods to give me the energy to keep going.

Next, when I looked at *why* I was doing these physical things to my body, the emotional reasons became clear. I found it very difficult to say, 'no' – to my children, my husband, business associates, etc. Out of guilt and some kind of 'strongman' complex, I was trying to do it all. Also, I must point out that extended sleep deprivation interferes with your ability to think and make decisions. It's very easy to get into an inefficient or damaging feedback loop and be too exhausted to see it, or figure out how to break it.

> We've been trained by the medical/drug system to expect instant relief (suppression of symptoms) and when we don't get it, we think the natural treatment method isn't working.

Jini Patel Thompson | **LISTEN TO YOUR GUT**

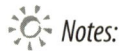 Notes:

After addressing the physical component of my healing path, I also had to address the emotional component, otherwise I wouldn't fully heal, or, I would be sick again fairly quickly. I had asked my mum to come out and help during my convalescence and I stayed in bed for two weeks, sleeping and allowing my body to heal. My mum also took my daughter at night and gradually (with no trauma, crying, etc.) taught her how to sleep through the night without breastfeeding, so as to provide a long-term solution to my sleep deprivation problem.

As I was lying there in bed recovering, having ample time to read, take a bath whenever I wanted to, having all my meals (shakes, broths & jello!) brought to me, I realized: I have a better life now! What motivation do I have to get well? So that I can return to the life of drudgery and exhaustion I've been living? How had my life become so pathetic? So my next line of thinking was, "Okay, what do I need to change in my life to make me want to get well, to make me look forward to getting out of bed in the morning?" As a result of that exploration, I hired one of my son's sports camp teachers to babysit two nights a week from 4 – 8 pm. Tuesdays became my night to myself or to go out with a girlfriend, and my husband went out to play soccer with his friends. Thursdays were designated date night with my hubby – we would usually catch a matinee movie and then dinner.

I also hired a cook/housekeeper to come in from 4 – 8 pm three nights a week (Monday, Wednesday, Friday) and what a difference she made! She did all the laundry, tidied up the house, made supper and a dessert (enough for two meals), then cleaned up after and left a sparkling kitchen. If one of the kids was grumpy during dinner, she played with them so that I could actually eat a full meal, undisturbed! I then also hired a cleaner to come in every Saturday morning to thoroughly clean the whole house, change beds, do laundry, etc. Could we financially afford all this help? Yes and no. But as my husband and I agreed, our children are our first priority. In order to take care of our kids properly, we both have to be healthy and happy. We decided that even if we have to go into debt for the next few years, it's worth it. Once the kids are in school, we'll have more time to work the hours necessary to pay off any debts. Then, to fully round out my healing,

I released the pain and trauma of the past few months and the bleeding episode from my colon with my bodywork therapist, whilst embracing and affirming the new knowledge and balance that had come into my life. I also had several sessions with a hypnotherapist to address the root issues involved.

Now, if I had taken my colonic bleeding as a sign that natural healing methods didn't work, and just gone on Prednisone or Remicade to suppress the symptoms, what a tremendous opportunity for learning and growth I would have missed – for myself and my family. And think of the extensive, systemic damage the drugs would have done and how long it would have taken me to heal from that. Instead I simply addressed the bleeding, and then determined and healed the root causes. Your body is *always* advocating on your behalf, it's up to you to decide what to do with the messages and opportunities it gives you.

> Your body is always advocating on your behalf, it's up to you to decide what to do with the messages and opportunities (i.e. symptoms) it gives you.

Symptoms Or Side Effects?

I've often received emails from people who are following the recommended treatments in this book, but still experiencing a particular symptom. One of the first things I've learned to ask is, "Which medications or other supplements are you also taking?" Usually, the person is also taking a drug (or in some cases a natural supplement) that causes the exact same symptom they can't seem to heal. As you read through the list of possible drug side effects listed below, you may also want to ask yourself, "What kind of damage is this drug doing to my body that it could produce these kinds of symptoms?" And is the suppression of symptom 'A' worth incurring additional symptoms 'B, C, D and E'? If I recommended an herb in this book that would stop diarrhea, but also cause nausea, gas, headaches and fever, would anyone want to take it? And wouldn't you think I was ridiculous for even suggesting you take it? In fact, wouldn't you think that a method of 'healing' that causes extensive, additional damage is a tad insane?

I was contacted by a medical doctor who was thinking about putting his daughter on 6-MP, but he was worried whether that would interfere with her hormonal system. However, his daughter had already been on

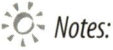 Notes:

Prednisone and Remicade – both of which completely impair adrenal gland function. The adrenal gland produces hormones that are inextricably intertwined with hormonal pathways and production throughout the body – and other glands require hormones from the adrenal gland as 'building blocks' for the hormones they produce. Her hormonal system had already been extensively damaged and 'interfered with'. This man is a medical doctor, he knows all this (and in much greater detail than me). But he too is blind to the reality of prescription drug use: Suppression of a particular symptom(s) simultaneously damages the body, with the subsequent damage often being worse than the original symptom you are seeking to suppress. Nothing in the body functions independently, everything is interlinked with far-reaching, or, domino-like consequences. Nothing in your body functions in isolation. When you look at the list of side effects for a drug, think about what system, glands, organs, etc. must be being damaged by that drug to produce such a symptom and think about the ramifications of that on your health and body.

Often when you present your doctor with your concerns about side effects, she'll pull up the pharmaceutical data on placebo-controlled trials and show you that the incidence of these side effects is quite low, so you don't need to worry. Firstly, you may be one of the minority that experiences those side effects, so it is a concern. Secondly, I have heard from too many people who are experiencing supposedly 'rare' side effects from particular drugs to conclude that the rates of incidence indicated in pharmaceutical trials play out the same way in reality. The reason for this disparity, I cannot say – although recent reports seem to indicate that pharmaceutical companies have not been totally honest in their drug reporting, and in some cases have deliberately misrepresented or suppressed studies/results that don't support their drug. Keep this in mind when considering a drug or when trying to sort out your own symptom profile – don't just look at the 'common' side effects, look at the ones designated as 'rare' too. For example, I have heard from dozens of readers so far who were following all the appropriate natural healing methods and still experiencing bloody diarrhea. However, once they discontinued taking Asacol, their bloody diarrhea soon disappeared.

You also need to read the complete 'side effects' list for drugs you may be taking for other conditions. One of my phone consultation clients was convinced her colitis started after she took Zoloft (an antidepressant) but all the doctors she'd told her theory to quickly dismissed her concerns. So I looked up the pharmaceutical information for Zoloft and sure enough – one of the "common" side effects listed was Gastroenteritis, and one of the "rare" side effects listed was colitis!

I can understand using drugs as a short-term, emergency therapy; when you're really scared and haven't yet discovered an alternative therapy that works. Sometimes we take drugs because we're simply not aware that there are effective natural alternatives. Other times we may take drugs because we are afraid, because someone else (a doctor, a family member) tells us we must, otherwise this or that terrible thing will happen. What they don't usually tell you, or even know, is all the terrible things that may happen to you because you're taking the drugs. Or perhaps we take the pills because deep down we're lazy, because we don't really want to expend the time and energy necessary to investigate why and how our bodies have become so pain-full, so full of dis-ease and it's so much easier to pop a few pills and hope that looks after it. As long as we're following an authority figure's direction for our health, we just need to do as we're told, right? Wrong. No one inherently possesses any authority except that which you give to them. You are still responsible for your own health, whether you appoint someone else as your authority, or whether you appoint yourself.

It's really important for you to take a balanced, discriminating look at yourself and your motives. Ask yourself, "Why am I taking each of these drugs?" If you discover you're taking drugs mainly out of fear, then your next step is to determine whether the time is right to face your fear, or whether it's best for you to keep using the drugs until you're in a stronger place. I'm certainly not advising anyone to discontinue their prescription drugs prematurely. You have to be ready, with an alternative plan in place, and the timing has to be right for you. I encourage you to look at the alternatives and then follow a course of treatment that feels right for you. Some of you may not feel safe tapering off your drugs until you've used the

> Often, people are simultaneously taking a drug (or in some cases a natural supplement) that is causing the exact same symptom they can't seem to heal.

diets, supplements and therapies in this book often enough to feel really comfortable and fluent with them. No problem, please always follow your own intuition and what you feel is appropriate and safe for you. Some people are also able to use drug therapy very sparingly and find it effective as a short-term or stop-gap measure. If you're one of these people and it's working for you then great, by all means continue with what feels right for your body.

Here are some of the common drugs used in IBD and IBS treatment protocols and some of the 'side effects' you may experience. This information was provided by registered pharmacists and/or the drug manufacturer. For a complete list of side effects, contraindications and drug interactions (harmful interactions when taken with certain other drugs), please see the package insert or your pharmacist's CPS (Compendium of Pharmaceuticals and Specialties) listing:

Azathioprine (also known as Imuran)
Nausea, vomiting, diarrhea, fever, leukopenia (reduction in circulating white blood cell count), bone marrow suppression, thrombocytopenia (abnormally low platelets), fungal, viral or bacterial infections, myalgias (muscle pain), immunosuppression.

Ciprofloxacin (also known as Cipro)
Pseudomembranous colitis, diarrhea, painful oral mucosa, gastrointestinal bleeding, difficulty swallowing, flatulence, thrush, tendon rupture (eg. achilles tendon), erosion of cartilage in weight-bearing joints, convulsions, increased intracranial pressure, toxic psychosis, photosensitivity, central nervous system stimulation; lightheadedness, dizziness, confusion. There have been deaths due to anaphylactic shock and cardiovascular collapse. Should not be used by anyone with seizure disorders.

Infliximab (also known as Remicade)
Tuberculosis (70 reported cases as of 2001 and four deaths), invasive fungal infections and other opportunistic infections, can cause death in people with congestive heart failure (seven deaths as of 2001), immunosuppression.

Mercaptopurine (also known as 6-MP, Leukerin, Mercaleukin, Purinethol)

Unusual tiredness/weakness, yellow eyes or skin, nausea, vomiting, mouth ulcers, diarrhea, skin rash, hepatoxicity (impaired liver function), fever, joint pain, loss of appetite, blood in stool or urine, unusual bleeding or bruising, painful or difficult urination, swelling of feet or lower legs.

Mesalamine (also known as Asacol, Pentasa, Canasa, Rowasa and Salofalk)

Gastritis, diarrhea, abdominal discomfort or pain, heartburn, back or joint pain, oral ulcers, bloody diarrhea, loss of appetite, hair loss, headaches, dizziness, runny or stuffy nose, sneezing, acne, erythema nodosum, urticaria (hive-like rash), pancreatitis, cholecystitis, neck pain, edema, Lupus-like syndrome, anemia, thrombocytopenia (abnormally low platelets), eosinophilia (abnormal chest X-ray findings), leukopenia (a reduction in circulating white blood cell count), lymphadenopathy (lymph nodes with abnormal size, consistency and number), gout, depression, confusion, pneumonia, asthma exacerbation, interstitial nephritis, dysuria (pain on urination), urinary urgency, hematuria (blood in urine), epididymitis (inflammation of the epididymis duct behind the testis, along which sperm passes to the vas deferens – leads to testicular pain and swelling), menorrhagia (excessive bleeding during menstrual periods).

Metronidazole (also known as Flagyl, Trichozole, Protostat)

Diarrhea, nausea or vomiting, loss of appetite, dizziness, abdominal pain or cramps, vaginal irritation, discharge or dryness, skin rash, hives or itching, sore throat and fever, dark urine.

Prednisone (also known as Apo-prednisone, Novo-prednisone, Deltasone, Orasone)

'Moon face', hump of fat on upper back, abdominal bloating, weight gain, burning/painful stomach, mood changes, depression, insomnia, shakiness, weakness of thigh muscles, interruption of menstrual cycle, increased risk of infections, easy bruising of the skin, stretch marks, excessive growth of body hair, cataracts, osteonecrosis or 'dead bone' (often affects the hip joint),

> No one inherently possesses any authority over you or your body, except that which you give to them. You are still responsible for your own health, whether you appoint someone else as your authority, or whether you appoint yourself.

osteoporosis (which often leads to fractures, particularly in the spine), heart attacks (if you also smoke and have high blood pressure and high sugar levels).

* A glucocorticosteroid called Budesonide (Entocort) also causes these same side effects.

Sulphasalazine (also known as Azulfidine, Salazopyrin)

Nausea, vomiting, gastrointestinal discomfort, flatulence (gas), rashes, allergies, irritability, headaches, insomnia, reversible reduction in sperm count, fever, fatigue, Lupus-like syndrome, blood count abnormalities (requires monitoring blood count every three months), hepatoxicity (requires monitoring liver function every three months at least).

Tegarosod (also known as Zelnorm)

The FDA has added new warning information to the label of Zelnorm. Patients are warned to stop taking Zelnorm immediately if they develop rectal bleeding, bloody diarrhea, or new or worsening abdominal pain. These are symptoms of intestinal ischemia in which the supply of blood and oxygen to the intestines are compromised. Zelnorm can cause severe diarrhea that can result in dehydration and a need for intravenous fluids. Therefore, Zelnorm also should be stopped if diarrhea occurs. Can also cause headaches and should not be used if you have bowel obstructions, abdominal adhesions, renal or hepatic impairment, or gallbladder disease.

Weaning Off Prescription Medication

If you decide to wean yourself off your drugs and your doctor will cooperate with you, excellent. But you may find that easier said than done. I was reading an Internet posting once from an American fellow and he mentioned that if you tried to diverge from your doctor's advice at all, he/she would notify your insurance company that you were behaving "AMA" (Against Medical Advice), and it would be very difficult for you to get insurance or a renewal. So if you feel that you should be off drugs, and your doctor disagrees with you, then find a new doctor who's more open-minded and willing to work with you, not against you. The following tapering off procedure is probably similar to what your doctor will recommend.

*Please remember that all the information in this book is simply my own opinion. I am not a medical professional, and you undertake all therapies and procedures at your own risk and liability.

Never just stop taking a drug. An abrupt change would be very stressful and probably trigger a flare in symptoms. Always gradually bring your body off the drug, giving yourself time to adjust, whilst simultaneously following the appropriate *Healing Diet*, exercising, taking care of yourself emotionally, using the appropriate herbal supplements, and getting plenty of sleep and relaxation time. If you've been on a mild drug, or haven't been on the drug for very long, e.g., two months, you can do a 'fast taper' in which you just halve the dosage every week until you're down to half a pill (which you take for a week), and then you stop. However, if you're on a stronger drug (like Prednisone) which you've been on for six months or more, you'll have to do a 'slow taper' similar to what's outlined below. You need to slowly taper off the drug in order to give your body time to kick in and re-start the functioning that was suppressed by taking the drug.

> Never just stop taking a drug. An abrupt change would be very stressful and probably trigger a flare in symptoms.

Slow Taper Procedure
e.g., Prednisone – Current dosage: 10 mg/pill, 6 pills/day.

Start by dropping to 3 pills/day (30mg.) for two weeks.

Week Three and Four:	1 ½ pills/day (15mg.)
Week Five and Six:	1 pill/day (10mg.)
Week Seven and Eight:	½ pill/day (5mg.)
Week Nine:	¼ pill/day (2.5mg.)
Week Ten:	¼ pill/every other day (2.5mg)
Week Eleven:	Nothing.

Keep in mind that the tapering schedules outlined here are simply guidelines for you to use and you should feel free to adjust them in whichever way you feel is best for your body. For example, using the Prednisone slow taper outlined above, you may want to reduce to the dosage listed in Week five and six and then stay at that for the next month before reducing your dosage again. Use your intuition (see *Dialoguing With*

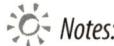 Notes:

Your Body in Chapter Six if you're not sure about how to listen to your body) and wean yourself off your drugs at the pace that's right for you. If you go too fast and don't allow your body enough time to activate and implement its own healing mechanisms, you'll only set your healing back. Also, you need to make sure you're simultaneously following the appropriate Healing Diet and taking whichever herbal supplements will help you at that time. Adding a bodywork therapy and emotional healing tool to your support structure (see Chapter Six) will also greatly aid you in your healing process. If your medical doctor won't work with you on this issue, then please find a naturopathic physician who will, as this will help you feel a lot more confident and secure through the ups and downs that will undoubtedly ensue.

Remember that most of the drugs used in treatment of IBD (and some for IBS) are very strong, systemic drugs. Therefore, they cause a great deal of damage and will also likely make you feel ill when your body starts to detoxify and flush out these drugs. Do not expect to stop your drugs, implement natural healing methods and just feel better with every day that passes. When you're weaning yourself off drugs – and during the root-level healing process that will follow – go back and read Chapter One again, so you have a better idea of what to expect on your healing pathway. Expect ups and downs, expect short-term recurrences or periodic worsening of symptoms (healing crises). But know that if you stay with your body during these times and allow it to detoxify itself, or give you additional messages about what needs healing, then you will reap the rewards in abundance. If you stay tuned and connect with your body during these healing crises, you'll know what you need to do next. Don't give your authority away to me, or your doctor, or anyone else during these times. You are the only one who knows what's best for your body and you may feel led to do something that I disagree with, or your doctor, or family disagrees with, stay with your own body and follow its guidance above all else.

Follow your own path and only do what you feel is right and safe for you. You may choose to combine elements of what's listed in this book with drug therapy, if it works for you, great! You may also want to take a long time and wean yourself off each of your drugs very, very slowly. You know what's best for you, so check in with yourself and your body regularly and follow your own intuition.

If you've been on drugs for longer than six months in a row, please make an appointment to see a naturopath to find out which organ and gland functioning is being interfered with as a result of the drugs you're ingesting. Your naturopathic doctor can then prescribe you the appropriate herbs and vitamins necessary to reduce toxicity and stimulate normal functioning in the affected glands and organs. But remember to follow the guidelines in Chapter Two when introducing new supplements. Acupuncture is also very effective for stimulating organ and glandular functions.

Immunosuppressive Drugs & Hormonal Health
If you've been taking any of the immunosuppressive drugs (like Prednisone, Remicade, Imuran, etc.) for three months or longer, your hormonal (endocrine) system will most likely be out of balance and this can cause far-reaching consequences in the body. Immunosuppressive drugs can suppress the function of the adrenal, thyroid and pituitary glands, thus interfering with normal hormone production. However, as hormonal health is still a relatively new field, you need to find a physician (MD or ND) who specializes in hormones and has lots of experience reading and interpreting hormone tests combined with symptom profiles.

I had two doctors (an MD and an ND) tell me my hormone levels were normal, when I knew intuitively there was something wrong with them. I was eating three meals plus two protein shakes per day and I was still losing weight. I was freezing cold all the time and even when I used a hot water bottle or bath to warm up, I wouldn't stay warm afterwards. I was very irritable and felt depressed many days, and I was usually very tired. I finally found a doctor who specialized in hormone health and she ascertained that indeed, my thyroid was low, my cortisol levels very high, and my estrogen, progesterone and testosterone were all very low

☼ Expect ups and downs, expect short-term recurrences or periodic worsening of symptoms (healing crises). But know that if you stay with your body during these times and allow it to detoxify itself, or give you additional messages (symptoms) about what needs healing, then you will reap the rewards in abundance.

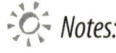 Notes:

as well. I began supplementing with raw adrenal gland extract, thyroid extract, DHEA, and natural progesterone cream. From my *second* day of supplementation, I was no longer cold and I began gaining about three pounds per week. My mental/emotional symptoms also subsided very quickly and my energy increased proportionately.

If you're a woman over the age of twenty, I highly recommend you purchase a book called, *What Your Doctor May Not Tell You About Premenopause* by John R. Lee, MD and Jesse Hanley, MD. Don't let the title mislead you, this is the best book on hormonal imbalances I have read, and all the factors – from birth control pills to synthetic clothing to emotional/lifestyle factors – that contribute to hormonal imbalance are covered. The book also goes into hormone testing and therapy in detail so it's an invaluable resource guide if you suspect your hormone levels are off, or that your adrenal or thyroid are not functioning properly. Men who've been on immunosuppressants will also find this book helpful. As well, there's a booklet (geared more specifically to men) available in most health stores called *Natural Progesterone Cream: Safe and Natural Hormone Replacement* (A Keats Good Health Guide) by C. Norman Shealy, MD, PhD, that is helpful – particularly if you have, or your family has, a history of prostate gland problems.

Most hormonal supplements your naturopath prescribes can just be added to a daily protein shake along with the rest of your supplements, if you prefer. DHEA is tasteless, raw adrenal extract is pretty bland as long as it doesn't have other substances added, raw thyroid extract (like Armour Thyroid) is a very small pill that can be swallowed or chewed easily. Do not take synthetic hormones as they do not have the same holistic, supportive effect on the body – make sure all hormones and thyroid or adrenal supplements are 100% natural. You may also want to try homeopathic thyroid and adrenal support medicines. During my second pregnancy, I used a homeopathic formula that provided support for my liver, spleen, thyroid, pituitary, pancreas and adrenal glands and found it effective. We monitored my thyroid levels (TSH) throughout my pregnancy with blood tests, and the homeopathic remedy alone (along with good diet, nutritional supplements and exercise) resulted in consistent, marked improvement throughout the pregnancy. A hypothyroid condition can cause mental retardation in the fetus so it's not something you want to take chances with! Above all, if you suspect you have a hormonal imbalance the important thing is to find a doctor who *specializes* in hormones – an ordinary medical doctor (MD) or naturopathic doctor (ND), or gastroenterologist, will not be skilled enough to interpret your test results and symptoms accurately. You need to find a medical doctor or naturopathic doctor where the majority of their practice consists of people with hormonal (endocrine) problems.

SURGERY

Regarding surgery, I maintain a similar stance to drug use – not for me, thanks! Prior to my departure from the medical system, my doctor was insisting that I *must* have gastrointestinal surgery. Sure I've gone through some pretty rough periods since, but I'm still here and doing quite nicely, in fact, much better than the people I know who've had the recommended surgery (or five). My resolve did falter at one point and I gave in to having surgery to remove some external perianal skin tags back in 1988.
They weren't bothering me at all, but the doctor was worried they might be malignant. Not surprisingly, they were benign and promptly grew back in six months. What a waste of time, trauma, pain, and damage that was! Like drugs, surgery for inflammatory bowel disease does not address the root cause, it merely cuts out the section of the body that is displaying the symptom. Surgery does not heal, it just temporarily removes the symptom. Like drugs, it is a short-term solution that often escalates over time as the body is increasingly damaged. Obviously, like drugs, this is also an area where you'll have to make your own decisions based on what you feel is best for your body.

I have managed to stay so strong in my resolve to avoid internal surgery at all costs, because of the research I did prior to making my departure from the medical establishment. At that time (1988), every textbook I read on Crohn's stated that when surgery was performed, the disease, for some

> Immunosuppresive drugs can suppress the function of the adrenal, thyroid and pituitary glands, thus interfering with normal hormone production – causing far-reaching consequences.

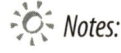 Notes:

unknown reason, jumped to a minimum of three new sites. Again, this struck me as the same flawed reasoning that was behind drug therapy; short-term relief at a tremendous cost and worsening of the condition long-term. More recent reports indicate there is a 40-80% chance of the disease recurring close to the resection (the statistics vary depending on which study you read), with the number of years between surgery and recurrence being roughly proportionate to the severity of the initial condition.

I once read a report of a woman with Crohn's who was so ill she was close to death, so her doctors felt she might as well try a risky, untested surgical procedure in the hope it might prolong her life. Thus, she received a complete intestinal (small and large intestine) transplant. Even on massive doses of immunosuppressive drugs, her new healthy intestine had Crohn's throughout within seven months. This is further evidence that IBD is a whole-body phenomenon, as the author of the report concludes:

> "The findings in this case suggest that factors other than immune mechanisms are involved in the pathogenesis of this disease and support the theory that Crohn's disease may be an exaggerated response to environmental triggers such as infection, enteric microflora, nicotine, or drugs in genetically susceptible individuals." [6]

I often consult with readers whose colitis has progressed to the point where they are seriously considering a colostomy (complete removal of the colon). Their doctors often tell them that their problems will be over and they'll be pretty much disease-free after a colostomy. However, if you go to the support-group websites for people who've *had* a colostomy or J-pouch surgery, you get a completely different story. There, you will discover that 45% of the people who've had a colostomy suffer recurrent, ongoing infections of their J-pouch. And many of them report that this causes symptoms similar to, and in some cases worse than, their original colitis! So if you are considering a surgical procedure, make sure you visit a few support-group or message board type websites for people who've already been through the procedure. And don't focus on the ones who've recently had surgery, but listen to what the people are saying 6 months or one year following the surgery.

Personally, I believe we will have much better results if we treat and heal the whole mind/body rather than just try to medicate or cut out the currently affected part. No matter how bad my condition has become, I have always been able to heal it naturally using the *Healing Diets*, herbal supplements, bodywork therapies and visualization techniques listed in this book. Yes it can be scary at times and it can also take a lot of work and self-discipline, but it is so very much worth it. I also make extensive use of spiritual and energy healing therapies, because contrary to popular belief, 'miracles' are not so few and far between. If you feel you're inevitably headed for surgery, why not see an energy or spiritual healer and ask for a miracle. What have you got to lose?

When Is Surgery *Really* Necessary? – Holistic vs. Medical Parameters

Another factor that's helped me to avoid surgery is the fact that I don't have colonoscopies or sigmoidoscopies, barium enemas, upper GI tract x-rays, or any other exploratory procedure done. Aside from the initial set of exploratory procedures done for my diagnosis nearly 20 years ago, I've had no further testing or exploratory procedure of any kind. Therefore, I have no idea how 'bad' my condition has been at times and I believe this has helped me to not be frightened into having surgery, but rather to stay focused on healing myself. When I was first diagnosed, the doctor couldn't even do a complete colonoscopy since she couldn't get the tube through a part of my intestine that was narrowed – even though she tried to ram it through six times (oh yes, I was counting!). I continued to have terrible abdominal pain periodically for a few years following, along with bleeding, diarrhea and severe anemia. But I never had surgery and I never went back for another colonoscopy. I know the symptoms to watch for that would indicate intestinal perforation or rupture (very rigid abdominal wall, no bowel movements, intense pain and fever or chills) – which are critically life-threatening events and require hospital treatment. But I do know how to stop colonic hemmorhaging and small intestine bleeding using

> Like drugs, surgery for inflammatory bowel disease does not address the root cause, it merely cuts out the section of the body that is displaying the symptom. Surgery does not heal, it just temporarily alleviates the symptom.

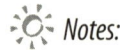 *Notes:*

natural methods (see Chapter Two). Therefore, in the absence of a truly 'life-threatening' condition, I prefer to use natural methods to heal my body rather than surgery. Keep in mind that a medical doctor's assessment of an exploratory test result is based on his experience and what he believes is possible within the parameters of his profession. Unfortunately, since most medical doctors are not educated about alternative healing therapies or procedures they will honestly tell you that there's nothing else you can do and you must have surgery. In their experience, they're speaking the truth.

I received an email from a woman who resisted surgery for a long time until her husband convinced her she was endangering her life. After the surgery, her doctor told her that the section of the intestine they removed was so narrowed there was no way it would have ever returned to normal. In the doctor's experience, there was nothing he could do to restore her intestine. However, our bodies are capable of 'miraculous' regeneration, change and healing once we give them the right tools and conditions. Until you utilize the bodywork therapies (including EFT, hypnotherapy, and energy/spiritual healing), herbal treatments, *Healing Diets*, and lifestyle guidelines listed in this book, you really have no idea of what your body is capable of.

I currently have either a narrowing or a stricture in my throat and my rectum. For years I've been purposely keeping my stool loose so as not to tear the stricture upon defecation – which then causes it to bleed. I eat slowly, taking small mouthfuls and chewing well to avoid choking. A fellow I know has the same problem with his throat and he's had it ballooned open twice so far (which is very painful and traumatic). Each procedure lasts about six months and then he's back to square one. Or is he? We don't know the deeper damage this violent, abrupt procedure could be doing to his throat tissue, visceral membrane and musculature in the area.

I've chosen to address my condition holistically. I've discovered that the amount of narrowing in my throat is directly related to my stress level, whether I'm upset, and whether there's something I need to be saying that I haven't said. Addressing the applicable factor causes my throat to relax and open up so at times I don't even notice anything wrong with my throat. I've recently felt ready to address the stricture or narrowing in my rectum in sessions with my craniosacral therapist, Lori Main. When we first began working with the area, I could barely insert my pinkie finger through the stricture and then it would bleed afterwards. By the second session, Lori could insert her index finger (past the second knuckle) with no bleeding following. She's also not sure that the narrowing is even a stricture and we're now thinking that it may just be a traumatized internal sphincter muscle. I'm also noticing changes in my hips, knees, back and throat as she frees up the restrictions in my rectum and releases the emotional trauma stored in the tissue. I've also started working on the emotional factors underlying my choking problems with a wonderful EFT therapist named Aileen Nobles. See Chapter Six for more detailed descriptions of these types of therapy and what they can do for your body.

So you see, when a medical doctor says this or that is or isn't possible, he is only speaking from his narrow band of experience. Most medical doctors do not receive any training in the dozens of very effective alternative therapies available for healing and releasing the body. I encourage you to educate yourself on what options are available to you and try the gentler, root-level, long-term forms of healing first. The emergency surgical procedures will always be available to you. And in truly life-threatening conditions they do have their place. It's up to you to connect with your body and discern, truly, how serious the problem is and what will benefit you most at this time. You cannot rely on anyone else to do this for you with the same degree of truth or accuracy, for no one (no matter what their professional qualification is) knows your body better than you do.

You may have already had a few surgeries by the time you read this book; that's fine. Find out exactly which sections of your intestine were removed (get a copy of the report from your file, if possible) and make an appointment to see a naturopathic doctor. Your naturopath will be able to work out which, if any, nutrients you're unable to absorb properly, and then you can take the vitamin or mineral in sublingual, transdermal, or lozenge form. Following is an illustration that shows you some of the nutrients absorbed at different places in the gastrointestinal tract. Take this in to

☼ We will have much better results if we treat and heal the whole mind/body, rather than just try to medicate or cut out the currently affected part.

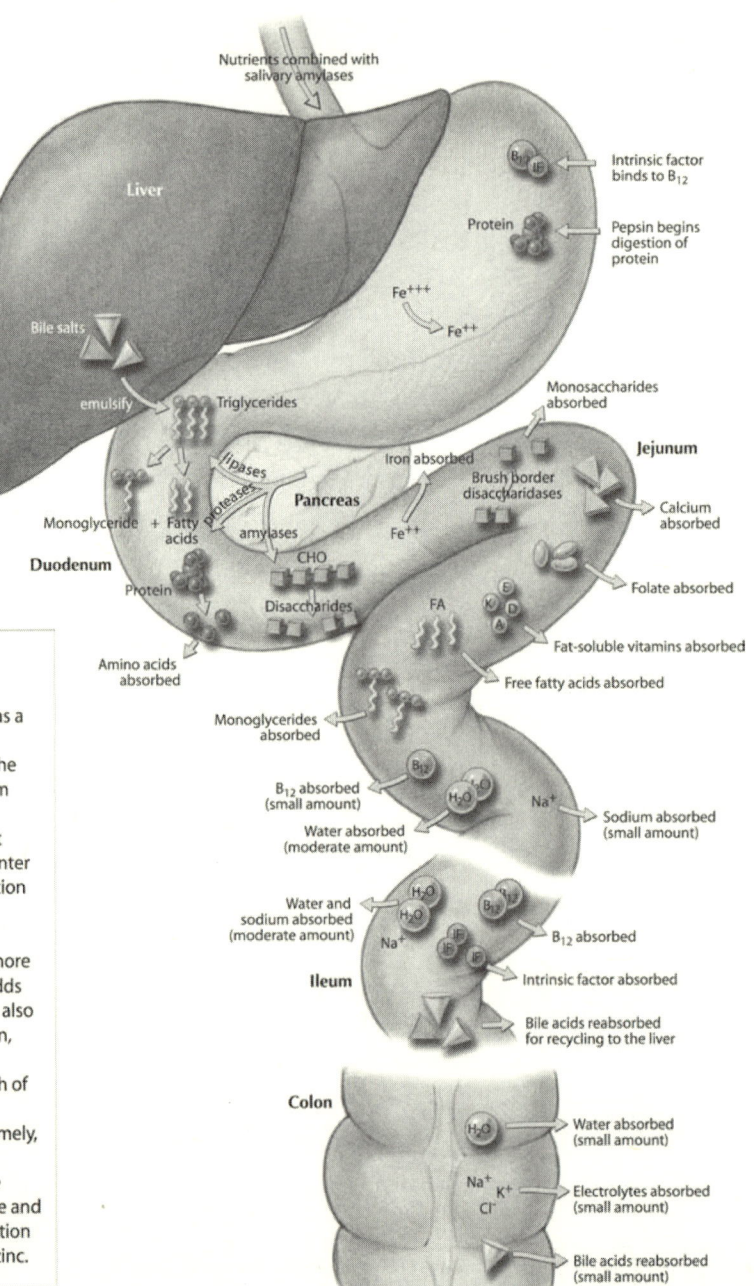

Short bowel syndrome

The short bowel syndrome resulting in dehydration and malabsorption occurs as a result of massive intestinal resection, especially of the ileum with or without the colon. Resection of up to 100 cm of ileum causes diarrhea, because there are progressively greater degrees of bile salt malabsorption. Malabsorbed bile salts enter the colon where they cause water secretion by activating cyclic adenosine monophosphate. When the resection exceeds 100 cm, there is progressively more fatty acid loss in the colon, which also adds to water secretion and diarrhea. There is also malabsorption of vitamin B_{12}. In addition, there is loss of energy in the form of increased fat loss. However, as the length of the resection increases, there is malabsorption of all macronutrients, namely, fat, carbohydrate and protein. The malabsorbed carbohydrate entering the colon is fermented to produce flatulence and diarrhea. In addition, there is malabsorption of vitamins and trace elements such as zinc.

Fig.1: The relative locations of digestion and absorption of nutrients in the healthy gastrointestinal tract. CHO = carbohydrate.[7]

your doctor to work out which additional nutrients you should be supplementing with.

The important question to ask yourself is whether you're ready to get off the surgery cycle and, when things get difficult for you again, what are you going to do? When your doctor tells you that he thinks it's imperative that you have surgery, what are you going to do? You still have a choice; no matter what your doctor says or what scare tactics he may employ, you can still say yes or no. If you've been giving away this authority, then now is the time to take it back.

The next time your doctor tells you that you need to have surgery, question him extensively. Stay very logical and ask him detailed, specific questions as to what he feels is happening, why he feels you need surgery, what he thinks is likely to happen if you don't have the surgery and if he has any reliable statistical backing for his opinion. Take notes and write down everything pertinent he says. Then take some time, maybe a day or two, to think about his opinion and compare it with your own feelings. Take some time to be still and go into your body, open up a discussion with your intestines and see how your body feels about having the surgery and whether you feel it's necessary (See *Dialoguing With Your Body* in Chapter Six). It can also be very effective to ask your subconscious to give you a dream to help you decide what would be best for your body. Ask for a dream for guidance when you go to bed at night and keep a pen and pad of paper beside the bed to record anything you can remember upon waking, whether in the morning or in the middle of the night. You may receive guidance or feel strongly that surgery is the best course for you – in that case, by all means proceed with it. Ultimately, only you can and should decide whether having surgery is right for you. You are the one who knows the best treatment for your body.

> When a medical doctor says this or that is or isn't possible, he is only speaking from his narrow band of experience. Most medical doctors do not receive any training in the dozens of very effective alternative therapies available for healing and releasing the body.

GASTROINTESTINAL EXPLORATORY PROCEDURES

Some gastroenterologists feel it's necessary to have regular internal scopes to monitor your disease. Personally, I think colonoscopies, sigmoidoscopies,

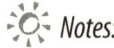 Notes:

gastroscopies, barium enemas, etc. are overrated as a disease-management tool. They are unnecessary in many cases, and also very damaging to the mucosal lining and bacterial flora. Please go back and re-read the section on probiotics in Chapter Two to find out how integral a healthy gut flora is to your health. When you have a colonoscopy or barium enema, it completely disrupts (and sometimes wipes out) the bacterial flora in your bowel. Any kind of upper-GI exploratory procedure is going to have a negative effect on the bacterial flora in your stomach and small intestine. If these procedures are not followed with a long-term, high dose course of probiotics, then your gut is left wide open to damage and infection from bad bacteria, yeast, parasites, viruses, etc.

However, although gastroenterologists know that these procedures seriously disrupt the bacterial flora of the gastrointestinal tract, most do not follow exploratory or diagnostic procedures with probiotic (good bacteria) supplementation. This is ludicrous! Some of the top research presenters at probiotic conferences are gastroenterologists. Are members of the profession not in communication with each other, or is there another element or motivation at work? I don't know. What I do know is that any exploratory gastrointestinal procedure (particularly colonoscopies and barium enemas) should be followed with *Jini's Probiotic Retention Enema* and at *least* three months of full-spectrum, high dose, oral probiotic supplementation. Again, see Chapter Two for full instructions on taking probiotics.

Colonoscopy Screening For Colon Cancer

For the past few years in America, there's been a massive advertising push urging people over age 50 to have yearly colonoscopies to screen for colon cancer. Not surprisingly, I've begun to have an increasing number of people over the age of 50 contacting me for advice. The last woman I talked to was 74 years old and until that year, had never had a gastrointestinal problem in her life. She was dealing with a widespread and debilitating case of ulcerative colitis when a mutual friend passed on my phone number to her. One of the first questions I asked her was whether she had a colonoscopy prior to her colitis problems? "Why yes," she said, "my doctor suggested I have one to scan for colon cancer and then a short while later I began having problems…." Well, that was worthwhile! Now you know that you don't have colon cancer, but we'll set you up for ulcerative colitis instead!

If you look at cancer in holistic terms, it is not something that suddenly occurs, it's usually at least a five or ten year accumulation of unhealthy practices. You'll hear people say so many times, "He was perfectly healthy, nothing wrong with him, and then the next day he had cancer!" These are people looking at the body through an allopathic (western medicine) viewfinder. If you were to look at that person from a natural, holistic perspective, you would find many factors that have contributed over the years to the gradual degradation of health that results in cancer. And although there will be clear physical factors that have contributed to such an illness, there will also be emotional factors.

Dr. Gabor Mate (MD) has written a fantastic book that I strongly urge everyone reading this to get, called, *When The Body Says No – The Hidden Cost of Stress*. The book describes in detail exactly how emotions and feelings can produce illness.

> "Our immune system does not exist in isolation from daily experience. For example, the immune defences that normally function in healthy young people have been shown to be suppressed in medical students under the pressure of final examinations. Of even greater implication for their future health and well being, the loneliest students suffered the greatest negative impact on their immune systems. Loneliness has been similarly associated with diminished immune activity in a group of psychiatric inpatients. Even if no further research evidence existed – though there is plenty – one would have to consider the long-term effects of chronic stress. The pressure of examinations is obvious and short term, but many people unwittingly spend their entire lives as if under the gaze of a powerful and judgmental examiner whom they must please at all costs. Many of us live, if not alone, then in emotionally inadequate relationships that do not recognize or honour

☼ Any exploratory gastrointestinal procedure (particularly colonoscopies and barium enemas) should be followed with *Jini's Probiotic Retention Enema* and at least three months of full-spectrum, high dose, oral probiotic supplementation.

> Drugs, surgery and exploratory/diagnostic procedures put the responsibility for finding out what's wrong with your body and helping it, onto someone else. It's much more difficult to take this responsibility ourselves. It's easier to look to someone else to help you, rather than look to yourself.

our deepest needs. Isolation and stress affect many who may believe their lives are quite satisfactory." [8]

So you see, if you're concerned about the possibility of colon cancer, then begin preventive measures. Implement the guidelines in Chapter Four and eliminate all the carcinogens from your food supply and environment. Use Chapter Two to heal your colon and stop the physical damage that predisposes people to colon cancer. Use the emotional healing techniques in Chapter Six to fully heal your mind/body, and recognize that emotional health is just as crucial as physical health – and indeed, the two cannot be separated. However, if you have a strong intuition that you should have a colonoscopy to screen for colon cancer (or for any other reason), then by all means do so! You know your body the best and you should definitely listen to what it tells you.

The Wales Day Centre (a colo rectal and proctology clinic in Sydney, Australia) has an excellent website giving good descriptions and full color pictures of many exploratory/diagnostic procedures, so it's a good place to go for general information if you're considering any of these procedures. Click on both their patient and practitioner information sections: *http://www.wales.com.au*. The pictures may also be useful for you to use during healing visualizations (see Chapter Seven).

Colonoscopy As A Tracking Or Confirmation Tool

Please realize the seriousness of these procedures and don't undertake them lightly, or because your doctor is pressuring you to. Another reader who had achieved full remission underwent a colonoscopy to confirm that she was indeed completely healed. However, shortly thereafter, she experienced a flare and asked me whether I thought the two (colonoscopy and subsequent flare) were related? Of course they were! Please don't do this to yourself. If, for some reason, you feel you must have an invasive, damaging procedure done to confirm your healing, then please follow it immediately with *Jini's Probiotic Retention Enema* and three to six months of full-spectrum, high dose, oral probiotic supplementation.

We can get into a fascination or 'information addiction' with our bodies. So much of our life seems unstable and frightening, full of shifting sands and precarious perches. We can feel like we're always on the edge of a precipice, in constant fear of the element that's going to bump us off the edge and send us hurtling downwards. And anyone who's gone through a 'flare', where one day you're feeling fine and the next day you're two feet from the grave, knows exactly what I'm talking about! So we seek to gather as many hard facts as we can, hoping to allay our fears and be able to say 'this is what's wrong with me'. So many people with non-specific symptoms talk of the relief they feel when they're finally diagnosed. This is due to the paradigm of medical/pharmaceutical healthcare that we've been brought up with. We think that if we can only pinpoint, specifically, what's wrong, then we can take that specific drug or surgery to cure it. But as we've already discussed, each step along this thought sequence is erroneous. Drugs and surgery don't cure. And having a label to assign to your set of symptoms does nothing to heal you. Natural, root-level healing involves breaking out of this mindset and simply connecting with your own body. Your body can tell you everything that's wrong with it and everything you need to do to heal it. You just have to listen. Of course, connecting with and listening to your own body is harder initially than taking drugs, having exploratory procedures, or even surgery. Drugs, surgery and exploratory/diagnostic procedures put the responsibility for finding out what's wrong with your body and helping it, onto someone else. It's much more difficult to take this responsibility ourselves. It's easier to look to someone else to help you, rather than look to yourself.

Here's another way of looking at the whole exploratory procedure issue. The average length of life for an intestinal cell is three days. Technically, this means that the gastrointestinal tract is capable of complete regeneration, or degeneration, in three days time. So, let's say you had a colonoscopy that revealed you had extensive ulceration along your descending colon. If you did everything required for complete healing (emotional, physical, spiritual), you could potentially turn that around and have a completely healed intestinal surface three days later. Likewise, if your colonoscopy

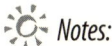 *Notes:*

showed that everything was fine, in only three days time, you could have ulceration or inflammation present throughout. If the test results can be so transient, how meaningful are they?

Some of you may have heard of a newer technology for scoping the upper gastrointestinal tract called Capsule Endoscopy. This involves a test preparation procedure to clear the tract and then swallowing an encapsulated camera that takes photos as it travels along the small intestine. In a drug trial that utilized this procedure, researchers were surprised to discover that 13.8% of the *pre-screening group* (healthy people with no history of IBD, IBS, etc.) had ulceration present in their small bowel![9] So what does that mean? Does it mean that 14% of the population, with no symptoms whatsoever, actually have IBD but just don't know it yet? Or does it mean that the intestinal wall and mucosal lining degenerate and/or regenerate much more quickly and/or frequently than previously supposed? We really don't know enough to draw a conclusion. I'm providing these examples merely to make you question the inherent value of exploratory procedures, and whether they're worth the damage they do to your intestinal lining, mucosa, and bacterial flora.

I rather like the approach of a gastroenterologist I know in Vancouver, Canada. He asks the question, "Will performing a scope at this time change the existing course of treatment?" If the answer is "No", then he doesn't suggest doing one. Many doctors use scopes out of fear, worried that something bad *might* be going on. Others like to do them as a form of research or on-going data collection. Many do them as a preventive measure against potential malpractice suits – if you do develop cancer in your colon and your doctor has not suggested yearly scopes, then he's in big trouble. So when a doctor is pressuring you to have a colonoscopy, you need to take his position and fears into account.

Think back over all the scopes you've had. Did you learn anything new about your condition? Did the information result in a better, more effective

> **Fecal Occult Blood Test**
> Since it screens for blood in the stool, don't take the test during your period and avoid red meat for three days beforehand – both may cause a false positive and lead your doctor to order an unnecessary colonoscopy or sigmoidoscopy. Turnips, cauliflower, broccoli, bananas, melons, beets, radishes and vitamin C and iron supplements can also skew the results. So can drugs: In the week leading up to the test, you shouldn't take anti-inflammatories like Advil or more than one daily dose of aspirin.
>
> Sari Globerman, *Oprah Magazine*, March 2005.

course of treatment? Did you find that after each stint of testing you were weaker and sicker, and it set your healing back significantly? Did you suffer psychological and emotional trauma as a result of the scope(s)? In my view, these procedures are simply too invasive and damaging to the body and can result in long-term damage and imbalance to the intestinal lining and bacterial flora. In addition, my mother's doctor once told her about some of the "complications" a colonoscopy can result in, like perforation through the intestinal wall and even a ruptured spleen in one case. At present, there isn't even an effective method for completely sterilizing colonoscopy equipment (please see references in Appendix D for substantiating data) – so think about the implications of that for disease transmission (IBD, cancer, AIDS, hepatitis, etc.). There are disposable sigmoidoscopes available now, so if you're going to have a sigmoidoscopy, insist on a disposable one to avoid risk of contamination.

I haven't had a colonoscopy since my very first one used to determine the medical diagnosis of my condition. Why do I need another one? I know when my intestines are bleeding, I know when they're spasming, I can feel if a portion is thicker than elsewhere. I live with my intestines every day, I do not need a gastroenterologist to do a scope to tell me that there's "a significant increase in ulceration of the bowel wall, a fissure in your rectal canal and increased production of mucus". I can tell all that from my bowel movements: How I feel when I'm having them, and what shows up in my stool and the surrounding liquid.

Also, if you're going to use the techniques and diets in this book, and follow a pathway of natural healing, your gastroenterologist's assessment of your current condition is not going to make much difference to your treatment. If you're experiencing blood with your bowel movements or mixed in with your stool, the *Healing Diet* to follow and herbal supplements recommended are similar regardless of whether the bleeding is from ulceration of the bowel wall or your rectal canal. Try to trust your body and learn to read the signs it gives you, rather than resorting to a damaging procedure to give you that same information. I'm not saying that colonoscopies and other exploratory procedures are never appropriate or helpful. I'm just suggesting

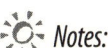 Notes:

you think very carefully before submitting to one and ask your doctor the key question, "Will the results of this procedure change the course of treatment?" Again, we get to the same point as when considering surgery: Take your doctor's opinion as simply that, his opinion. Compare it with your own opinion and gut feelings and decide whether or not you really need yet another scope or scan and whether that will actually benefit you in any significant way. Weigh up the possible risks and subsequent damage the procedure will cause and ask yourself whether it's worth it. Don't be surprised if you find the answer is no.

A large part of the reason we submit to unnecessary scopes and surgeries is because of fear. Be aware of, and make sure you're not taking on the fear of your doctor or family members. Fear-based decisions are never optimal, so if you find yourself making a decision largely due to fear, take some time out. Slow it down (your doctor and family may try to make you feel like everything is extremely urgent! Just ignore them) and take some time by yourself to relax, meditate and get in touch with yourself. Take a walk out in nature and read some uplifting, expanding books – anything by Deepak Chopra, Andrew Weil, Caroline Myss or Bernie Siegel will help you get back your power and strength and separate yourself from your fear. Then, when you're in a more balanced, centered frame of mind you can make your decision as to whether you want to have that surgery or exploratory test done.

YOUR DOCTOR AND YOU

I spent eight years without a gastroenterologist or even a regular GP (general practitioner) because I couldn't find a doctor who was willing to work with me and support me in the way that I wanted to treat and heal my body. Instead I encountered scorn, hostility, doctors who were intimidated by me, and doctors who thought I was naive and stupid. It was simply more trouble than it was worth. As a result, I frequented the walk-in medical clinics where I was able to just show up from time to time, request a prescription for folic acid, or get some blood work done, or testing for hormone levels, etc. This worked well, for a while.

☼ We can get into a fascination or 'information addiction' with our bodies. We seek to gather as many hard facts as we can, hoping to allay our fears, and to be able to say, 'This is what's wrong with me.'

However, as time wore on I felt an increasing need to balance out my relationship with modern medicine and perhaps seek a more integrative approach to my health care. Fortunately, there has been such a growing awareness of alternative health and healing in the last few years, that it has affected and influenced even the medical profession. Indeed, some of its loudest proponents are medical doctors themselves (Christiane Northrup, Deepak Chopra, Andrew Weil, Bernie Siegel, etc.). More and more medical doctors are also training as naturopaths, acupuncturists, homeopaths, etc. I was able to find a medical doctor whose approach to health is fairly open-minded and inclusive. She is also fairly comfortable with me not following her advice and is simply there to provide medical information and treatment protocols. In her words, "Try to think of me as just another resource. I'll give you my opinion on what I think is best and why, and then you put it together with your other knowledge and resources and make a decision as to what you feel is best for you". It makes a tremendous difference to have a doctor who supports and is willing to work with you and with what you feel is best for you. If you're looking for a medical or naturopathic doctor, or a gastroenterologist in your area, go to my website: *www.JiniPatelThompson.com*, and check out the Healthcare Professionals section. Here you'll find other readers' recommendations for doctors they have found to be good and/or open to natural healthcare methods. Also, if you have a doctor you think is doing a good job, please post their name and contact information on the site, so others can benefit too.

If you do not have an affirming, supportive doctor, please start looking for one. The last thing you need is a doctor who disagrees with the way you wish to manage your health. She/he will only give you negativity, undermine your efforts and use scare tactics to get you to do what she/he believes is best. None of this will support you in your efforts to heal yourself. Try to find a doctor with additional holistic healing qualifications, or one who has a reputation for being a non-traditionalist. They are out there and it is so important to have a doctor who supports you and is willing to work with you in the way that you want, or one who is simply happy to let you do your own thing. Still, remember to not give your power away no matter how

> The last thing you need is a doctor who gives you negativity, undermines your efforts, and uses scare tactics to get you to do what she/he believes is best. None of this will support you in your efforts to heal yourself.

safe or knowledgeable you think your doctor is. Always maintain yourself and your own gut intuition as your final authority and decision-maker.

If you absolutely cannot find a supportive doctor in your area, then find a supportive natural physician – naturopath or homeopath. Follow your appointments with your medical doctor with an appointment with your naturopath. Your naturopathic physician will help balance out the negativity you receive from your medical doctor and will help you combat any fear or scare tactics that may have thrown you into despair. Your naturopathic physician can also help you with natural methods for addressing health concerns that may have shown up in your medical tests.

My main point regarding the medical profession and the tools it has to offer (drugs and surgery) is simply this: Treat it as an option. It is one path out of many and not necessarily the best one. Use the procedures and tools that are useful to you, when they're useful, and don't worry about the rest. Drugs and surgery are usually invasive, traumatic ways of treating the body and they don't tend to support holistic, long-term healing. If there's a kinder, gentler way to accomplish the same end, then even if it takes longer and is more work, take the gentle, healing path. It's time to start working *with* your body; loving, supporting and nurturing it on a gentle, deep-level, long-lasting healing path.

NATUROPATHIC MEDICINE

In my opinion, having a good naturopathic doctor that you see regularly is just as important as regular visits to your allopathic doctor (GP). Their training consists of four years of specialized, intensive training in natural medicine at a college or university that's accredited by the CNME (Council on Naturopathic Medical Education). The CNME in turn is regulated by the U.S. government. Be sure and ask your naturopath which college he/she went to and how long the course was, as there are numerous non-accredited colleges selling mail-order degrees. See Appendix B for referral information to an accredited naturopath. A registered naturopathic physician is able to work with you in all facets of treating and maintaining

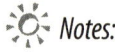
Notes:

health using a range of natural, herbal and homeopathic methods. And I'm not just referring to the treatment and management of your IBD or IBS. Use your naturopath for all aspects of your health – if you get a cold or the flu, arthritis, or an irregular period, for example.

There are also an increasing number of medical doctors who also have a naturopathic degree or integrative medicine qualification, and they can be very helpful since their knowledge covers the whole spectrum of treatments and testing procedures available in both modalities. But again, you have to make sure the doctor is skilled, respectful and that you 'click' with him/her.

> Make sure your doctor is skilled, respectful, and that you 'click' with him/her.

Natural Diagnostics

I once went to my naturopath simply because my intuitive feeling was that I was deficient in some mineral. After asking me a series of questions, he determined that I was deficient in magnesium. One of the main clues was that my throat was spasming occasionally and making it difficult for me to swallow sometimes. A few days after starting the magnesium supplementation, my throat was fine – because magnesium relaxes smooth muscle tissue (which is why it can also cause diarrhea in high doses). Now, can you imagine if I'd gone to my allopathic doctor complaining of a spasming throat and trouble swallowing? I don't even want to think of the barrage of tests that would have been ordered, probably including a gastroscopy! How long do you think it would take an allopathic doctor to discover the problem was due to magnesium deficiency? Most likely, it would not be discovered. Experience has taught me to always take the gentler, less invasive path first. If you're having a health problem, seek out the natural forms of healing first.

A naturopathic doctor is not only well trained in a wide variety of natural treatments, but is also excellent as a resource and reference guide to other forms of non-invasive testing or therapy that may benefit you. Again, use the same discretion you would when choosing any doctor or practitioner. Ask around for someone with a good reputation, phone your local association of naturopathic physicians for a referral of doctors in your area (see Appendix B) and don't be afraid to keep looking until you find the right doctor for you. Finally, use your naturopathic doctor the same way you use all your doctors, healers and practitioners – as a resource. Don't give your power away and always follow your own intuition above anyone else's advice or opinion.

Turn now to the *Healing Journey Workbook* and complete the section for Chapter Five.

6

Mind/Body Therapies

"When someone comes to me for healing or help, the first thing I do is to examine the overall pattern of the person's life. This usually reveals certain blocks that are holding him or her back from being healed.

These blocks may be present on both a physical and a spiritual level. From the spiritual standpoint, the most common blocks are the negative attitudes and emotions that a lot of people carry around all the time.

These blocks must be overcome for healing to occur. In working with people who have cancer or other serious illnesses, I find that unless they can learn to let go of negativity, their sickness comes back."

Sun Bear, Medicine Chief of the Bear Tribe Medicine Society

There are many wonderful, healing bodywork and treatment therapies available and each one has its own particular benefits to offer. I have tried enough different types of therapies over the last twenty years to fill a small encyclopedia (and spent tens of thousands of dollars doing so!), so rather than go into everything I've tried, I'm just going to present you with those therapies I've found to be the *most* helpful and healing.

Three Types Of Useful Bodywork Therapies

There are three types of bodywork for people with IBS or IBD that are particularly useful. These are loosely defined categories, and as you go through this chapter, you'll notice there is a definite overlap between the three categories. Or, the therapy can fit into different categories depending on the skill and/or intent of the practitioner.

The first category of bodywork therapies focuses primarily on the physical tissues, bones, organs, etc. where the problems are occurring and the therapies are designed specifically to release and heal the problems in the physical body. This category includes acupuncture, acupressure, massage therapy, visceral and myofascial release, rolfing, craniosacral therapy, etc.

The second category of bodywork therapies offers an integrated mind/body approach, where you address the physical restrictions, trauma and malfunctioning, and at the same time access the emotional and spiritual bodies to release the emotional pain, trauma and anger that is stored in those tissues, organs, bones, etc. This is called a somato-emotional approach ('soma' means 'body') to healing. These therapies include many of the therapies mentioned above, but the practitioner has gone to the advanced levels of the modality, or received additional training in somato-emotional release. So again, this category of therapies includes advanced craniosacral therapy, advanced rolfing (practitioners at this level in rolfing are rare), acupuncture and acupressure.

The third category of therapies involves interpreting, or getting to the underlying emotional root of the physical problem by addressing the

---

☼ In my experience, there is *always* an emotional component to any physical problem. Many times the physical problem/symptom will just disappear once you address the underlying emotional component, but at other times you need to address *both* the emotional and physical bodies.

emotional component first. By releasing and healing the emotional trauma, the corresponding trauma in the physical body can be automatically and simultaneously released. Keep in mind that psychotherapy and other forms of 'talk' therapy are not sufficient to effect root-level, long-term healing in the physical body. You need a form of emotional therapy that also *integrates* with the physical body in some way (like EFT or hypnotherapy). In my experience, there is *always* an emotional component to any physical problem. Many times the physical problem/symptom will just disappear once you address the underlying emotional component, but at other times you need to address both the emotional and physical bodies.

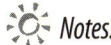 Notes:

Practitioner Skill Is Paramount

However, you do need to keep in mind that each of these therapies is only as good as the individual practitioner. For example, I once went to two massage practitioners with identical training and background, and one was fabulous and the other fair to middling. So, unfortunately, finding a good practitioner can sometimes be a difficult, costly, and time-consuming task – but definitely well worth it. When locating a practitioner, ask around all your friends and family and see if anyone knows of someone with a good reputation. Pick up the local, free metaphysical/new age publications in your city and see who's advertising. Above all, go with your gut and let your intuition guide you as to which type of therapy you'd like to try, and which practitioner(s) to make an appointment with. It's also useful to call a number of therapists first and just have a quick chat with each of them. You'll get a sense of who you like or 'click' with just from the phone conversation and then you can try those first.

ACUPUNCTURE

Acupuncture (and at a gentler, slower rate, acupressure) is excellent for balancing the energy flows in your body and stimulating the healthy functioning of all your glands and organs. I found the main benefit derived from this type of treatment was stress control and pain reduction. It is also excellent for maintaining and promoting overall, holistic health and

> Acupuncture is excellent for balancing the energy flows in your body, stimulating the healthy functioning of all your glands and organs, and reducing stress and pain.

supporting proper organ and gland functioning. However, in my opinion, there is a big difference between Chinese and Japanese acupuncture.

With Japanese acupuncture, I have never even felt the needles going in, much less felt any pain or twinges as a result. I have only ever felt relaxed and nurtured during and after a session. With Chinese acupuncture, the needles used are much larger. I could feel every one going in and some of the insertions were even painful. After the needles were in I felt hot rushes up my legs, parts of my body went numb, other parts felt ice cold and in one session it felt like my arms had separated from my body.

So, unless you prefer more aggressive, dramatic treatments, I definitely recommend seeing a Japanese acupuncturist rather than a Chinese acupuncturist. Try to find a practitioner who is actually Japanese and has undergone their training and certification in Japan. If the practitioner is non-Japanese, be sure and find out the length of their course and how long it took them to receive their certification. The acupuncture I received in Tokyo was at a Zen monastery and each practitioner was deeply immersed in training for about four years. Unfortunately, I've seen numerous Western practitioners advertising who've just done a two to four week course in acupuncture in China or Japan and come back to practice as a certified acupuncturist (question MDs in particular). Likewise, if you do decide to go for Chinese acupuncture, try to make sure the practitioner is Chinese and/or has received their training and practiced in China first.

There are certain acupuncturists who have also trained in somato-emotional release, so if your practitioner has this training, then acupuncture or acupressure can be a gateway to accessing the emotional body as well.

BIO-KINESIOLOGY

Bio-kinesiology, or applied kinesiology (sometimes called Touch For Health), is basically a system of testing and asking your body directly what's wrong with it and what it needs. The practitioner first sets up a control, say an amount of pressure on your raised arm that you can easily resist. Then, she will proceed to ask your body a series of questions whilst applying pressure to your arm. When she asks something to which the answer is "yes", your arm will collapse, unable to resist the pressure. Some practitioners will also combine this with stimulating acupressure points to test the functioning of glands, organs and various bodily systems.

After your body has outlined where it's malfunctioning, or in need of support, the practitioner will select some possible herbal or homeopathic remedies and then proceed to ask your body which of them it wants and in what dosage. This is done by laying the remedies on your stomach and asking via the muscle-testing procedure (pressure on the arm) whether this particular remedy will help and in what dosage.

Practitioner Energy Interference

I know several people personally who've had excellent results using this method of diagnosis and treatment, both for one-time illnesses and also as a system of ongoing healthcare. I myself was introduced to both liquid chlorophyll and homeopathic iron as a result of a session. My only reservation about this method of treatment is that I wonder how much of the practitioner's energy and intent is involved in the testing process. For example, let's say I have a practitioner who feels that yeast is a really bad thing and that most people have an overabundance of yeast in their system. When she is asking me the question about yeast, she will simultaneously be projecting a very strong energetic thought or intent about yeast into the feedback loop – and she is part of the loop because she is touching my body and also asking the question. So when my arm collapses, signifying that I have a yeast problem, how much of that response is mine and how much is hers?

So, again, my position regarding this type of therapy is that it can be very helpful and useful, but do not give your power away to it. Your body may test positive for something during the session, but afterwards when you're back at home you may get a strong intuitive feeling that you don't actually have that problem or need to avoid that food. In that case, definitely go

☼ My position regarding bio-kinesiology is that it can be very helpful and useful, but do not give your power away to it.

with own body and intuition. You being directly in tune with your body is the clearest channel of information and communication there is. Use your applied kinesiology practitioner and the testing process as a resource, as an opinion, as a source of information, but not the only one and not necessarily the best one.

MASSAGE THERAPY

I saw a therapeutic massage therapist regularly for about ten years (sometimes once a week, sometimes once every ten days) due to the scoliosis in my spine and multiple injuries from car accidents and martial arts. Now, I have a fantastic yoga instructor (Sandra Sammartino – she's 63 years old and has been teaching for over thirty years), and as a result my neck and spine are gradually straightening and I'm learning how to unlock and release tissues, bones, etc. myself. As a result of her training and classes, I no longer need to have massage therapy, although I'll occasionally go for a treat or stress relief.

During the decade I did need regular massage, every time I moved to a new city it was a real hassle finding a good practitioner. When I moved to Vancouver I tried six different therapists before finding someone I was happy with. My advice to you is: Don't give up. Keep trying until you find a practitioner who's so good that they make a significant difference to your body and wellbeing. I walk out of one hour sessions with my massage therapist feeling like I've got a new lease on life and my body feels completely unblocked, fluid and expansive. In short, I feel wonderful and any pain or tightness in my body is relieved.

Benefits Of Massage Therapy

Researchers at Miami's Touch Research Institute (TRI) found that premature infants who received three massages a day over 10 days gained 47% more weight than preemies who weren't massaged. According to *Family Therapy Networker*, TRI has also documented the benefits of massage in treating everything from colic and bulimia to chronic fatigue syndrome

---

☼ Keep trying until you find a practitioner who's so good that they make a significant difference to your body and wellbeing – your body should feel unblocked, fluid and expansive.

and back pain.[1] Massage also raises immune-system cell levels in people who are HIV-positive.[2]

Look for a certified or registered practitioner who specializes in therapeutic as opposed to relaxing massage. Practitioners who also have additional qualifications like craniosacral, visceral manipulation, myofascial release, or applied kinesiology will be able to give you a better treatment; the more training the better. My massage therapist has been able to help me with diverse problems such as relieving me of heartburn, stimulating my appetite, releasing a stuck ileocecal valve (between small and large intestine) and improving my breathing (by releasing and freeing-up my diaphragm). Massage also stimulates the blood flow, cellular exchange, and elimination of toxins from the body. I cannot recommend the benefits of a good massage therapist highly enough. If cost is a big issue with you, remember that the training colleges for certified practitioners always offer sessions at greatly reduced rates and going only once a month is certainly better than nothing.

CRANIOSACRAL THERAPY

Craniosacral therapy is a bodywork therapy that can be just a straightforward physical therapy whereby the practitioner facilitates deep-level release of muscle tissue, connective tissue, and various internal valves, tissues and organs. Or it can be a therapy that goes that next step further into the release of traumatic memories and emotions that are being stored in the physical body. It's really up to you which level you wish to go to and how you would like your practitioner to treat you. You're usually fully clothed throughout the session. Practitioners who are only trained in the first or second levels of the therapy will only use it as a physical therapy tool. The ones who've pursued the higher levels of training will utilize it as a somato-emotional release tool as well. It's up to you to discuss with the practitioner your needs and wishes and specify what you feel comfortable with prior to the session beginning.

☼ Emotional wounds, or trauma, are also stored in the physical tissues of our body. Thus, healing your emotional issues through counseling or psychotherapy is not enough. You must also go into the body itself, and release the pain and trauma that is stored there.

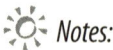 Notes:

Craniosacral therapy was originally developed by an osteopath (akin to a MD and chiropractor rolled into one) named Dr. John Upledger. It focuses on the energy, vibrational and fluid flows and rhythms around the brain and spinal cord. In this way it is a physical therapy. However, depending upon the intent and skill of the therapist, craniosacral therapy can also facilitate what is called somato-emotional release. This technique is based on the premise that emotional/spiritual trauma is also stored in the physical tissues of our body. Thus, healing one's emotional issues/traumas through counseling or mental self-realization is not enough. One must also go into the body itself and release the pain and trauma that is stored there (hence somato(body)-emotional release). Somato-emotional release can also be facilitated by other types of therapy such as Reiki, Pranic or energy healing, Qigong and Therapeutic Touch – all of which I would also recommend.

Traumatic Memories Stored In The Body
Every craniosacral session I've had has been different. In the first one, Brian Finnie (the therapist) was massaging and moving my neck around and as he moved my neck a particular way I would have certain memories spring large-as-life to my mind. If the memory got to be too overwhelming (because I was actually re-living these memories) he would move my neck slightly out of the position and the memory would fade away and I'd be instantaneously normal and happy again. Then, after giving me a few moments to rest, he'd move my neck back into that position and whoosh, I'd be right back in the technicolor memory and emotion immediately, sobbing my eyes out, or incredibly angry, or whatever. As I re-lived these memories from my current position of increased strength and maturity (that is, stronger and more mature than when the incidents actually occurred), I was able to see them in a new light and with new understanding. I was able to place the events within a context and somehow, in the accessing of these memories within my body, I was able to release them and their accompanying emotional state. Needless to say, being able to release these experiences and emotions at such a deep level feels absolutely wonderful. I could literally feel the tightness and heaviness being released from my body.

Finding My True Voice

I had a most remarkable experience with another practitioner, Ruth Redekop, who is trained in both craniosacral and energy healing. I went to see her because a month previously I'd had an eruption of mouth ulcers all over my tongue, lining of my mouth, gums and the lining of my throat. I'd spent the month using all my physical-level cures for mouth ulcers (non-acid diet, DGL licorice extract tablets, aloe vera juice) that usually worked, but they just kept getting worse.

I explained all this to Ruth and said, "I know it's something else, but I've just been unable to get to it, I've tried going into the problem when I'm meditating, but haven't been able to turn up anything." So, she started the session with some craniosacral therapy on my bowel and then moved up to my jaw and mouth. After about 5 minutes (with her hands on my jaw) she said, "Ok, can you tell me what's going on in here". I started to talk and as I talked I realized that for the past year or so, I had given up my "Voice".

About a year previously, my husband and a close friend had said that they were really hurt by my usual direct manner of communicating and they had asked me to change the way I speak, to make it a kinder, gentler way of communicating. Appalled at the thought of hurting anyone, I complied. Well, they were happy and I became someone who didn't sound at all like me. Interestingly, over the year both my friend and husband became more and more blunt and direct in their manner of communicating, while I sounded more and more like a counselor, couching and talking round everything. In fact, as I talked to Ruth, I realized that I had become one of those namby-pamby, mince-words, talk-round-the-issue type of people that I can't stand! I also realized that I was not responsible for other people's feelings or reactions to who I am. If people can't handle my truth, then don't ask me for it!

It took me about ten minutes to realize and verbalize all this to Ruth. She then asked me how my mouth ulcers were. I kid you not, they were 90% gone, as in *disappeared*. That evening I went home and told my husband and friend about the session and about how I was going be from now on: Me. The next morning I woke up and the ulcers were 100% gone. So, there

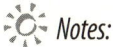 Notes:

you have it. Take it or leave it. I will also say that this healing is the most dramatic that I've ever experienced. Usually, I find healing occurs in layers or stages and takes place over several sessions.

Your Body's In Charge

A woman I know in Israel goes to a spiritual/energy healer there and she says she doesn't even know what it is that he does, but she feels her colon is linked to her inner child. She says she cries through every session and for an hour or two afterwards, and then for the next few days her colon is perfectly fine, as if her ulcerative colitis didn't even exist. Yes, our emotional body is inextricably linked and intertwined with our physical body and when you start to explore this link and heal the emotional body, some of the physical results are truly amazing.

The really important thing to keep in mind about this kind of therapy is that your body is in charge of what emerges in the session, and yes, it may be emotionally difficult, but your body knows your limits and will not take you where you cannot handle it. It will not take you beyond your limits, so you don't have to fear having something occur that is unmanageable. If you feel unsure about going to the somato-emotional level, you can start with a craniosacral practitioner who uses the therapy at a purely physical level (without the somato-emotional release), which is also very valuable and healing for the body. Then after you're comfortable with the therapy modality, if you wish, you can seek out another therapist who can take you a little deeper.

For those of you that tend to suffer from heartburn, even though you don't eat a lot of acidic foods and you don't lie down right after eating, you'll probably find tremendous relief from seeing a craniosacral therapist. When you go to the therapist, tell him/her that you've been having a lot of heartburn and your solar plexus and diaphragm need releasing. Of course, make sure that you're not taking a drug that's known to cause heartburn as a side-effect. For myself, whenever I've had heartburn, one 10-minute session of craniosacral therapy has usually eliminated it.

> ☼ Being able to release these experiences and emotions at such a deep level feels absolutely wonderful. I could literally feel the tightness and heaviness being released from my body.

Internal Craniosacral Therapy

Having physical-level craniosacral therapy to release your tailbone (coccyx) and rectal canal can also make a tremendous difference to people with irritable or inflamed bowels. I know of one woman who was cured of thirty years of diarrhea using this therapy. The practitioner accesses these areas internally, either through your vagina or your rectal canal, so it has to be someone you trust and feel comfortable with. Most osteopaths are also trained in un-jamming or releasing the tailbone, so if you're already seeing an osteopath you may want to discuss this with them. If the practitioner is skilled and sensitive, you should feel minimal to no real discomfort throughout the procedure. You can also bring a family member or spouse with you to remain in the room while the treatment is being carried out if you feel vulnerable.

Craniosacral Therapy For Babies / Children

There are certain hospitals in the UK (England, Scotland, etc.) where every single newborn receives an osteopathic treatment that includes craniosacral therapy. There is inevitably trauma to the cranium (head), body and emotional body of a baby born via vaginal or caesarean birth. If this trauma or damage is unresolved, it can lead to a host of problems for the person, both in infancy and as it grows to a child. These problems can include headaches, vision problems, chewing and swallowing problems, sitting, crawling and walking problems, projectile vomiting, colic, lack of balance/coordination, etc. There are so many problems treated with invasive medical procedures – like surgery for blocked tear ducts, orthotics or braces for feet and walking problems – that are simply unnecessary if the baby/child is taken for craniosacral therapy. If your child is accident-prone it may be because their balance and coordination are being hindered – craniosacral treatment can re-balance accident-prone babies/children and help them avoid so much damage and trauma.

I have lots of stories of 'miraculous' occurrences following craniosacral for babies or children and if you're interested in hearing them, or if you have a baby/child, then pick up my video called *BABY FART AEROBICS: And*

> Yes, our emotional body is inextricably linked and intertwined with our physical body. When you start to explore this link and heal the emotional body, some of the physical results are truly amazing.

Other Natural Treatments for Colicky Babies (available at www.ColicInfant.com). There is a large section in the video where I show a live craniosacral treatment on my daughter Zara (then eight weeks old) accompanied by a fascinating, in-depth interview with craniosacral therapist Lori Main.

Craniosacral is such a wonderful, completely nurturing healing therapy, that I believe every child and/or baby should have at least a couple of sessions to set them up for unrestricted growth and development. Babies and children should also be treated with craniosacral after any violent fall or accident that causes jarring to the body, especially if their head was knocked or injured at all. I firmly believe that if I had received craniosacral therapy as a baby and child, then I would not have developed scoliosis by the age of twelve.

Craniosacral Therapy Or Surgery?

I once had a phone consultation with a woman who had given birth four months previously, and ever since had heartburn so severe that even the prescription medications weren't working. Then an ultrasound showed an unidentified mass the size of a baseball in her abdomen, so the doctors were now wanting to do a full panel of gastrointestinal exploratory tests and possibly surgery. Understandably, she was very worried and coupled with the stress and sleep-deprivation of a newborn, you can just imagine this poor woman's state. After a thorough discussion with her, I presented her with my opinion in which I summarized, "You're understandably very scared right now and receiving a lot of pressure from doctors to proceed with the exploratory tests/surgery as soon as possible. However, you are faced with a choice. You can pursue the non-invasive healing methods first and see if that works. If it doesn't, the exploratory tests and surgery are always going to be there for you. If you take two weeks to explore kinder, gentler methods of healing, is that going to make so much difference to your prognosis?" I told her about the kind of things that craniosacral therapy can help with and especially since she'd just been through pregnancy and childbirth (which can really move around the internal organs and intestines), I suggested she start with that first. Luckily, she was in a city close to mine so I was able to refer her to a top-notch craniosacral therapist named Henry Epp (in Vancouver, Canada). I also suggested she simultaneously see a naturopath, just to cover all possibilities.

After only two sessions with Henry, she discontinued her heartburn medication and had no remaining heartburn whatsoever. In fact, she felt such a change in her body that she had her doctor re-do the ultrasound. The baseball-sized mass had completely disappeared and no further testing or surgery was required. Needless to say, she was overjoyed. Now just imagine the incredible amount of illness and trauma she saved herself by pursuing a natural path of healing first.

The possibilities for healing of IBS and IBD-related conditions through craniosacral therapy are so immense, that I recommend everyone reading this manual to find a good practitioner and have at least one or two sessions to see for yourself the relief possible through craniosacral therapy. To find a practitioner in your area, use the search tool at *www.upledger.com* and specify a practitioner at Level II or higher.

 Notes:

EMOTIONAL FREEDOM TECHNIQUE (EFT)

I've spent the last few years learning about and experimenting with a body/mind healing tool called EFT (Emotional Freedom Technique). EFT is derived from a centuries-old Chinese acupuncture meridian tapping practice called Neigong. The founder of EFT, an engineer called Gary Craig, used the principles of Neigong, but adapted it for the western mind.

EFT works by tapping on a series of acupuncture (meridian) points whilst a) talking out loud about the problem, b) re-framing the problem in a way that sets you up for a positive or alternate experience concerning the problem and c) choosing or affirming that you're willing to move into a new reality with this issue. Tapping on the acupuncture points whilst talking frees or releases the problem/negativity/trauma etc. from your energy body and your physical body. In this way it is a healing therapy that effectively integrates and effects change in the mind, body and spirit.

LISTEN TO YOUR GUT

EFT works extremely well when applied correctly. The key is being able to figure out what is at the root of your problem/issue/symptom and then tapping effectively on that. In certain circumstances, there can be a number of roots, or layers to the problem, which all have to be addressed to see resolution in your physical body. EFT is my favorite body/mind healing tool for the simple reason that once you learn how to do it effectively, you can do it yourself and take it with you anywhere. You may need a therapist initially, to guide you through your complicated, many-layered issues, but thereafter you'll probably be able to address most problems on your own. Some people are able to reach this level of proficiency on their own, without any outside help, but others need several sessions with a skilled therapist to become fluent in the technique. Alternatively, you can purchase instructional videos from Gary Craig's website to help you (they're very reasonably priced). You can find out all about EFT, sign up for his free newsletter (which is excellent) and download a Basic Training Manual for free by going to *www.MeridianTherapyTechniques.com*. Gary Craig makes all this information available without charge because his ultimate vision is to have one person in every family trained in EFT and thus able to alleviate so much avoidable suffering.

For myself, I downloaded the basic, free training manual, read the newsletter regularly and had a mild degree of success using EFT on my own, but nothing noteworthy. However, I kept at it since it really 'clicked' in my gut that this *should* work really well, and I just hadn't figured it out yet. Then I tried a very expensive PhD psychotherapist who was EFT certified, but again, $400 later I can't say a whole lot had changed. I must point out though, that I didn't really 'click' with this therapist. Although he was a nice enough fellow, I found him to be quite egotistical and at one point he even said, "You're going to think that I'm God." Uhh...I don't think so, buddy! Yes, I know, I should have listened to my gut and walked out right then.

Despite my disappointing experience with this high-profile therapist, my gut kept urging me not to give up and a year later I found a really good EFT therapist named Andy Bryce. I have had excellent results from my sessions with Andy – with clear, measurable results. And not just for me, but there's been a domino-effect for my husband and kids too – as we heal ourselves, the people connected with us shift and are healed too, if they're open to it. I had many sessions with Andy and worked mostly on money, career, issues with my mother, and my own parenting. Andy started off as a massage therapist, then moved into energy (pranic) healing and became a Reiki Master, hence his intuitive abilities are quite high and this really helps in being able to get to the root of an issue.

When I began my sessions with Andy I was at a very low point, feeling absolutely swamped and in serious financial debt. In fact, after the first two sessions I didn't re-book, because I couldn't afford it. But Andy, bless him, said to me, "No, Jini, I *see* who you are and you are so close. Just pay me whatever you can afford, and if you can't pay me anything, then no problem, we're going to keep going. Because once we get you free of this stuff, money is not going to be an issue for you." So I worked out what I could afford, and we kept going. Things kept improving with each session, and I actually kept a written record of the all the positive financial events and shifts that occurred (and continue to occur!) By the fifth session, I sent Andy a cheque for the balance owing on all my discounted sessions.

EFT is such a wonderful therapy because it illustrates so perfectly (and quickly) that when you change energy/thought/feeling, you change reality. I'll just give you one example of how this works. Andy and I worked directly with my money issues for three sessions. When I first went to see him, we were absolutely bottomed out financially from raising our children ourselves (no daycare), and funding the growth of a new business. We had no assets left, were deeply in debt and it looked like we would have to sell our house in the next two months. During the sessions, I discovered that my money issues were also linked into parenting issues – prior to having children I'd had no trouble making money and could make things happen very quickly. After our kids were born, both my husband, Ian, and I felt like we were moving through mud, trying to make things happen.
Every day, every project, was such a struggle – with none of the ease and flow we'd both experienced before having children. During my sessions with Andy, I discovered clear psychological/emotional blocks I had to

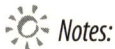 Notes:

becoming wealthy, and I also realized that my extreme love for my children combined with my fear that I "must not screw them up" caused my energy to seize up (as fear usually does). Energetically, I was contracting and stagnating, rather than expanding, flowing, and opening.

As I cleared these blocks using EFT, everything started to shift financially, for both myself and Ian. Previously, we had applied to every bank we could think of for some sort of financing, re-mortgage, second mortgage, line of credit, etc. – anything that we could use to fund us until our new business was generating sufficient revenue. Every financial institution, including aggressive banks like ING Direct, turned us down. Your debt ratio is too high, they all said. Well, after my third session with Andy, tapping away on money issues, Ian phoned up our bank manager again – and the bank agreed to re-mortgage our house for another $50,000! Now, you see, this is the beauty of EFT – absolutely *nothing* had changed with our physical situation. We still had the exact same debt ratio. Our bank manager had refused to loan, re-finance, or re-mortgage our house only six weeks prior. The only thing that had changed was the energy. Our physical reality was the same, but our energy reality had changed completely. So we got the money we needed to fund the next stage of the business, and we didn't have to sell our house! As I continued to work with Andy on my financial issues, things like this happened one after the other.

I've included this financial example of EFT's effectiveness because sometimes with 'miraculous' physical healings, people will come up with all kinds of reasons to explain it away, or they'll attribute the healing to some other factor. However, with a hard topic like money, where all the factors have stayed the same, it's pretty hard to dismiss the evidence. It may take some time to work through all the layers of an issue (or illness), and it may take some experimenting to find the right practitioner, but EFT definitely works very well – and it works long-term.

I then felt my gut urging me to contact another EFT therapist named Aileen Nobles (I had read an article she'd written for the EFT newsletter). Aileen has been a psychic hypnotherapist for the past 28 years and her clientele is

> ☼ EFT is such a wonderful therapy because it illustrates so perfectly (and quickly) that when you change energy/thought/feeling, you change reality.

extensive, including celebrities and political figures. She has her own cable television show called *Light Transformation*, where she will often do EFT sessions on air. She was also *Psychic to the Stars on Leeza Gibbon's Top 25 Countdown Show* – a syndicated weekly music radio show. She was filmed having a session with a client for The Learning Channel's *All About Angels*, and she gave predictions on NBC's *The Other Side*. Aileen also talked about her experience working with angels on the *Susan Powter Show*, and consulted for CBS' *Angels Among Us*. In spite of being a well-known psychic in the U.S., Aileen is so gentle, friendly and caring, I felt immediately safe and relaxed with her.

My gut was telling me that Aileen was the person to work with on long-standing physical problems I'd had with choking and an extremely tight internal anal sphincter muscle. I'd had choking problems since birth, and my internal anal sphincter had been malfunctioning ever since I had rectal surgery to remove some perianal skin tags in 1988. As I've written throughout this book, physical problems are rarely (if ever) just physical problems. And with chronic issues/symptoms you can be sure there are multiple layers and many causative events involved. This is why it is so helpful to find a therapist who is also highly spiritually intuitive, psychic, etc. Not only will they come up with things that instantly 'hit home' with you, but they will ask you the right questions to stimulate buried memories, forgotten hurts or vows, and make connections between separate events that you may have missed. Needless to say, my sessions with Aileen were profound, healing, and transformative. I highly recommend both Aileen and Andy to anyone doing this program.

You can find a complete listing of EFT therapists in your area by going to: www.MeridianTherapyTechniques.com. You can also have EFT sessions by phone and this is equally effective (all my sessions with Aileen were by phone and some of my sessions with Andy). To find out more about Andy Bryce and/or book a session with him, go to: *www.spiritcoach.ca*. To find out more about Aileen Nobles and/or book a session with her, visit: *www.aileennobles.com*.

> ☼ It may take some time to work through all the layers of an issue (or illness), and it may take some experimenting to find the right practitioner, but EFT definitely works very well – and the results are long-term.

Before you book an EFT session, I recommend you go to this website *www.MeridianTherapyTechniques.com* to download the free Basic Training Manual and learn the EFT tapping points first. This will save you some money, as you won't have to spend your session time learning which points to tap on. For your first few sessions, it's also handy to keep the diagram of meridian tapping points in front of you, in case you can't remember exactly where they are. It's also useful (but not necessary) to have a speaker-phone for phone sessions, so you can have your hands free and really relax.

HYPNOTHERAPY

I've had many sessions of hypnotherapy throughout the years and they have definitely contributed to my healing. Hypnotherapy is useful for addressing not only current issues and symptoms, but also if you want to explore your infancy, early childhood, or even past life events that you think may be negatively influencing your health. Again, the skill of the practitioner is of paramount importance here. Make sure the person possesses legitimate accreditation and that you also 'click' well with them on a personality level. You need to find a practitioner that you feel very comfortable and safe with, otherwise you won't be able to relax fully.

Hypnosis is simply being in a state of deep relaxation – similar to meditation, or that zone where you've just woken up in the morning and are still kind of 'floaty' and relaxed. There's nothing scary or voodoo about it at all. You remain in complete control at all times and can talk or end the session if you wish. Some people who are able to relax completely, very quickly, enter a state of supreme relaxation referred to as 'deep trance'. In a deep trance state it's like you're asleep, and upon 'awakening' you may or may not have any conscious memory of what's happened. However, even for people who don't remember anything, once someone starts talking about the session and what happened, the person will usually start to remember.

However, whether you're in a light trance or deep trance, there certainly is a measure of 'giving up control' that takes place. This has to happen in order for true relaxation to take place and for the session to be successful.

> Hypnotherapy is useful for addressing not only current issues and symptoms, but also if you want to explore your infancy, early childhood, or even past life events that you think may be negatively influencing your health.

Choosing a practitioner who gives you a good gut feeling is your first step towards ensuring you're with someone who is safe. Other things you can do to ensure your safety (and thus enable yourself to fully relax) is to make sure the session is tape recorded from beginning to end. Or, you can set up your own video camera at the start of the session and then stop it at the end. Another alternative is to have a close friend or family member come in to the session with you the first few times, until you feel comfortable. This can be difficult though, as you'll need to have someone who is truly supportive, non-judgmental, and able to accept whatever might come up during a session. Also, you may find yourself editing what you say because of your friend/family member in the room, and that won't be very helpful. For these reasons it's best to go with a tape or video recording if you can.

Hypnotherapy (like EFT and Craniosacral therapy) is very helpful for people with IBD and IBS because it taps into the realm of healing possible within the brain-gut axis (see Chapter One). By addressing mental/emotional issues that are adversely triggering the autonomic nervous system, hypnotherapy can resolve or at least help conditions like diarrhea, constipation, cramping/spasming, pain, heartburn, and faulty digestion and absorption. Remember, that these are all functions that are directly influenced by the autonomic nervous system (see Chapter One). So if you resolve the malfunctioning of your nervous system, you will automatically resolve (or at least improve) the functioning of your digestive system.

Hypnotherapy has been extensively studied for its positive effects on people with irritable bowel syndrome (IBS) and the studies have been published in prestigious medical journals like *Gastroenterology, Gut* and *The Lancet*. I have excerpted some of these studies in Appendix D for those of you who are interested, or want to do further research. The research to date shows that hypnotherapy is extremely successful in reducing or eliminating all symptoms of IBS, and that the results held during follow-up periods of 3 – 6 months. However the following parameters must be met for optimal results:

▶ You need to have at least seven sessions in a row to see a measurable effect that lasts.

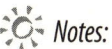 *Notes:*

- People with severe psychological problems or atypical symptom profiles showed lower rates of success.

- People over the age of 50 showed lower rates of success (perhaps because of mental barriers and an inability or unwillingness to fully relax?).

Personally, I believe hypnotherapy is so effective for people with IBS because their dis-ease has not become as systemic or entrenched as it is in people with IBD. Also, almost all people with Crohn's, colitis, etc., will have an infectious component to their illness. Altering/improving hormonal secretions and digestive function is not going to resolve an infection of pathogenic microorganisms (like yeast, fungus, mycoplasma, mycobacteria, parasites, bad bacteria, etc.). Therefore, for people with IBD, hypnotherapy is definitely effective and can provide substantial relief and healing, but it is not likely to eliminate your diarrhea (for example) or completely resolve all symptoms, as it can for someone with IBS. Obviously, people with IBS can also have an infectious component to their illness and perhaps these people comprise the 'atypical symptom patterns' referenced in the studies in Appendix D – for whom hypnotherapy helped, but was not nearly as successful as for those with classical symptom patterns.

If you have IBS, I strongly recommend you try EFT or hypnotherapy to address the emotional component of your illness. If you have IBD, I think you'll see better results from EFT or craniosacral therapy, or, find a hypnotherapist who's *also* certified in EFT (see *www.MeridianTherapyTechniques.com* for a list of practitioners) – this would be wonderful for people with IBD or IBS.

MEDITATION

Essentially, anything that puts you in touch with your intuitive self and plugs you into whatever it is you call "God", can be labeled a form of meditating. There are numerous beneficial techniques and it's simply a matter of finding what type of meditation suits you the best. A walk in the woods breathing in the wonderful fresh smells and feeling a part of the

Sidebar: Anything that puts you in touch with your intuitive self, and plugs you into whatever it is you call "God", is a form of meditation.

mental chatter and activity often find it helpful to use a mantra when meditating. Repeating a phrase (mantra) over and over again gives their mind something to do so they can focus on their breathing and allow themselves to become calm and still. Transcendental Meditation and Primordial Sound Meditation are both forms of mantra meditation. Simply sitting in a pool of sunlight, breathing deeply and opening yourself to receive the healing rays of the sun is a form of meditation. If you're a Christian who likes to pray, then just sit or lie down somewhere and instead of you talking to God or Jesus, let them talk to you – stay quiet and peaceful and simply listen, open yourself to receive.

If you practice some of the healing visualizations listed in this book, as you become more and more fluent with them you will find yourself in a deeply relaxed, meditative state. If you find it difficult to relax and meditate on your own, your local metaphysical bookstore should sell a selection of guided meditation cassette tapes – just pop one in your tape deck and follow the directions. Meditation helps you to develop your intuition and your ability to listen to and understand your body. There are also direct health benefits derived from regular meditation including stress reduction, lowered blood pressure, improved mental functioning and an improved immune system. Following is a simple meditative technique I enjoy.

Cultivating Stillness

Sit down on the floor (if possible; or in a chair) with your back straight, and shoulders relaxed. Keep your eyes open and focus your attention on your ajna chakra (also known as "the third eye", located midway between your two eyebrows). If you lick your finger and dab some saliva on your ajna chakra it will help you to know and focus on where it is. Focusing your attention on your ajna chakra will cause your vision and attention to shift into soft-focus, like when you're staring absentmindedly at something. Sit there for as long as you can and just do

> **Level of Chronc Stress predicts Clinical Outcome in irritable bowel syndrome**
> In the majority of patients with irritable bowel syndrome (IBS) and functional dyspepsia (FD), life stress contributes to symptom onset and exacerbation. One hundred and seventeen outpatients who satisfied the modified Rome criteria for IBS (66% with one or more concurrent FD symptoms) participated in a trial to test the relation of chronic life stress threat to subsequent symptom intensity over time. It was found that chronic life stress threat was a powerful predictor of subsequent symptom intensity, explaining 97% of the variance on this measure over 16 months. No patient exposed to even one chronic highly threatening stressor improved clinically (by 50%) over the 16 months; all patients who improved did so in the absence of such a stressor.
> Bennett, E.J. et al. *Gut* 1998, 43 (2) 256-61

nothing. Be with the stillness. If you have thoughts, just let them come and then let them go. You can have thoughts constantly coming into your mind, but you don't have to pay them any attention. Don't fight your thoughts, don't try to stop thinking, simply allow them to come and allow them to go. Try to be with your stillness every day.

DIALOGUING WITH YOUR BODY

I advise numerous times throughout this book to "follow your intuition" or "listen to your body". For those of you who want a little more guidance in exactly how to go about this, you can develop your awareness and intuition by using the following simple technique:

1. Use whatever method you currently use to get still and peaceful. This could be praying, walking through the woods, soaking in a bubble bath, lying down and breathing deeply, or various forms of meditation. Use your method to become relaxed and still.

2. When you're fully relaxed and peaceful (or as near as you can get), and your breathing is deep, place your hand on your abdomen and simply allow the feelings and thoughts from your tummy/bowels/gut to flow into you. Allow yourself to feel whatever comes up, no matter how trivial or stupid or painful it may be. You will not be hurt by allowing yourself to feel. You will be healed. Just stay here for a while, allowing yourself to feel and acknowledge whatever comes up for you. The first few times you do this, you may want to stop after this point, or you may want to continue on to the next step. Do whatever feels comfortable for you.

3. After you've allowed some of your feelings and thoughts to arise, begin a dialogue out loud with your tummy/bowels (wherever you sense the feelings and thoughts are coming from). This could involve simply repeating out loud whatever feelings you're having: "Yes, I'm feeling angry that my girlfriend went away for the weekend...Yes, I'm very worried about my deadline for this work project". Or, you may find

> Meditation helps you to develop your intuition, and your ability to listen to and understand your body.

yourself perceiving your guts as a helpless baby, or your own inner child, and your dialogue may involve things like: "Oh my poor sweetie, it's okay, you're safe, mummy/daddy is going to look after you now...Yes, I know, you've been so hurt." The important point is simply to allow whatever you feel like saying, don't judge it, don't think about what it might mean, don't worry that you're sounding ridiculous, simply allow.

4. Continue breathing deeply. If you have any questions for your bowels or stomach, ask them now, and trust whatever you feel is the answer. The feeling may be quite faint in the beginning, but you need to trust it and act upon it in order for your feeling (or intuition) to grow stronger. The more you trust those vague feelings or sense that you should or shouldn't do something, the stronger the feelings and sense will become. Intuition is like a muscle, the more you exercise it, the stronger it gets. When you have nothing more to say, continue to lie or sit quietly for a while, breathing deeply.

☼ You will not be hurt by allowing yourself to feel. You will be healed.

After you've done this technique numerous times, you'll get to the point where you can pretty much instantly access whatever's going on in your gut at any given time. You'll be able to still yourself and connect with your digestive system in a matter of moments anywhere you might be. If you want to connect with another part of your body that's in pain or distress, simply follow the same procedure but place your hand on whichever part of your body you wish to access. A little tip here: When you're asking your digestive system what kind of food it wants, or whether a particular food is safe to eat, make sure you're asking and receiving an answer from your stomach/intestines, rather than your taste buds. Your taste buds may want beer and pizza – but your stomach/gut wants grilled fish and butternut squash. Often I feel like eating something and when I check in with my body I realize it's my taste buds that want that food, but my stomach actually doesn't. There was one time I craved sugar a couple of times a day for two weeks, but every time I checked in with my stomach, it didn't want sugar, it wanted water. So I would drink a glass of water and presto, no more craving for sugar! I tell you, the body is a strange and wonderful thing.

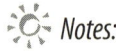 Notes:

COLONIC MASSAGE

Colonic massage is extremely helpful whether you're experiencing gas, bloating, diarrhea, constipation or blockages. As the parent of a child with IBD or IBS, this can be a very meaningful way to connect in a soothing, loving way with your child. Most, if not all, of the medical treatments your child has been subjected to are invasive and traumatic. Alternatively, colonic massage is a very helpful treatment that you can administer gently and lovingly. A couple of years after I had taught this massage technique to my brother (who is a medical doctor), he taught it to the mother of one of his patients in hospital with ulcerative colitis. The next day while he was doing rounds with a couple of other doctors, the woman came rushing up to him and thanked him profusely for teaching her the technique. She said her child had slept through the night for the first time and that it had helped him more than anything else they had done. A tip: Make sure you're in a loving, calm state of being before massaging your child, and keep your movements gentle and sensitive throughout.

When doing the colonic massage technique on the toilet, experiment with different sitting positions; lean forward or lean back. Breathe deeply into your diaphragm (you'll see it expand just under your ribcage), and the pressure from the air you've inhaled will often be enough to move some stool along.

Another technique is to sit back against the wall or back of the toilet, keep your abdomen completely relaxed and grab the tops of your knees with your fingertips. Use your arms to rock your torso gently back and forth – don't use your abdominal muscles! Breathe deeply and relax. Alternate these techniques with colonic massage and you'll soon find the combination/sequence that works best for you.

You can also get a child's stepping stool (available very cheaply at Ikea), or use a couple of phonebooks and place them under your feet whilst sitting on the toilet. Raising your knees up higher than your hips more closely approximates a squatting position – which is the best way to facilitate the passage of stool since it aligns and opens your rectal canal. However, if you have internal hemorrhoids, or a rectal fissure, you may not want to use the stepping stool under your feet. Properly aligning and opening your rectal canal can cause the stool to come out too quickly for those with hemorrhoids or fissures, or it may be okay/beneficial. Test it and see if it works for you.

If you use these techniques combined with colonic massage, rather than pushing and straining, you'll greatly reduce your chances of developing hemorrhoids and if you have some already, you'll be giving them the best chance to heal.

Blockages & Constipation

A self-administered colonic massage can really help if you're experiencing constipation, blockages in thickened areas of your colon, or blockages in diverticulae (hollow pouches that occur when the inner intestinal lining has pushed through weakened areas of the colon wall), where food is getting stuck and causing a lot of pain.

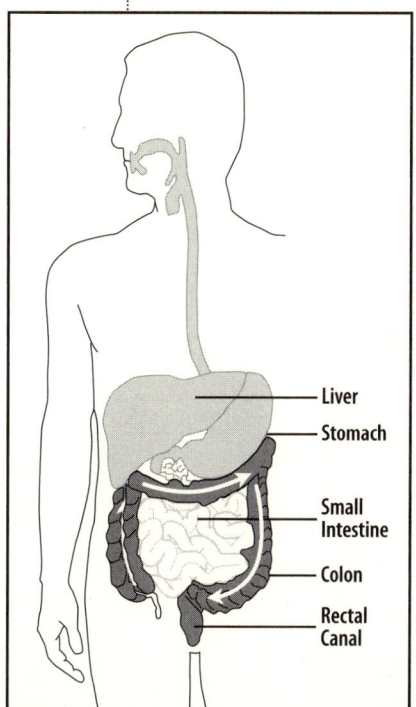

1. Lie down on your bed or the couch with your knees bent and the soles of your feet on the bed/couch. Take several slow, deep breaths to relax and calm yourself. Lift your shirt up, undo your pants and start at the lower right quadrant of your abdomen. Stroke your fingertips upwards until you reach the bottom of your ribcage. Now stroke your hand left across the underside of your ribcage and then down again to the lower left quadrant of your abdomen. You've just roughly traced the path of your colon, starting at the end of the small intestine in a horseshoe shape until it joins the rectal canal.

2. Follow the path of your colon in a soothing, stroking motion (always in the same direction as described) and notice as you become more sensitive to where it is and how it feels.

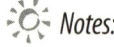 *Notes:*

3. The next step is to apply a bit of pressure with your fingertips and move them in a circular, probing motion as you follow the colon around. Experiment with both the probing motion and the amount of pressure you use.

4. As you get to know your colon better, you'll be able to notice any areas that feel harder and/or thicker than the rest. If you've got stool stuck in a diverticula (intestinal pouch), the pain and irritation should tell you where it is. Focus on this area now and gently massage in and around it with your fingertips. Imagine yourself gently breaking up the stool clogged there and helping it move through the thickened section, or out of the pouch, and stroking/massaging it along the path towards the rectal canal.

5. When you think you've cleared most of the blockage from the problem area, go back to the lower right quadrant and begin massaging the colon, moving upwards toward the ribcage, across, and then down to the lower left quadrant. When you get to the blockage again, spend a little more time, massaging the food through there and then continuing on the path to the rectal canal.

6. At any point in this process, you may feel the need for a bowel movement. If so, go sit on the toilet and continue with the massage. Remember to take deep breaths and stay relaxed. Keep your abdomen and anal sphincter muscle loose, open and relaxed.

For a diverticulitis blockage, perform the massage on an empty stomach and experiment with drinking two glasses of warm spring water fifteen minutes before your massage, and then two more glasses immediately following, to try and further help flush out the stool particles.

Gas & Bloating

A similar colonic massage technique can also be used when you're feeling bloated and experiencing cramping from gas.

1. Begin the massage sitting on the toilet. Take deep breaths and relax the abdomen and anal sphincter muscle, allow yourself to make as much noise farting and crapping as you want. Don't tense or hold anything back.

2. Use the same technique as described above – following around the path of your colon from lower right, up, across to the left and then down the left side – but instead of using your fingertips, use the heel of your right hand in a kind of digging, circular motion and follow the colon around to the rectal canal.

3. When you get to the bottom of the lower left quadrant, dig/press a little deeper and massage towards the center of your groin (where your rectal canal is). Sometimes you may want to hold the pressure there for a few moments and rock gently back and forth.

4. Again, experiment with the massage motion and the amount of pressure you use. Be patient as it will take you a while to develop your technique to maximum effectiveness.

5. Keep massaging along the colon until you feel the pressure is relieved and there's nothing more in there that wants to come out.

This technique is especially effective after surgery (or a colonoscopy) as your colon will be full of air and causing you a great deal of pain. Get up and start walking around as soon after you come out of the anesthetic as possible. If you need two nurses to support you in case you faint – get them. Walk around until you feel the pressure building, then go sit on the toilet (again, a nurse may need to come in with you in case you faint – don't worry, they've seen/heard everything and this is no time for modesty) relax your abdomen and anal sphincter muscle and begin the colonic massage. It will probably hurt like crazy but try to continue (of course, if you've had surgery on your colon, go *very* gently and carefully). When you've farted out as much as you can, go back to bed. Rest for about 15 – 20 minutes (more or less, whatever feels right), then call the nurse and go for another walk and massage session. Keep repeating this procedure until you have no more

> Most of the medical treatments your child has been subjected to are invasive and traumatic. Colonic massage is a very meaningful way to connect in a soothing, loving way with your child, whilst assisting their physical body.

air to get rid of. This will speed your recovery considerably because not only will it ease the pain, but you will also resume normal urination more quickly, feel stronger, and be in better spirits overall.

Cramping & Diarrhea

If you tend to get attacks of cramping where you have to run for the toilet and then sit there for the next hour or two, because every time you try to get up, you have another bowel movement, then this technique will also be a big help to you.

1. Begin your massage sitting on the toilet. Remember to breathe deeply and relax. As you perform the massage, you'll basically be helping to move the separate little stool deposits that are dotted throughout your colon around and out of your rectum in a much shorter period of time than if you relied on your own peristalsis (rhythmic contractions of the intestinal wall), which is obviously not getting the job done.

2. Start at the lower right quadrant of your abdomen. Stroke your fingertips upwards until you reach the bottom of your ribcage. Now stroke your hand left across the underside of your ribcage and then down again to the lower left quadrant of your abdomen. You've just roughly traced the path of your colon, starting at the end of the small intestine in a horseshoe shape until it joins the rectal canal.

3. Follow the path of your colon in a soothing, stroking motion (always in the same direction as described) and notice as you become more sensitive to where it is and how it feels.

4. The next step is to use the heel of your right hand, or your knuckles, in a kind of digging, circular motion and follow the colon around to the rectal canal. Experiment with both the motion and the amount of pressure you use.

5. When you get to the bottom of the lower left quadrant, dig/press a little deeper and massage towards the center of your groin and down as far as you can go (this allows you to massage your rectal canal). Sometimes

you may want to hold the pressure there for a few moments and rock gently back and forth.

6. Again, experiment with the massage motion and the amount of pressure you use. Be patient as it will take you a while to develop your technique to maximum effectiveness.

7. Keep massaging along the colon until you feel the pressure is relieved and there's nothing more in there that wants to come out.

EXERCISE

It's imperative that you exercise at least three times a week. I cannot stress the importance of regular exercise enough. If all you can manage is to go outside, walk down the block and back – great! Do it. And if you can do it every day, even better. Any amount or level of exercise will help your circulatory system get rid of toxins and will put your mind and emotions in a healthier state, so they can then help your body.

Mobilizing Your Lifeforce Energy

If you can manage more, exercise to whatever level is comfortable for you, but not beyond it. The goal of your exercising is to nurture and strengthen your body, not test it and challenge it. Hard, challenging workouts lead to immune system suppression – not a good thing for people who are already ill! Excellent workouts that are strengthening, but not too hard on the cardiovascular system, include weight training, walking, yoga and tai chi. The extra benefit of yoga, tai chi, chi kung and other 'soft' meditative martial arts is that these forms of exercise don't just affect and improve the physical body. They are doubly beneficial because they also liberate and activate the chakras (energy centers) and the overall energy flow (chi or ki) within the body. By doing them you are activating and stimulating your body's chi (lifeforce energy), which your body uses to heal itself. You don't have to join a class or turn this into an expensive endeavor, as there are many videotapes available for all levels of yoga and tai chi. Stay away from power yoga, Bikram's yoga or other strenuous styles. Choose yoga that is

> Yoga and Tai Chi are doubly beneficial because they also liberate and activate the chakras (energy centers) and the overall energy flow within the body.

described with words like 'gentle, relaxing, restorative', etc. I especially like using videos because then I can work totally at my own pace, in the comfort of my home.

If it's not automatically included in your exercise regimen, you should also do some sort of stretching routine every day (or as often as you can). If our musco-skeletal frame is cramped and tight, how can we expect our insides to be relaxed and easy? You don't even need to start a formalized program of calisthenics or a particular stretching routine. Just clear yourself some space on the floor and simply let your body move, twist, bend and reach in whatever ways and whatever direction feels good to you. As I've said before, your body knows exactly what it needs at all times, so just trust it and allow yourself to go with it. Remember to take deep breaths throughout and relax.

Yoga Videos

I'm hoping to do some yoga videos with my yoga instructor, Sandra Sammartino, in the near future, specifically for people with Crohn's, colitis, diverticulitis and irritable bowel syndrome. And who knows, by the time you're reading this program, maybe they'll already be available! Relaxing the abdomen, spine (and related areas) via yoga, massage, or craniosacral therapy can completely change your digestion, bowel movements, and quality of sleep. The night of my yoga class, I sleep 7 – 8 hours in a row completely uninterrupted – I don't get up to pee or poo for the whole night (usually I wake once). For those of you having 15 bowel movements a day, imagine how that would feel and how healing and restorative for your body it would be!

At the time of writing, my yoga instructor Sandra Sammartino is 63 years old and she's been teaching for over 30 years. Her yoga is so wonderful because she has an immense knowledge of the interrelatedness and intricacies of the human body and in each session we work with the energy body (prana, lifeforce energy) as much as the physical body. This really mobilizes your body's self-healing ability and produces profound nurturing and relaxation. In the videos with Sandra, we're going to focus specifically on freeing-up and relaxing both the small and large intestine and also

> The great thing about a yoga video is you can do it in the privacy of your own home – very useful if you're having frequent bowel movements, or if you wish to do it right before bed, to help you have a deep, healing sleep.

addressing all the varied parts of the body that refer or tie in to the gut. The great thing about having it on video is you'll be able to do it in the privacy of your own home – very useful if you're having frequent bowel movements, or if you wish to do it right before bed to help you have a deep, healing sleep. To see if the yoga videos are available, go to my website: www.ListenToYourGut.com

Exercising With Anemia

For an outline of an exercise regimen to help you either gain or lose weight, or for those of you with Osteoporosis who need to strengthen your bones, see the section on *Malnutrition* in Chapter Two. Remember, just because your hemoglobin levels are low, it doesn't mean you have to give up exercise. Doctors may try to panic you with tales of an impending heart attack if you exert yourself with a hemoglobin level of 7 (or 70 depending which measurement they're using) or lower. Now if you're a 40 year old couch potato, 50 lbs. overweight, who's never done a day of exercise in your life – the doctor is probably right (but there's still no excuse for you not to get out for a walk every day). However, as with all things to do with the mind/body, everything is relative.

> If all you can manage is to go outside, walk down the block and back – great! Do it.

I've enjoyed good cardiovascular and muscular fitness my whole life, so I was able to do 3-hour kickboxing classes with a hemoglobin level of 7.2 (or 72). At a hemoglobin level of 6.2 I could no longer do the high-energy cardio workouts but I could go for 2 hour walks or do an hour of yoga.

Again, listen to your body, it will tell you what it can and can't do. Check your pulse frequently or place your hand over your heart to feel how hard it's working. If your pulse is too high or your heart feels like it's pounding like a jackhammer, then you're doing too much, too fast. It's better to go slowly and gently than to trigger a backlash reaction in your body because you've pushed it too far. Remember that nurturing and relaxation are the primary goals of exercise whilst your IBS or IBD is active. It takes a tremendous amount of energy to heal, so use exercise to nurture and support your healing process, not exhaust it.

Overcoming Reluctance

We've covered a lot of important mind/body healing tools in this chapter, and in the very next chapter I'll get into specific mental exercises or techniques that you can use to mobilize your lifeforce healing energy as well. Remember that to achieve healing in your physical body, you must also heal/resolve your emotional issues and stressors. This may be a hard road for many of you to take, and some people have a lot of resistance to seeking outside help for their emotional problems – or even admitting they have any emotional problems! I understand your reluctance, mistrust, stubbornness, etc. But you must believe me: No one achieves deep-level, long-lasting healing without healing their emotional body.

Even the medical profession has come to realize this and has established two fields of specialty to deal with this: Psychoneuroimmunology and Neurogastroenterology. So no matter how difficult it is for you, and how alien it feels to you, just push yourself through it and book yourself a session with whichever therapy you feel drawn towards. My consultation clients who see the best results are the ones who are simultaneously having EFT or craniosacral sessions. I have also had clients who were absolutely stuck in a symptom pattern, or escalating condition and refused to address their emotional issues. In these cases, they are either eventually forced by their declining health to finally seek emotional healing, or they abandon holistic healing altogether. You don't need to let your health deteriorate any further, or endure any more needless suffering. Pursue emotional as well as physical healing and you will heal yourself in the shortest amount of time, improve your quality of life and relationships, and experience wonderful aspects of yourself you didn't even know you had.

Turn to the *Healing Journey Workbook* now, and complete the section for this chapter – Chapter Six.

> I have had clients who were absolutely stuck in a symptom pattern, or escalating condition, and they refused to address their emotional issues. In these cases, they are either eventually forced by their declining health to finally seek emotional healing, or they abandon holistic healing altogether.

7

Use Your Mind To Help Your Body

"My colleague, Dr. Rachel Naomi Remen, has said that illness could be considered a Western form of meditation. In the West, where the meditative tradition is not strong and people are not in the habit of stopping periodically to become quiet and reevaluate their lives, an illness – and sometimes only a serious illness such as a heart attack or cancer – stops a person so he can step back and have an opportunity to take stock of what is important to him."

Dr. Martin Rossman, MD

Much has been written about the interplay of the mind and body. Modern science has now discovered that thoughts and emotions produce actual chemical reactions or changes in the physical body (thoughts and feelings create physical states). Dr. Candace Pert has proven that neuropeptides are the result of thoughts and emotions being translated into physical matter.[1] If you'd like more information about this, Bill Moyers' book, *Healing and the Mind*, has a whole section of him interviewing medical and scientific professionals at the forefront of this new field of knowledge called psychoneuroimmunology.[2] If you want a simpler term, you can just call it mind/body medicine. The fact is that you can use your thoughts to create or determine your reality.

> Scientists have now discovered that thoughts and emotions produce actual chemical reactions or changes in the physical body: You can use your thoughts to create your physical reality.

AFFIRMATIONS

Positive affirmations are a powerful tool you can use to help yourself achieve everything from athletic excellence, to financial success, to excellent health. I suspect they're underrated because people feel stupid doing them initially. An affirmation is basically a positive statement that you repeat aloud in the present tense whilst looking at yourself in the mirror.
You can make up your own affirmation, or any book by Louise L. Hay contains many good ones.[3] Combining affirmations with EFT increases their effectiveness exponentially and will greatly reduce the time necessary to achieve the desired result.

The key to using affirmations is to keep them positive and in the present tense as though the situation/state already exists, "I am strong, I am healthy and I love my body", or, "My colon is healthy and absorbs all the nutrition I give it". Affirming is a way of programming your subconscious to do your bidding, or look after something for you. The message is delivered in three ways; you say the words, you hear the words, and you see yourself speaking. Simultaneously using EFT to integrate the affirmation with your physical and energy body is even more powerful. Saying something in the future tense, for example "I will be healthy", is not very effective. Your mind won't do anything now, in the present, as it will be locked into waiting for the future as you directed it. Also, an affirmation needs to be a positive, pro-active statement to work best. Negative statements, e.g., "I do not snore" can work, but not nearly as well as the positive statement, "I sleep on my side. I sleep peacefully and quietly". My husband used that statement every night before going to sleep to ensure he didn't wake me up with his snoring! The affirmation worked about 98% of the time and after a few months he didn't even need to say it anymore.

Think about some mental roots, beliefs, or thought patterns that you currently have that do not serve you. For example, you may have a root-level belief (absorbed from a parent or your culture) that says something like, "Life is a series of sorrows interrupted by fleeting joy". Spend some time thinking about this thought pattern; how does this thought serve you, is it life-affirming, does believing this lead you to a fuller and richer experience of life? If you realize that a thought pattern is life-minimizing, or life-destroying, then you may want to change that thought pattern. In order to start re-programming this mental pattern, you have to get to the root of what's underneath this thought. I find that the common element under any thought or pattern that's negative, or defeatist, or less-than, is simply a form of fear. So, addressing the fear that's at the root of the above thought pattern could involve some of the following affirmations: "It is safe for me to live." "Life is wonderful. I love life." "Today is an expression of joy." "Life is so good to me. I'm glad to be alive." "I experience joy in all areas of my life."

Developing affirmations for yourself is going to involve a fair amount of time spent looking at your current thoughts, patterns and beliefs. Try to think of maxims you always heard your parents repeating, you'll likely discover these have infiltrated your mind-set in a most insidious way In order to heal yourself physically, you must also address your mental state. You need to let go of thought patterns that do not serve or help you and replace them with ones that do. You need to shift your mental state from one that is not affirming and serving you, to one that does. Yes, this first requires awareness, and then it requires discipline. Try to say your affirmations at least twice a day in front of the mirror, whilst tapping on the

☼ Combining affirmations with EFT increases their effectiveness exponentially and will greatly reduce the time necessary to achieve the desired result.

series of EFT acupuncture points and then say them out loud to yourself throughout the day whenever you remember and just tap on the 'karate chop' point. To download the EFT Basic Training Manual for free, go to: *www.emofree.com*.

HEALING VISUALIZATIONS

Visualizing means consciously imagining. It's the same thing you used to do so often as a child, except now you concentrate on imagining a specified thing, sequence, or result. You don't let your mind wander in and out of the scene, but hold it there as you "see" or imagine your chosen image or sequence occurring. If you find it difficult to concentrate and your attention wanders at first, don't worry about it. The more you practice visualizing, the better you'll become at it.

Visualizing also works on the premise that thought determines reality. Ask any top athlete, or member of the Chicago Bulls basketball team and they'll tell you how effective visualizing is. Any physicist will tell you that anything and everything in our universe is composed of energy. If you break anything down to its smallest unit, you'll have pure energy. Likewise, thought is also energy and therefore dynamic and capable of affecting change and altering physical reality. Your thoughts determine your beliefs, your beliefs determine your actions, and your actions determine and create your physical reality. Regular, concentrated visualization of a desired occurrence or process can produce very real, physical results.

There are many different ways to visualize healing. Some people like to visualize soothing colors (e.g., blue to calm inflammation), others visualize inanimate things such as a web of rubber bands stretching with each breath in and then sagging, losing their tightness as the breath goes out. There are many, many books available on visualization techniques for both direct healing and also relaxation, strengthening and energizing. I'm just going to describe three of my favorite techniques with you here, one for direct healing, one for overall healing, and the other for balancing and calming. I find it's best to visualize at night in bed, so you can drift off to sleep with

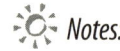 Notes:

the images and feelings still floating around you. Of course, you can do these visualizations ten times a day if you like, or do a main one at night or in the morning and return to it briefly to affirm your image(s) throughout the day. You may want to take some of these visualizations and record them, so that you can play them in your personal listenng device as you drift off to sleep at night.

Direct Healing

This technique has been extremely effective for me and I have used it on everything from healing bleeding intestinal wounds and ulcers to curing an ear infection overnight. Visualize the site you want to heal (your intestinal tract, ear canal, etc.) imagine how it looks in there and what needs to be done to clean it up and soothe the site and heal it. Then imagine a team of tiny little workers coming in and doing whatever needs to be done to treat, soothe and heal the area.

Here's an example of what I visualize to heal an ulcerated area of my intestine: First I look at the intestinal wall where it's ulcerated and I notice that it's swollen, puffy, and there's blood and pus oozing out. My little workers in their bright, clean overalls arrive and immediately go to work. They have little wings on their backs so they can fly up the sides of the wall and treat wounded areas without having to rest their body weight on the painful surface. First they cleanse the area with soft pressure hoses containing warm water which washes away a lot of the blood and pus. Next, they have super soft gloves which they rub in a circular motion to slough off all the dead, pus-filled tissue. They rinse again with the warm water. Now they have pots of herbal salve in their hands and they gently massage this in over the wounded area. I can see/feel how much better my intestine feels already. I stop visualizing at this point and leave the area alone for a day or so as I know the salve takes a while to sink in and go to work.

The next day/night I visualize the workers going back in and dousing again with warm water and gently cleaning with a soft, moisturizing soap. The wall looks much better. It has stopped bleeding and the wounds are in

> Any physicist will tell you that anything and everything in our universe is composed of energy. If you break anything down to its smallest unit or particle, you'll have pure energy. Likewise, thought is also energy and therefore dynamic and capable of affecting change and altering physical reality.

> Your thoughts determine your beliefs, your beliefs determine your actions, and your actions determine and create your physical reality.

the first stages of healing. I decide it's time to bring down the inflammation. My workers spread on a cooling, soothing herbal cream and set up a temporary wall at either end of the wounded area to seal it off from the rest of the intestine. Then they set up a cooling unit which acts like a fridge to bring down the temperature of the area until the wound is nice and chilled with no more redness. The workers then dismantle the walls and take them and the cooling unit away. I drift off into sleep knowing the coolness and soothing herbal cream are helping my intestine tremendously.

I keep going with the visualization, imagining whatever it is my intestine needs next until it is quite healed. Then I usually do a final cleansing followed by a coat of herbal salve for moisture and suppleness.

Take some time and don't be afraid to experiment to find out what kind of visualization works best for you. Listen to your body and adjust the length and frequency of your visualization accordingly. For example, in the visualization outlined above, I may want to visualize the first part (with the herbal salve) for four or five days consecutively until I feel the area is healed enough to move onto to the next stages of treatment. As with anything, you'll become more fluent and find it easier to concentrate the more you apply yourself to visualizing.

Also, different images work for different people. Go with whatever pops into your head. A six-year-old boy I know used to visualize dragons and a battle scene where whatever he felt was making him ill was killed off. A visualization like that would not work for me, but for him it was quite effective. Again, use whatever works best for you.

Overall Healing

You can do this visualization either lying down, or sitting up cross-legged, or propped against some pillows. Close your eyes and just breathe deeply for a few minutes. Concentrate on nothing other than your breath. Inhale and bring the breath deep down into your diaphragm, watch/feel your abdomen protrude as it fills with breath. Then slowly, evenly exhale all of the breath, push out even the last wisps of breath, then slowly, deeply, inhale again.

Stay like this for a few minutes, just inhaling and exhaling as deeply as you can. Feel your body sink and settle a little deeper with each breath in and out.

After a few minutes of breathing deeply and evenly, imagine the top of your head opening up like a flower whose petals bloom and unfurl in the sunlight. Above you is a great ocean of brilliant white light. This beautiful white light is God, or the Universal Energy, or the Divine Healing Light, or whatever name you feel comfortable with. Open yourself to receive this love and healing and feel the beautiful, brilliant white light stream in through the top of your head. It flows down in a river of white light, filling your throat, your chest and down both of your arms. Breathe deeply in and out as you see this lovely white, healing light fill your ribcage and abdomen and then flow strongly down through each of your legs.

Stay here awhile and breathe, seeing yourself filled by this brilliant column of white light from head to foot, that fills up your entire body, wraps around all your bones and organs and even permeates through to each and every cell in your entire body bringing love, nourishment and rejuvenation.

See the healing white light flowing through your entire digestive system, see your intestinal walls, both inside and out, awash in soothing white light. Feel the beautiful white light soothing and calming any wounds or inflammation, see the walls of your intestine becoming smooth and radiant in the healing white light. Stay here awhile and breathe, feel the soft white light cushioning and soothing every part of your precious tummy.

Now see the beautiful white light washing down all around you, surrounding you with a sea of shimmering whiteness. Feel yourself melting into that pool of white light. Feel the white light that's filling your body flow outward through your skin as you merge with the ocean of white light. Feel yourself melting and dissolving into this beautiful sea of brilliant white light, ebbing and flowing and becoming one with it. Stay here with this image and breathe deeply for as long as you like.

☼ Regular, concentrated visualization of a desired occurrence or process can produce very real, physical results.

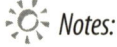 Notes:

Balancing / Calming

Lie on your back with your arms relaxed at your side. Close your eyes and imagine a big, round, pure golden ball of light in your abdomen (this is your Chi, your seat of energy and power located about two finger-widths below your belly button). Take deep breaths in and out of your diaphragm. With each breath in, see your golden ball expand and glow brighter, with each breath out it reduces a bit but the light is more intense and shimmering. Relax here and breathe for a while, holding the visualization with each breath.

Now imagine a huge brilliant cloud of this beautiful golden light above your head. This is your universal energy and it is always available to feed, nourish and connect with you. There is a stream flowing from this huge field of golden light and it flows in through the top of your head, imagine the top of your head opening to receive this beautiful light. The light flows down and pools pulsating in your throat, from there it flows to your heart and envelops it with soft, warm, soothing light. It flows now to your solar plexus as you take deep, relaxing breaths. The stream of golden light then flows down to your abdomen and joins with your own pulsating, brilliant golden ball of Chi. See it expand and glow brighter with each deep, relaxing breath.

Breathe for a while, seeing the stream flowing from the cloud throughout your body. Now see the stream flowing from your abdomen to the back of your spine, through your tailbone, out of your body and into the earth. You are grounded and centered. You are part of the heavens and part of the nourishing, soft earth. See the beautiful, warm golden light pulsating and radiating healing and peace as it streams from the universe around you, through your body and into the good, soft earth. Accept this light and healing as a gift from God or the universe. Rest here and breathe peacefully.

CONTROLLING YOUR BOWELS

Many people with IBD have, at one time or another, dropped their stool in their pants rather than in the toilet. I've heard numerous stories of unfortunate accidents from people stuck in traffic, or a long waiting line at a public bathroom, or some who have simply been unable to find a toilet in time. Yes, it's tremendously embarrassing and yes, you do eventually get over it. But the really good news is that you can train your bowels so that it never happens again!

Think of your bowels as a small puppy that you need to teach what is allowed and what isn't. Start the training at home where you have the time and privacy necessary to start pushing your boundaries and if you have an accident, it's not such a big deal.

Begin by learning how to close your anal opening. Closing your anus requires the same muscles and motion used to do Kegel exercises. If you're unfamiliar with Kegel exercises, then simply practice closing your anus periodically the next time you have a bowel movement. While the stool is passing through your anus, clench it shut by pulling up the lower pelvic wall and rectum. If you can't conceive of how to do this, then simply squeeze your bum muscles together, this should immediately stop the flow of your stool. Then relax and let the stool pass through again. As you do this several times, you'll begin to feel the actual muscles responsible for closing your anal opening and you won't have to clench your bum muscles together in order to close it. Practice this exercise not only during a bowel movement, but also throughout the day. Try to work up to being able to do 20 closings (and releases) in a row. Also, start trying to hold your anus shut for up to 20 seconds non-stop. Like any muscle, you need to strengthen, condition and develop your control over its movements.

Once you've developed your anal sphincter and the other muscles required to close your anal opening and hold it shut, you can begin the next phase of training. Do the following procedure at home initially.

1. Wait until you need to have a bowel movement quite urgently. Then stand very still, place your hand on your colon and clench your anus closed. Now here's where training the puppy comes in: You now need to talk to your bowel very sternly (but lovingly) and tell it out loud that, "I'm sorry, but we (meaning you and your colon) cannot have a bowel movement at this time." Then you need to tell your bowel when

☼ I have received many emails from readers thanking me profusely for this technique, saying this technique alone has changed their life. So congratulations to all of you, for being innovative, adventurous people who are willing to think outside the box!

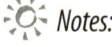 *Notes:*

it will be able to pass stool. Since you'll start by doing this training at home, begin with requiring your bowel to wait two minutes. Say to your colon, "In two minutes, and not a second sooner, we may have a bowel movement." Now try to stand quietly and breathe evenly whilst timing yourself. Sitting or jiggling around is not usually a good idea.

When the two minutes is up, walk quietly to the bathroom and say to your colon, "Ok, now we can have our bowel movement." If you can't make it and you have an accident, don't worry about it, just think how long it takes to toilet train children. Keep practicing this procedure, gradually expanding the waiting time until you've got it up to five minutes.

2. When you can hold your stool in for up to five minutes, you're ready to begin training your bowel to suck the stool back up the rectal canal. As many of you probably already know, merely keeping your anus closed will only hold back a bowel movement for a fairly minimal amount of time. However, by getting your bowel to move the stool back up the rectal canal, thereby completely relieving the pressure and urgency to void, you can go from thirty minutes to two hours without passing stool. Again, go through this procedure at home a few times first.

3. Wait until you need to have a bowel movement urgently, then go through the steps in point 1, above. But, do not tell your colon that you can have a bowel movement in a few minutes. After you've held your anus shut for a few minutes, begin talking to your colon. Again, you address your body as "we" because you're acknowledging that your mind/body/spirit is one entity and you're honoring the unity of yourself as whole; complete and working together. You are also recognizing that there is intelligence and awareness in every cell in your body, it is not just the brain controlling the body. It's using the awareness and intelligence of every part of the body to work together as a whole to accomplish what's best for the whole body.

4. Here's an example of what I say, "Ok darling, now we need to suck this stool back up, because we're in the middle of dinner and we are NOT going to have a bowel movement until we've finished eating, probably in about 45 minutes."

5. Then, with your hand still on your colon, begin clenching and releasing your anal sphincter whilst simultaneously pulling in with your abdominal muscles each time you clench your anus. This results in a kind of rolling or wave motion in your abdomen. At the same time, visualize, or imagine the motion results in your rectal canal acting like a pump that moves the stool back up the rectal canal. Also visualize your descending colon helping out by creating a vacuum effect that further helps to suck the stool up the rectal canal. As you're doing this, you'll begin to notice that your need or urgency to pass stool is lessening. Then rest for a bit, still holding your anus closed. If the pressure is not substantially relieved, begin the procedure of clenching and releasing your anus whilst contracting your abdominals again. You may want to alternate this procedure with rest periods several times.

6. The complete procedure, along with visualizing (imagining) should take about two minutes or less. Take a rest whenever you need it. Again, it may take a while for you to be able to perform the muscular movements continuously, whilst visualizing, so be patient with yourself. When you feel the pressure or urgency to void has decreased significantly (i.e. you're no longer in danger of soiling yourself) go back to whatever you were doing, or focus your attention on something else. Thank your bowels for their good work, and then leave them to look after themselves. Shift your attention and continue with what you were doing.

If you're on an anti-diarrhea drug or some other drug that directly affects the colon and its peristalsis, then I don't know how well this technique will work for you. This degree of cooperation with your bowels involves mind/body harmony and teaching your body to work with you. If you have a drug

☼ Think of your bowels as a small puppy that you need to teach what is allowed and what isn't. Start the training at home where you have the time and privacy necessary to start pushing your boundaries. and if you have an accident, it's not such a big deal.

interfering with the process, you may or may not be successful with this technique.

I definitely encourage you to put in the time necessary to master this technique as the freedom it will give you is glorious. There have been many times where I've been out shopping or involved in some activity and my colon has started spasming and I've felt like I was going to explode. I've then implemented this technique and been able to go two hours or more without having a bowel movement. I also don't like having a bowel movement in public washrooms, so I simply tell my bowel that we have to wait until we get home to our toilet where we can have a much nicer, more relaxing bowel movement. Then I continue with whatever I'm doing – having lunch, running errands, whatever – and I don't need to have a bowel movement again until I get home. At which point I feel like my puppy-colon must be one of Pavlov's dogs, because as soon as I turn the key in my front door I can feel the stool moving rapidly down my rectal canal in anticipation of the promised bowel movement!

When I first published *Listen To Your Gut* back in 2000, I thought that hardly anyone would try this technique. And indeed, I expected people to think I was quite loopy for even putting it into print. Much to my surprise, I have since received lots of emails from readers thanking me profusely for this technique, saying this technique alone has changed their life. So congratulations to all of you for being innovative, adventurous people who are willing to think outside the box!

> The primary factor that makes pain hurt, is fear.

TRANSFORMING PAIN

Most of the painful episodes associated with IBD and IBS are caused by the intestines cramping or spasming severely. Other causes include blockages in the colon (see *Colonic Massage* section in Chapter Six) or rupturing of the bowel. Often when your gut is spasming, you get hot, sweaty and shaky and it's so painful that you start to think your bowel or appendix is rupturing, but this is actually quite rare. If you are having a rupture or perforation take place, you will experience the following symptoms: Fever, very rigid abdomen, severe shaking or shivering, constipation – not passing any gas or stool. Otherwise, you're probably just having a spasm/cramp attack. If you suspect you're having a rupture or perforation take place, then you can still use the techniques listed below, but do them on the way to the hospital.

If you tend to experience these cramping/spasming attacks on a regular basis, then you may want to develop some tools to enable you to deal with and eliminate the pain – other than being rushed to the emergency room and pumped full of drugs. I strongly suggest you take up either meditation, yoga, or tai chi as any of them will give you a strong base for breath control. Being able to control your breath will help you to control both the feelings of 'pain' and your oxygen/carbon dioxide exchange, so you don't have to worry about passing out. You may also want to try drinking two glasses of spring or filtered water (fairly quickly, one after the other) as soon as you feel the pain begin – sometimes this alone can avoid or lessen an attack.

The best technique for pain-management does not involve ignoring or fighting the pain, but rather, moving into it. Instead of trying not to think of the pain, or rallying your body and mind to fight against it, you have to submit to it. Water is one of the strongest forces on our planet. Its supreme strength resides in the fact that it is completely malleable and therefore unstoppable. When you need an image or way to think of yourself during these attacks, think of yourself (your whole body) as water, unresisting, flowing. If you were to choose a traditional image of strength, like a rock for example, this would not be nearly as effective. Anything solid and rigid like a rock presents an ideal surface of resistance for other forces to slam up against, drill through, chip and crack, or, like water, to patiently and enduringly wear a path through. Whenever you resist something, you give it something to fight against, you provide it with the motivation to gather its strength and intensify against you.

The next time you have a spasm/cramp attack, either try to keep the image of water in your head, or repeat to yourself, "I am water." Then imagine the whole room is filled with pain, your pain, the pain you're experiencing, and let the pain completely overwhelm you. Let it take over and surround every

> Instead of trying not to think of the pain, or rallying your body and mind to fight against it, you have to submit to it.

part of you. Say to the pain, "Here I am. I am water. Come to me. I accept you."

This is where you need to have some practice and control over your breathing, so that you can imagine such a scenario whilst maintaining deep, even breaths. As you allow the pain to pervade every facet of your senses and as you accept it and welcome it, you will gradually pass through the panic and fear that you're going to die from the pain. It helps to remember that if the pain really does become more than you can bear, you will simply pass out, and then you won't feel any more pain. The body has this fail-safe mechanism in place for pain that truly is unbearable, so you don't need to be afraid you'll die from the pain, or that you'll be driven out of your mind by unbearable pain. As long as you're conscious, you can bear it. This really helped me during 44 hours of labor giving birth to my first child.

> Whenever you resist something, you give it something to fight against, you provide it with the motivation to gather its strength and intensify against you.

As you allow the pain to flood you, take you over, and pervade every part of your being, you will also gradually begin to observe it, you will also begin to realize that 'pain' doesn't have to hurt. As you let the pain take over and saturate every pore of your body, you will begin to recognize 'pain' as just another sensory input – a signal sent from your body to your brain to convey a message, no more, no less. You will then be able to sit there with the "pain" washing over you in waves, but yet it won't hurt.

The primary factor that makes pain hurt, is fear. The hurt we feel is not generated from the pain feeling itself, but from the fear that is its conductor. In and of itself, the nerve impulse that we have labeled 'pain' doesn't have to hurt. However, when it's delivered via a conductor such as fear, it feels very shocking and hurtful. Autopsies have shown that when people commit suicide by jumping off a high-rise building, or when they die in a plane crash, many of them are not killed by the impact of their body hitting the ground – they are already dead at that point. Their intense fear and horror of the coming pain or impact has already killed them by causing them to have a heart attack.

If during your next cramping episode, you walk into the center of your pain, and you face your fear of the pain and you say, "Here I am. I am water. I accept you. Come to me, here I am," you will discover, gradually, that your pain doesn't hurt anymore. You will master your fear of experiencing pain and you'll realize that being free from fear is the most liberating, healing state to be in.

If you have a spouse, partner, friend or child around while you're having the cramping, they can also assist you in the healing process. While you're going through the process outlined above, your helper can be giving you some direct healing. Have your helper place his/her hand about an inch or two above your bare abdomen (wherever you're experiencing the cramping) and have them visualize white and ice blue light flowing from the center of their palm into your gut. White is the divine healing light and ice blue is to calm and soothe inflammation and irritation. They then imagine/visualize this white and ice blue light flowing through and around every part of your intestine, wrapping around and permeating the intestinal walls, soothing and healing everything it comes into contact with. You don't have to do anything but allow and accept the healing.

Dependent upon your acceptance of this healing method and the fluency/concentration of your helper, this technique can stop the cramping in anywhere from 30 seconds to ten minutes. But remember, instruct your helper on what to do, or give them a copy of this section ahead of time, so that during the cramping episode your mind is able to focus completely on facing and accepting your pain. You don't even need to be aware of what your helper is doing for the healing to take effect, you merely have to accept it.

You can use this technique on your own for transforming all kinds of pain. I used it frequently during my martial arts career as I tore the cartilage in both my knees, had my left shoulder dislocated twice, severely damaged my neck, and suffered numerous sprains, wounds and hematomas. In spite of these injuries, by transforming the pain I was able to keep going and finish the fight or training regimen – don't ask me now why I wanted to! I guess I was going through a macho phase.

> If you take the time and effort to learn this technique, it is something you'll be able to use in various situations throughout your life. It is very liberating to know that no matter what happens, you have the strength and freedom in your own body to cope with it, and usually transcend it.

I also use this technique to have my dental work done with no anesthetic. Even when my dentist is drilling right on a nerve it doesn't feel painful to me. What freedom to have no residual discomfort or toxic side effects (from anesthetic) whatsoever, to walk out of the dentist's office after a filling and feel completely normal!

This technique was also invaluable during the births of my two children – 44 hours of labor for my son and 15 hours of labor for my daughter. I ran into one of the doctors who'd assisted at the birth of my son (my labor spanned two shifts) in a grocery store a year later and was very surprised that she remembered me. She said, "Of course I remember you, you're the one whose labor went on and on forever and you refused any painkillers. None of us could believe it!"

So you see, if you take the time and effort to learn this technique, it is something you'll be able to use in various situations throughout your life. It is very liberating to know that no matter what happens, you have the strength and freedom in your own body to cope with it, and usually transcend it. This knowledge and ability is very healing and the strength you manifest from this technique will pervade all areas of your life – both physical and emotional.

Turn now to the *Healing Journey Workbook* on the *Listen To Your Gut CD*, and complete the exercises for Chapter Seven.

8

Treatments I'm Often Asked About

"The human body has a remarkable built-in healing mechanism; it is constructed and programmed in such a way that it can heal itself.

In chiropractic we speak of an innate intelligence of physiological homeostasis that automatically strives to restore equilibrium in the body when an imbalance occurs in any of its many complex systems. This innate intelligence is the common basis for all healing.

People are healed by many different kinds of healers and systems because the real healer is within. The various healing modalities are merely different ways of activating that inner healer."

Dr. George Goodheart, DC
Founder of Applied Kinesiology

> Ayurvedic medicine has some very interesting, valid theories on the different types of bodies/personalities (doshas), how the seasonal changes affect the body, and how to live in balance and harmony.

I'm fortunate in that I have received (and continue to receive) a lot of feedback over the years from my readers. After a while, I noticed that people kept asking me for my opinion on the same products, diets and treatments – over and over again. Therefore, this chapter answers those very same questions and gives you my personal opinion on certain specific products, diets, etc. Please keep in mind that all the information following is my own, personal opinion only. I'm not trying to convince anyone of anything, and I'm not passing official judgment on anything. I'm simply giving my personal opinion because so many readers have asked me to.

AYURVEDIC MEDICINE

I have a lot of respect for this body of medicine, and a lot of what it has to offer is definitely valid and helpful. The daily practice of yoga and sesame oil massage are very beneficial to the body. Likewise, I think an Ayurvedic spa weekend comprising various panchakarma treatments would be relaxing and rejuvenating. I have had pulse diagnosis performed by the venerable Dr. Triguna himself (mentioned in Deepak Chopra's books as one of the best in the world) and his reading of my condition was 100% accurate. However, in my case, the products he prescribed for treatment were not very effective. I'm very sensitive to taste and consistency, and some of the remedies I simply could not swallow, others made me feel nauseous and irritated my bowel. Overall, at a total of $550, it was an expensive experience (Dr. Triguna's consultation fee alone was $350 for about a 10 minute diagnosis; ahh, the price of celebrity!). Anyway, any books you read in this field will not be wasted knowledge. Ayurvedic medicine has some very interesting, valid theories on the different types of bodies/personalities (doshas), how the seasonal changes affect the body, and how to live in balance and harmony. My only caution would be regarding taking the remedies themselves, particularly if you have a squeamish or sensitive palate. Be sure to follow the guidelines in Chapter Two for introducing new supplements.

TRADITIONAL CHINESE MEDICINE

I really like the theoretical paradigm underlying Chinese medicine; the balance of yin and yang, the relating of the body to the essential elements, the concept of having too much or too little heat, cold, water, etc. Like Ayurvedic medicine, there is a tremendous body of knowledge here, both interesting and applicable, that will only contribute to your understanding of your body.

Regarding the actual treatment and application of remedies, personally, I found it much too aggressive for my body. Chinese herbal medicine is based upon a process of cleansing, toning and strengthening. I could handle the toning and strengthening part of the therapy, but the cleansing part really knocked my system out of whack. I lost seven pounds, my digestive system was aggravated and it took me a good six months to regain my balance and strength. Unless your body responds well to aggressive treatment, it may not be such a good idea to see a TCM (Traditional Chinese Medicine) doctor. Also, some of the herbal mixtures are absolutely foul, and the smell alone can be enough to trigger your gag reflex. I don't know how I managed to consume mine for a whole month. The first two weeks I drank the teas, I had to go outside to drink them so the wind could blow away the smell and I could gulp in fresh air between sips.

Chinese medicine is also not usually a good idea for people with IBD or IBS because it tends to use multiple-herb remedies. Therefore, your chances of having an adverse reaction are much higher. And like Ayurvedic medicine, some of the remedies can irritate the gut and exacerbate symptoms. If you want to pursue Chinese medicine, then use single herbs only and introduce them one at a time, leaving 2 – 3 weeks in between each one to check for adverse reactions.

I like to experiment with individual Chinese herbs (like the Astragalus listed earlier in this chapter) that I can safely trial-test and monitor individually. In my experience, Chinese herbs in general tend to be far more potent then their western equivalent, so I usually start off with half the

> If you want to pursue Chinese medicine, then use single herbs only and introduce them one at a time, leaving 2 – 3 weeks in between each one to check for adverse reactions.

recommended dose and that's often enough to achieve the desired result. So, as per usual, if you feel this is an avenue you should explore, by all means go ahead. But stay really tuned to your body and don't be afraid to stop treatment if you don't feel it's helping you. Remember to follow the guidelines in Chapter Two for introducing new supplements.

THE BLOOD TYPE DIET

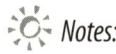 Notes:

This is the diet presented in Dr. Peter J. D'Adamo's book, *Eat Right For Your Type*. The basic premise of the diet is that your blood type indicates your ancestry in terms of where your originating group of humans lived and what they ate. Therefore, your blood type will indicate which type of diet is most compatible with your body and digestive system.

An interesting feature of the Blood Type Diet is that nearly everyone is advised to eliminate wheat, dairy and tomatoes. Since wheat and dairy products are the primary culprits in most people's food allergies and intolerances, it's not surprising that people who follow the diet experience substantial relief. Also, as I've said previously, North Americans in general consume far too many tomato-based, acidic foods – one of the main causes of heartburn and aggravation of the intestinal lining. If most people were to cut down or stop eating tomatoes, they would experience significant relief. Whether and how much all the additional guidelines in the diet contribute to digestive health, I can't say. They may contribute substantially, or their effects may be minimal, especially compared to the benefits reaped by eliminating wheat, dairy and tomatoes.

I personally know three people with IBS and one with Crohn's who have tried this diet plan and experienced a lessening of symptoms as a result. I've gone through the recommendations for my blood type (AB) and for the most part found them consistent with what I've discovered already. However, during a flare-up or acute phase of IBD or IBS, I don't think the Blood Type Diet guidelines are strict enough to address or alleviate the symptoms particular to IBD/IBS; diarrhea, bleeding, malabsorption, bloating, etc. I also have questions as to the scientific validity of the premise upon which the diet plans are based.

My personal opinion on this diet is that if you feel drawn to implement it, then please do so, but implement it in conjunction with the appropriate *Healing Diet* (see Chapter Three). For example, if the Blood Type Diet says you can eat lemons, but the *Healing Diet* says 'no lemons', then don't eat lemons. If the *Healing Diet* says you can eat avocados, but the Blood Type Diet says 'avoid avocados', then don't eat avocados.

Keep in mind that whatever diet you choose to implement, the most effective way to eat right for your body is still determined by individual trial-testing of foods (see Chapter Three). When all is said and done, your own body knows exactly what it wants and needs for optimal functioning and healing. Always listen to your body above and beyond any diet guidelines (see *Dialoguing With Your Body*, Chapter Six) and your body will always give you the best diet to follow.

I've found for myself that my body wants and tolerates different foods at different times. For example, occasionally, my body wants milk and I will drink up to four glasses of milk per day and feel great. At other times, my body will go through periods where it doesn't want any dairy products for a month or two at a time. If I drink milk during one of these periods, I will instantly experience bloating and sometimes diarrhea along with excessive mucus production. Your body is not a machine, there isn't some pre-set formula that will ensure optimum performance for the rest of your existence. Your body is a fluid, dynamic, responsive, variable wonder and the best way to feed yourself is simply to stay open and tuned to what your body wants and needs each day.

SPECIFIC CARBOHYDRATE DIET

This is the diet outlined and advocated in Elaine Gottschall's book, *Breaking the Vicious Cycle* (originally titled, *Food And the Gut Reaction*). It took me seven years after first reading this book to gather up the self-discipline

> An interesting feature of the Blood Type Diet is that nearly everyone is advised to eliminate wheat, dairy and tomatoes. Since wheat and dairy products are the primary culprits in most people's food allergies and intolerances, it's not surprising that people who follow the diet experience substantial relief.

necessary to give the diet a try. When I finally did embark on it, I adhered to each and every guideline meticulously for one year. I saw real improvement in the first 3 months, but it was downhill from there, and when I assessed myself at the end of the year, my symptoms were actually much worse than when I had started. The reason I stuck with the diet for so long was because I wanted to give it a good, fair trial.

Now, I know there have been many people helped and even completely healed from using this diet. Although I think most of those people have to stay on the diet indefinitely and cannot eat normally, or else they will experience a resurgence of symptoms. To be honest, I think the reason it didn't work for me was largely a matter of personality. The diet has tremendously rigid guidelines and you have to prepare all of your food from scratch. You have to bake all your own bread out of special nut flours and bake all your snacks or desserts yourself. Eating out becomes an ordeal in itself and almost not worth enduring. Now here's the kind of person I am: I don't like being forced to cook, I love eating out, I hate being controlled and regimented in anything in my life, I typically derive extreme enjoyment from my food and am considered something of a gourmet. Can you see where the clash between this diet and my personality would come into play? I went on the Specific Carbohydrate Diet and I was in the kitchen cooking for eight to nine hours every single weekend, preparing my food for the week and baking my bread and snacks. I hated it! As a result I became an irritated, angry person and I felt unbearably controlled and non-spontaneous from the time I got up till the time I went to bed.

☼ I would love to see Elaine Gottschall add probiotic supplementation to her diet program as I think it would raise the success rates even higher.

This is where the interplay of the body/mind schemata kicks in. I think that whatever good the diet did my physical body was counteracted by my emotional/mental state. Our mind and emotions can affect and produce results or consequences in our body just as much as what we do physically to our body. This is why I say numerous times throughout this book to always follow your intuition and do what you feel is right for you, make only the changes you feel you need to make, and proceed at whatever pace of change is comfortable and positive for you.

The body/mind interplay was really evidenced for me when I had a blood test to measure antibody response to certain foods (as a method of determining food allergies) over ten years *after* being on the Specific Carbohydrate Diet. When the test results came back, I saw that I had tested positive (antibody response) for many of the staple foods I had consumed whilst on the Specific Carbohydrate Diet! Now, I'm not actually allergic or intolerant to any of these foods – I know because I've tested all of them using the far more reliable method of food clearance and reintroduction (see Chapter Three). But, I think the antibody response was a sign that my body was still registering the stress and negativity associated with eating those foods over and over again for a full year and hating every minute of it! So then I had to do some EFT tapping (see Chapter Six) to clear the emotion/trauma still retained in my body from following this (for me) very stressful diet.

> Our mind and emotions can affect and produce results or consequences in our body, just as much as what we do physically to our body.

If you feel your gut leading you to follow The Specific Carbohydrate Diet, and if you're a structured, love-to-cook kind of person (or you have someone else to do all your meal preparation for you) then I think you'll probably see some good results from it. Personally, I would love to see Elaine Gottschall add probiotic supplementation to her diet program, as I think it would raise the success rates even higher, and after a year or so of supplementation, people could probably start introducing 'forbidden' (but otherwise healthy) foods again.

DETOXIFICATION PROTOCOLS

Most herbal detoxification (detox) programs are simply too harsh and damaging for people with Crohn's and colitis. If your diverticulitis is in an acute phase, then likewise abstain from any detox or cleanse protocols. For people with mild to moderate IBS, you may be able to follow a detoxification program and benefit from it, but remember to follow it immediately with probiotic supplementation. For people with severe IBS, again, I feel herbal detoxification programs are too intense and may damage an already inflamed mucosal lining.

☼ It's best to wait until you're fairly healed and at a normal weight before beginning a detoxification program, and choose treatments that are gentler and perhaps take longer, to avoid triggering an adverse reaction.

If you have Crohn's or colitis and you are underweight and/or suffering from diarrhea, then you will probably experience negative results (a flare, severe weight loss, bleeding, etc.) from a detoxification protocol. Keep in mind that the very nature of detoxification involves cleansing, or expelling various substances from your body. And your body has prescribed ways of expelling or detoxifying: Diarrhea or increased bowel movements, vomiting, pushing things out the skin, increased mucus production and expulsion, and urination. So, as you can see, if you're already in a weakened, ill state, then experiencing these things suddenly and abundantly is going to be very stressful.

In my opinion, it's best to wait until you're fairly healed and at a normal weight (or overweight) before beginning a detoxification program and to choose treatments that are gentler and perhaps take longer to avoid triggering an adverse reaction. I don't even like the idea of juice fasts for people with IBD and IBS, unless you consume primarily non-sweet vegetable juices and no fruit juices. Otherwise, the natural sugar in the juices can cause *Candida* (yeast) to flourish and may trigger a flare-up of symptoms. I had a phone consultation with a client once whose colitis was triggered by a water and juice fast. On the first day of the fast he was out driving around on errands and forgot to drink enough water and by day three he experienced a surge of abdominal pain and bleeding. Remember that IBD and IBS are triggered by stress. So if a detoxification protocol is going to stress your body, then either make sure you just stay home resting in bed or on the couch the whole time, or don't do it.

There are also many protocols outlined in this book that are automatically detoxifying and they include:

▶ Drinking 8 – 10 glasses of water per day

▶ *Jini's Wild Oregano Oil Protocol*

▶ Bentonite Clay

▶ The IBD Remission Diet

- High dose probiotic supplementation
- *Jini's Probiotic Retention Enema*

So, like anything else, follow your gut and if you do go on a detoxification program then make sure you're supported during the detox by getting lots of rest, drinking lots of water and taking probiotics. I would also drink ½ cup of George's 'Always Active' Aloe Vera Juice, three times per day, during the protocol to help prevent damage to the intestine.

COLON CLEANSING

Many sources insist that colon cleansing is integral to bowel health. This cleansing can take the form of a course of herbs to cleanse and detoxify, a special diet and fasting, or manual flushing of the colon using a saline or herbal solution, or some combination of any of the above. Personally, I don't feel these procedures are necessary for anyone who has already been through the medical exploratory or diagnostic tests. After you've been through a barium enema followed by a colonoscopy, your colon is about as clean as it's going to get! Colonoscopies in particular cannot be successfully performed unless the intestinal wall is completely clear of fecal matter, so rest assured that the test preparation for a colonoscopy is an extremely thorough cleanse.

I also don't feel it's a good idea to cleanse your colon regularly as it disrupts the bacterial flora in your bowel. A major premise of the healing plan in this book involves allowing the body to heal and balance itself and this includes helping your body to develop a natural, healthy bacterial balance. If you have chronic constipation as a feature of your Irritable Bowel Syndrome, then you may wish to have one or two colonics done initially to clear out any impacted fecal matter that may be compounding your problem. But then you must follow these colonics with *Jini's Probiotic Retention Enema* to immediately replace the flushed good bacteria and then continue for three months with oral supplementation (see Chapter Two). For most

> After you've been through a barium enema followed by a colonoscopy, your colon is about as clean as it's going to get!

conditions, I view colon cleansing as a fairly invasive therapy and I don't recommend doing it more than once (and then only if you feel you need to).

BACTERIAL SOIL ORGANISMS

Bacterial soil organisms (often referred to as SO's, HSO's, SBO's, etc.) are currently being marketed as probiotics. However, probiotics have traditionally referred to food-cultured bacteria (e.g. *Lactobacillus, Bifidobacterium*), whereas bacterial soil organisms (as the name suggests) are found in the soil. Common species of bacterial soil organisms marketed as probiotics include *Bacillus cereus* and *Bacillus licheniformis*. Food-cultured bacteria have a record of safety for human consumption that spans thousands of years (e.g. kefir, yoghurt, miso, natto, etc.). Bacterial soil organisms have only recently (in the last ten years or so) been consumed directly by humans, and people ingesting them should be made aware that they are participating in an experimental therapy. Popular products currently containing bacterial soil organisms include Royal Flora, Primal Defense, Nature's Biotics, etc.

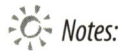 *Notes:*

The CEO of one of the main manufacturers of bacterial soil organisms sent me an email, since he'd heard I was advising my readers not to consume bacterial soil organisms. He sent me their company literature supporting the use of soil organisms and suggested I revise my opinion. I then emailed him back and asked him to send me any long-term studies (i.e. 20 years or longer) he had on the safety of human consumption of soil organisms – I never heard back from him (even after emailing him again twice). Please remember that it's very easy for supplement companies and pharmaceutical firms to simply pay a doctor to endorse their products, write articles for them, etc. It's a common marketing practice, and unless the 'research' is published in a well-known, long-standing scientific publication (one that's been in existence for five years or more), the information may be little more than propaganda.

I've done some fairly thorough research on bacterial soil organisms and I've listed some of the relevant articles in Appendix D for those of you who want to do your own research. To summarize the available research to date, I don't recommend anyone consume bacterial soil organisms for the following reasons:

- Soil organisms are spore-formers and they make good competitors for yeast, fungus and other pathogens. This is why many people taking soil organisms may initially experience very favorable results. However, these spores are extremely difficult to kill – surviving commercial sterilants, disinfectants, acceleration forces, heat, pressure, radiation and many antibiotics.

- Strong antibiotics – like Vancomycin – can suppress certain spores. But the spores are so persistent that another round of germination may occur after the drug is stopped.

- Soil organisms can also adapt loose genetic material and incorporate it into their cellular structure – the ramifications of which are as yet unknown.

- Various soil organisms can produce harmful peptides, affecting hemoglobin in the blood.

- It's important to keep in mind that virtually all antibiotic drugs were initially developed from soil organisms, and as new antibiotics become more potent, they cause more damage to the host, not just in the immediate gut environment, but systemically as well.

- In the EU (European Union) the use of soil organisms in *animal* feed is being stringently controlled and questioned at this time – but there's no monitoring of human use in North America.

- There are simply too many questions and unknowns to sanction the use of soil organisms for human consumption and one certainly cannot qualify them as "safe" at this time.

If you've already taken a product containing bacterial soil organisms (and read all supplement labels as they're being added to everything from protein shakes to dog food), you may be worried about consequences.

> Bacterial soil organisms have only recently been consumed directly by humans, and people ingesting them should be aware that they are participating in an experimental therapy.

> ☼ There are simply too many questions and unknowns to sanction the use of soil organisms for human consumption and one certainly cannot qualify them as "safe" at this time.

Unfortunately, since this is such an experimental therapy, there's not a lot of research available. I have heard from several readers who developed swelling and tenderness in the lower right quadrant of their abdomen after ingesting bacterial soil organisms for two months to a year – whether this is coincidental is very hard to say.

I had a phone consultation client who used a popular bacterial soil organism product to completely clear all his symptoms of Crohn's Disease. However, a few months later Oliver developed a rectal infection, abscess and two fistulas (he'd never suffered from these before) that were so painful he wound up completely bedridden – he couldn't even walk. By the time Oliver contacted me, he'd already had surgery twice for the fistulas and been on both Flagyl and Levaquin to try and eliminate the infection. He'd been completely bedridden for two months, on prednisone and massive doses of painkillers when he called me. Following our consultation, he discontinued ingesting the soil organisms, began *Jini's Wild Oregano Oil Protocol*, went on the IBD Remission Diet for two weeks, and started craniosacral therapy. We had another consultation seven weeks later and Oliver was off prednisone completely (for the first time in about ten years), had not had a single painkiller in nine days, the abscess and fistulas were much improved, and he was going out every day for at least a ten minute walk in the sunshine. Needless to say, Oliver was absolutely thrilled with his progress.

I've heard from many readers who had very good results initially (including complete remission) from ingesting bacterial soil organisms. However, up to a year later they experienced flare-ups or new symptoms that were often worse than their original condition. I suspect this is because bacterial soil organisms are very aggressive competitors in the gut and as a result they probably wiped out the yeast, fungus, bad bacteria and other pathogens that were causing the initial IBD or IBS. However, they will also wipe out your good bacterial flora, colonize your gut, form spores, and then what? This is the problem: No one knows. I have also heard from readers who've ingested bacterial soil organisms and experienced no unusual effects. Again, because there is no long-term research, it's very difficult to say at this point whether bacterial soil organisms (and which ones) can benefit human beings, or not. Dr. Glenn R. Gibson, a world-renowned researcher of probiotics (PhD Microbiology, University of Reading, UK), emailed me this statement: "Selection criteria show that best probiotic success arises when the strains are isolated from the same species as their intended use. Hence, I currently do not see the advantages of using soil derived organisms."

If you've ingested bacterial soil organisms already, you may be concerned about eradicating them and their spores from your gastrointestinal tract. Personally, I think Wild Oregano Oil is your best chance of killing these bacterial soil organisms and if you have ingested them, I strongly recommend you follow *Jini's Wild Oregano Oil Protocol* in Chapter Two. Again, there's currently no research or information available on the efficacy of Wild Oregano Oil against bacterial soil organisms in vivo (in the body), but since it kills all other known microorganisms, I'd say the odds are pretty good that it would work well. There are studies – like the one referenced in Chapter Two – showing Wild Oregano Oil is very effective at killing certain bacterial soil organisms (like *Bacillus cereus*) in vitro (outside the body), so again, I feel the odds are pretty good it will work effectively in the gut as well. Since bacterial soil organisms are spore-formers, you may need to repeat the Protocol in cycles for two or three years to completely rid yourself of the soil organisms – again, at the time of writing, there's no information on this topic available, so follow your gut and take the Wild Oregano Oil as needed.

PLANT STEROLS/STEROLINS

Plant sterols are simply plant fats that have been shown in repeated, reliable, scientific trials to boost immune system function. I have taken plant sterols/sterolins in the form of a product called Moducare for up to two months at a time, but seen no discernible difference. An honest health store owner I know swears by Moducare and says feedback from customers has been really good, but you have to take it for at least three months continuously to see good results. A naturopathic physician I know, who has a lot of cancer

> Plant sterols are simply plant fats that have been shown in repeated, reliable, scientific trials to boost immune system function.

patients, says she hasn't seen results that justify the price of the product – i.e. it helps, but it's not that great.

My opinion is that this is a natural product that is highly unlikely to aggravate anyone's gut, so if you feel led to take it, then do so. Even though I haven't seen any great results from it, the research is compelling enough that I continue to take it sporadically. If you have a baby who is not being breastfed, then I would definitely put ½ capsule into each formula bottle to make up for the lack of immune system factors naturally present in breastmilk (see Chapter Nine).

KOMBUCHA TEA

This tea has gotten a lot of press as an anti-inflammatory and excellent immune system strengthener. I trial-tested a bottle of it (imported from Germany and bought at a natural pharmacy) and it tasted quite good (kind of like a cross between apple cider and beer). I felt good during the two weeks it took me to finish the bottle, but didn't notice any significant change – although at the time I was also not experiencing any symptoms! However, I did see a posting on the Internet once from a woman who said she used it solely to heal her ulcerative colitis and continues to take it for maintenance. She said if she stops taking it, her symptoms return. It can be quite expensive to buy a prepared bottle of it from your health pharmacy, so keep in mind that you can order your own kombucha mushroom starter, and then grow it and make the tea yourself. However, you must make sure your growing environment is as sterile as possible. The amount of tea you should drink will depend on which preparation you get, so just experiment with whatever the recommended guidelines are and use your intuition as your guide. Refrigerate after opening. If you have any liver problems or damage, do not consume kombucha as there have been a couple of reports of liver failure due to kombucha.

As a much milder form, the Yogi Tea Company makes a green tea with kombucha and Chinese herbs that I find is excellent as my daily tea -both delicious and beneficial for the immune system. Although green tea does

> ☼ You can order your own kombucha mushroom starter, and then grow it and make the tea yourself. However, you must make sure your growing environment is sterile.

contain theophylline (a close relative of caffeine), it is minimal and the positive effects of the catechins (a group of compounds that lower cholesterol, improve lipid metabolism and have antibacterial properties) outweigh the presence of theophylline – in my opinion. Also, if you just dip the tea bag quickly 2 – 3 times you won't get much theophylline in your tea. The kombucha and Chinese herbs however, will be released immediately upon contact with the hot water as they are sprayed on the tea leaves in a preparation designed to dissolve immediately. The longer you let the tea steep, the higher the caffeine content will be.

MSM

Methyl-sulfonyl-methane (MSM) is a sulfur compound that is touted as being an excellent anti-inflammatory. For this reason, it is commonly used in arthritis treatment and often added to intestinal healing formulas. However, since MSM is a sulfur-based substance, it usually causes gas and bloating in people with IBD and IBS. Therefore, I do not recommend you consume it. I tried it myself numerous years ago and it did indeed cause bloating and increased my bowel movements. Again, read labels carefully as it's added to all kinds of products.

> Since MSM is a sulfur-based substance, it usually causes gas and bloating in people with IBD and IBS.

MOLOCURE A.M.P. ALOE VERA

Molocure is a very expensive brand of Aloe vera in freeze-dried powder form. I've heard from readers who've had good results from it, readers who've had no results from it, and only one reader who had a bad reaction to it. I haven't tried the product myself, but from the manufacturing process described on their website, it seems to be a good Aloe vera product. As the powder is processed from the inner leaf only, it contains no aggravating ingredients and therefore should be safe for people with IBS and IBD. However, keep in mind that you may see the same results from using George's 'Always Active' Aloe Vera Juice, which is a lot cheaper.

ASHWAGANDA

Ashwaganda (*Withania somnifera*) is an Indian plant in the same family as the tomato. Some herbalists call ashwaganda 'Indian ginseng' since it is used in Ayurvedic medicine in the same way that ginseng is used in traditional Chinese medicine.

Ashwaganda is an adaptogen herb. It is rejuvenating, balancing, strengthening, and calming to the nervous system. It's useful for relieving fatigue, nervous exhaustion, and memory loss. This herb also has a reputation as an aphrodisiac and is believed to help prevent sterility in males and sexual ailments. A mild sedative, ashwaganda also reduces mental chatter and promotes sleep. It also promotes tissue regeneration and slows the aging process.

Ashwaganda is available in capsule form, the whole plant is usually used and the product you choose should be standardized for withanolides. Do not use a product called ashwaganda oil internally – this is a combination of ashwaganda, almond oil and rose water that is meant to be used as a facial toner. Do not eat ashwaganda berries, as they can cause severe gastrointestinal pain. You should avoid this herb if you are taking prescription drugs for anxiety, insomnia, or a seizure disorder.

If you're sensitive to tomatoes, then test this herb carefully. Otherwise, if you want to try this herb, then try it in isolation (i.e. do not take any other supplements at the same time) and see how you tolerate it before adding any other supplements. I have not tried this herb myself, so I can't offer any comments on it. If you want to use it, then test it and see how it goes. Again, follow the guidelines in Chapter Two for introducing new supplements.

> A mild sedative, ashwaganda also reduces mental chatter and promotes sleep.

SEACURE

Seacure comes in capsule form and it is a combination of fish protein and fish oil. I tried the product but as I can't swallow pills, I had to open the capsules. At which point I realized it has a very strong fishy odor! I mixed the contents of a few capsules in juice and drank it down, but I simply could not face ingesting it again after that.

My personal opinion is that this is a harmless product, but it may be cheaper to just ingest fish oil (in odorless liquid or capsule form). As for the protein component, you'd have to ingest a lot of capsules to get a significant amount of protein and it's probably a lot easier to just eat the fish, or have a whey protein shake.

BC-9 HOMEOPATHIC REMEDY

This is a combination homeopathic remedy specifically formulated for people with Crohn's disease or colitis. A homeopathic doctor I spoke to said it works better for people with colitis than for those with Crohn's. I heard from one reader with colitis who tried it and she said it worked like a charm for about two months, then all her symptoms returned. I tried it and it had no effect on me whatsoever. However, the great thing about homeopathic remedies is that they are completely harmless, and probably the safest supplement to test or experiment with. So, again, if you feel your gut urging you to try this remedy, by all means go ahead, and hopefully you'll get some good results from it.

TRYING NEW PRODUCTS

Remember that before trying any new remedy, you need to test the product in isolation and introduce it according to the supplement guidelines in Chapter Two. Also keep in mind that the remedies recommended in this program have already been trial-tested by thousands of readers and everything you need to heal yourself is here. In almost every phone consultation I do, I find out the client is taking an herbal supplement(s) that is directly aggravating their condition. Please remember that even health professionals (like medical and naturopathic doctors, herbalists, etc.) are not fully aware of how extremely hypersensitive the gastrointestinal tract becomes in people with IBD and IBS, and their recommendations are not

> The great thing about homeopathic remedies is that they are completely harmless, and probably the safest supplement to test or experiment with.

always reliable. I strongly suggest that you at least wait until your condition is fairly stable (no bleeding or diarrhea, normal weight) before testing supplements other than the ones recommended in this program.

Now turn to the *Healing Journey Workbook* and do the section for Chapter Eight.

9
Pregnancy & Breastfeeding

*"Do you know why my body is special?
I think it's a present."*

Oscar Patel Thompson, age 4

☀ Be gentle and compassionate with yourself, and just do the best you can at the time.

Pregnancy, breastfeeding and the rigorous demands of parenting present a special challenge for people whose bodies are not strong and healthy to start with. In this chapter I'm going to outline all the special physical and emotional challenges in store for people with IBD or severe IBS, who choose to have children. I'm also going to give you some ideas on how to plan to meet these challenges successfully, without risking your health. I have two children (aged two and a half, and five years, at the time of writing) and have had my health crash several times from the rigorous demands of parenting. My goal in this chapter is to pass on to you the benefit of my experience, so hopefully you will be able to parent more successfully (during the early years) and keep your health intact, as much as possible.

Childbearing and parenting are somewhat difficult to write about because you cannot separate goals and beliefs about parenting from implementation. For example, if I believe that my child's health and welfare are number one, then that belief is going to shape and influence everything I do. If, however, I believe that my needs come first, and my child's needs are secondary – I will then respond differently in almost all situations.

My goal in this chapter is not to tell you which belief to hold or how best to care for your child. However, you need to know that I'm automatically going to be writing from my belief system – there is no such thing as an unbiased opinion! So, if you find yourself disagreeing with my position or assumptions, no problem, please just take the information and ideas that are useful to you and fit in with your philosophy, and ignore the rest.

Balancing Baby's Needs & Your Needs
Personally, I believe in an amalgamation of the two parenting positions outlined above. On the one hand, if you are sick or in the hospital, you are not going to be able to take care of your child anyway. So in that respect, you have to take care of yourself first. On the other hand, there is no way to adequately meet the needs of a newborn and infant without substantial self-sacrifice. The degree of physical energy required to effectively parent

an infant (especially 0-5 months) will most likely involve a degradation of your health. And this is the juncture where each of us has to make our own decisions about how far we're willing to go to meet our children's needs.

One of my goals for my children was to breastfeed them for as long as possible, but at least for one year. Ideally, I wanted to allow each of them to wean themselves, at whatever age they wanted to. I believe very strongly in the importance of breastfeeding, both from a health perspective and a spiritual/emotional perspective, so breastfeeding for a minimum of one year was an imperative for me. With my first child, Oscar, I was able to breastfeed him for 20 months and then my health became so precarious that I had to wean him. By that time, I was about 15 pounds underweight, very hormonally unbalanced, and bleeding from my colon. Some people may feel I sacrificed far too much and I never should have let my health degrade to such a level just to nurse my son. However, I still stand by my decision because I was taking into account who my son is, and his unique needs. He was a child for whom breastfeeding was his lifeline. Every time he latched on to my breast, his eyes would roll up from the pleasure of it, and his whole body would release with a huge sigh. Whenever he was emotionally or physically hurt, nothing could soothe him other than breastfeeding. Breastfeeding was an absolutely crucial need for his psyche and development. For myself, I took it as far as I could go to what I knew were my limits. I already had my treatment plan lined up and knew exactly what I needed to do to heal myself and roughly how long it would take. So I let him breastfeed until I (according to my limits, not someone else's) knew I then had to switch and take care of myself. We went down to my parent's house in Arizona so I could have help and support during my healing and I went on the IBD Remission Diet for two weeks. I did a gradual food reintroduction combined with shakes for the next ten days, and by the end of it I was up in my normal weight range again with no bleeding. It then took a few more months to sort out my hormonal problems.

With my second child, Zara, I was not as strong right from the beginning of my pregnancy – because I got pregnant only five months after weaning Oscar! When I weaned Zara, after breastfeeding her for 13 months, I was in

☼ Unless you get one of those rare children that automatically sleeps through the night, there is no way you can meet the needs of a newborn baby without sacrificing yourself to some degree.

> I believe very strongly in the importance of breastfeeding, both from a health perspective and a spiritual/emotional perspective.

a similar state of health as to when I had weaned Oscar. Again, I went on the IBD Remission Diet for two weeks and immediately began hormone supplementation to balance my endocrine system. I was also okay with my decision to wean Zara sooner because, although she really enjoyed breastfeeding, it wasn't an absolutely crucial thing for her, as it had been for Oscar. And she didn't derive the same sort of 'lifeline' comfort from it that Oscar did.

So, with both my children, I didn't manage to meet my goal of letting them wean themselves. And I do feel a bit sad about that because I think it would have been wonderful from an emotional/spiritual point of view. However, taking into account the person I was at that time, the knowledge I had, where I was on my Healing Journey, and my physical constraints at that time, I know I did the best I could. I sacrificed as far as was safe for me and I don't regret one minute of it.

Personally, I think our western world places too much importance on the 'take care of yourself first' concept and not enough importance on self-sacrifice (of sleep/health, money, autonomy, etc.) to meet your child's needs. And I don't care what anyone says, unless you get one of those rare children that automatically sleeps through the night, there is no way you can meet the needs of a newborn baby without sacrificing yourself to some degree. What we can do, however, is to get a generous support network in place so that the parents (and especially the breastfeeding mother) are supported to such an extent that the sacrifice required is minimal. I'll discuss setting up this network later in this chapter and hopefully you can learn and benefit from my mistakes/experience. If I'd had a sufficient support network in place with my two children, my health would not have deteriorated to the level it did, I would have been able to breastfeed longer, and I would have been able to enjoy those early years a whole lot more. Who knows, if I ever have a third child, maybe I'll finally be able to get it right! Parenting is a huge learning curve, and I hope each of you can shortcut this process by learning from the mistakes I've already made. If you get your support network in place, then hopefully you'll be able to keep your health intact throughout. Keep in mind that the protocols and concepts presented in this chapter are ideal scenarios. As any parent knows, we can't always fulfill our ideals! So again, be gentle and compassionate with yourself and just do the best you can at the time.

BIRTH CONTROL

Before you're ready to conceive, after you've given birth, and when you don't want to have any more children, you're going to be faced with the question of birth control. I am strongly opposed to any form of hormonal birth control (including birth control pills, transdermal patches and implants). Hormonal birth control methods will unbalance your endocrine (hormonal) system and destroy the good bacteria in your gut (by creating an alkaline pH). These are very unhealthy conditions – particularly for someone with IBS or IBD.

If you're using birth control pills for acne control or period regulation – again, you're just suppressing the symptoms of an imbalance, you're not resolving the actual problem. Acne can be healed using Wild Oregano Oil internally and externally, followed by high dose probiotic supplementation (follow *Jini's Wild Oregano Oil Protocol* in Chapter Two). Menstrual irregularities signify an underlying endocrine problem – perhaps your thyroid, pituitary or adrenal glands are not functioning properly and/or you're doing other things that are leading to a hormone imbalance. See *Immunosuppressive Drugs & Hormonal Health* in Chapter Five, and the section on *Plastic & Xenoestrogens* in Chapter Four for more information on resolving hormonal imbalance.

You also should not use any kind of spermicidal cream, jelly or condom lubricant because this will also disrupt your bacterial flora. So what's left? You can use condoms lubricated with KY jelly or a natural, herbal lubricant, but as we know, condoms can tear. IUD's (Intrauterine Devices) are not always recommended for people with IBS or IBD as they can trigger cramping, aside from other complications that may result. A diaphragm (but no spermicide) combined with a condom may work well – but make sure you use the regular, thicker condoms and if you're having vigorous or

> There are two methods of entirely natural birth control that have prevention rates similar to the birth control pill, when used correctly.

prolonged intercourse, then change the condom periodically for a fresh one to reduce chance of tearing.

> **GI Symptoms vary with Menstruation**
> A review of the literature was carried out regarding the effect of the menstrual cycle on bowel symptoms in women with and without irritable bowel syndrome. The studies surveyed suggest that gastrointestinal symptoms do vary with the menstrual cycle. One-third of otherwise asymptomatic women may experience gastrointestinal symptoms at the time of menstruation, and almost 50% of women with functional bowel disorder report an increase in symptoms during menstruation. In addition, women who suffer from dysmenorrhoea are more likely to have functional bowel disorder. The physiological basis of these phenomena is unknown. It has been suggested that raised serum progesterone levels in the luteal phase may be one of the mechanisms responsible but little is known of the physiological effects of sex hormones on the gut in vitro. It has also been suggested that prostaglandins released by the uterus at the time of menstruation might cause diarrhoea. Further research is needed to explore what common hormonal or neurological pathways may underlie the covariance in gastrointestinal and menstrual symptoms.
>
> Moore, J. et al. *BR. J. Obst.Gyn.* 1998, 105 (12) 1322-5

There are two methods of entirely natural birth control that have prevention rates similar to the birth control pill, when used correctly. The first one uses a daily saliva test to monitor hormone levels – the pattern formed by the saliva indicates your pre-ovulatory phase, ovulation, and then post-ovulatory phase. Scientists found that saliva mimics cervical mucus, so instead of having to swab the cervix and examine the specimen, you can just spit onto a slide and examine that under a microscope. This is the method I use and it's very simple. I just leave the kit on my bedside table and every morning, before I get up (I find the results most accurate and consistent then) I just dab my tongue onto the slide. I let the sample dry while I'm getting ready, then I take a look under the little microscope and in three seconds I know whether it's okay to have sex that day, or not. Of course, this same handy device can also be used for when you are trying to conceive – since it tells you exactly when you're ovulating. You can buy a saliva method kit or find out more about it at: *www.lunafertility.com*. Your kit will come with complete, detailed instructions. Obviously, if you're not in a monogamous relationship, then you still have to use condoms as well, to protect against sexually transmitted diseases. One word of caution: Do not use natural progesterone cream (or other natural hormone supplements) whilst using the saliva method of birth control, as it will obscure the results.

The other effective natural planning method also works on mapping your ovulatory cycle, but instead of monitoring your saliva, you monitor your basal body temperature. Or, some methods combine monitoring your basal body temperature and cervical mucus for maximum accuracy. If you're interested in this method of birth control, type in 'basal temperature birth control' to your Internet search engine, as there are many different methods and programs available.

NATURAL MENSTRUAL PRODUCTS

Since we're on the topic, I also want to discuss the importance of using natural, unbleached menstrual products. Like diapers, many commercial menstrual pads and tampons use a very harmful chemical called Dioxin to bleach them white. They are also composed of synthetic (i.e. plastic) materials and these can also leach harmful chemicals into your body – remember that mucous membranes (mouth, intestines, lining of your nose, genitals, anus) have the highest absorption capabilities of any tissue in the body. So you should make absolutely certain you're not using products that contain harmful chemicals in these areas. Which reminds me, for your baby, you should use cloth diapers or natural disposable diapers like Tushies (*www.tushies.com*) or Seventh Generation (*www.seventhgeneration.com*).

Currently the only disposable natural menstrual products I've seen are Natracare Brand (*www.natracare.com*) and they're available in many health stores. You can also get washable, re-usable, organic cotton menstrual pads from a variety of suppliers online and in health stores, and obviously this is better for our environment than using disposables. But the absolute best natural menstrual product I've come across is a device called the Diva Cup. It's a cone-shaped, silicone cup that you insert mid-way up your vagina and it collects your menstrual blood as it drains from your uterus. You then carefully pull it out, empty the blood into the toilet, rinse it out in the sink (or just wipe it with toilet paper) and then re-insert it. It holds one ounce of blood, so you may only need to empty it twice a day. After you buy the Diva Cup, there's no ongoing expense, no laundry to do, no adverse effects on the environment, and it's the easiest thing to use when you're traveling, swimming, etc. I strongly encourage you to give it a try. It's available online at *www.divacup.com* and they offer a one-year guarantee, so there's no risk. If you don't like it, just send it back. It's also available in health stores.

> A menstrual cup is inserted mid-way up your vagina and it collects your menstrual blood as it drains from your uterus. You then carefully pull it out, empty the blood into the toilet, and then re-insert it. There's no ongoing expense, no laundry to do, no adverse effects on the environment, and it's the easiest thing to use when you're traveling, swimming, etc.

If you don't like silicone, there's another menstrual cup product available called The Keeper that's made out of natural rubber (but some people don't like the rubber smell), it's available at: www.keeper.com.

PRIOR TO CONCEPTION

Ideally, it's best if you can follow the *Listen To Your Gut* healing program to get yourself off all drugs for at least three to six months before conceiving a child. Your husband/partner should also be off all medication and following the *Maintenance Diet* for three to six months prior to conception, to ensure the health and vitality of his sperm. The health of your baby begins in utero and you want to do everything you can to give it the best conditions to flourish.

Prescription Drugs

I don't care what your doctor may say about the 'safety' of being on steroids, Asacol or immunosuppressant drugs whilst pregnant. If a pregnant woman is not even supposed to drink alcohol or dye her hair because of possible damage to the fetus, how can these incredibly strong drugs possibly be safe? For example, as I wrote in Chapter Five, when Prednisone was released onto the market it was mandated to be used *only* in 'life-threatening conditions'. Subsequent research has shown that it causes significant damage to the eyes, bones and lungs of developing children.[1] If it can damage a child's organs *outside* of the womb, how can it not do any damage to an extremely vulnerable, developing fetus? We already know that numerous pharmaceutical companies have misrepresented drug trial data to the FDA in order to get approval for pending drugs (they leave out data from any trials showing negative results that do not support their FDA application). So how can you trust any data or trial results sponsored, indirectly funded, or otherwise linked to a pharmaceutical company? Instead, use your common sense and your intuition.

My personal belief is that it would be far less harmful to use any of the natural supplements listed in this book, rather than a prescription drug.

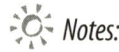 *Notes:*

Even in the case of potent herbs (like Wild Oregano Oil) that have not been tested on pregnant women, they are still plant substances, and therefore will be more compatible with your body, and will likely be metabolized more easily than a synthetic compound. If you have a severe flare-up, or distressing symptoms that you need to address during pregnancy, I believe it's far better for you (and your baby) to address these problems naturally – as long as you don't have other, complicating conditions. A good naturopathic physician can guide you in the use of untested herbs during pregnancy or breastfeeding. Towards the end of this chapter, I'm going to discuss the use of an elemental diet during pregnancy for people in dire circumstances and give you a few anecdotal examples of using an elemental diet to get through a severe flare-up, rather than resorting to medication.

Avoiding Morning Sickness

Depending on your health, you may want to do a gentle detox (or use the therapies in this program that are naturally detoxifying – see Chapter Eight) to reduce the likelihood of first trimester nausea. My naturopath told me about a patient of his who'd had two children already and suffered terrible 'morning sickness' with both. He told her that if she detoxified her body first, then her liver wouldn't have so much to cope with whilst pregnant (the liver automatically carries an extra load during pregnancy). So she underwent a course of herbal and infrared sauna detoxification prior to conceiving her third child. She then had absolutely no nausea during that pregnancy. Apparently he had numerous other patients who followed this practice of detoxifying before conceiving and all of them experienced minimal to no nausea during pregnancy. If you've taken prescription medication and been eating a 'normal' diet, then your liver function is likely to be weak. If you've been off drugs for a few months and continue to follow the protocols in this program, you may be okay without additional detoxification. But it would be a good idea to supplement with Milk Thistle (cleanses and strengthens the liver) prior to conceiving. Test it according to the procedure in Chapter Two for introducing new supplements.

> If a pregnant woman is not even supposed to drink alcohol or dye her hair because of possible damage to the fetus, how can strong prescription drugs possibly be safe?

I had been on the IBD Remission Diet for seven weeks prior to conceiving my first child, Oscar. So this provided me with an excellent detoxification and strengthening program before I got pregnant two months after finishing it. I experienced maybe seven incidences of very mild nausea lasting about 30 – 60 minutes each episode, during my entire pregnancy with Oscar. When I got pregnant with Zara, I'd only weaned Oscar five months prior and had gone on the IBD Remission Diet for two weeks to build myself up because I was so run down. I had wanted a whole year to build up my stores, detox and strengthen myself, but, the romance of Hawaii….! Thus, I had mild nausea briefly periodically at night, during the first trimester I was pregnant with Zara. Luckily it didn't interfere with my nutrient intake since I'd finished eating for the day by the time it hit.

SUPPLEMENTATION

It's vital for women to supplement with additional nutrients prior to conception, during pregnancy, during nursing, and then for at least three months following weaning. This holds true for any woman (due to average sub-standard nutrition and toxic environment), but especially so for women who've been diagnosed with IBD or IBS. Your body is already in a weakened, compromised state and most likely coping with additional drug residues (or ongoing drug toxins), so it's imperative that you supplement with additional nutrients and healing substances during this very important time in your and baby's life.

Probiotic Supplementation Is Crucial

Women with IBD or IBS who are planning to conceive should also be on high dose probiotic supplementation for three months prior to conception, throughout pregnancy, and throughout breastfeeding. It would also be ideal if you could do *Jini's Probiotic Retention Enema* (see Chapter Two) prior to conception as well. Mothers with IBS or IBD should also give Natren's Life Start (*B. infantis* probiotic) directly to their infants from three weeks to one year of age. When giving probiotics directly to an infant, *only* give Life Start (*B. infantis*). Once your baby begins eating regular foods you can start with

---

> Mothers with IBS or IBD should also give oral *B. infantis* probiotic directly to their infants from three weeks to one year of age.

the other species of bacteria – but not before. Studies have shown that even healthy mothers in the western world do not have sufficient 'good bacterial' populations and therefore cannot pass on a good bacterial flora to their babies.[2] Many theorize that this is at the root of the explosion of allergies in the Western world.

A baby receives its primary implantation of good bacteria as it passes through the vaginal canal – the bacteria enter through orifices like the ears, nose and mouth. Thereafter, it continues to receive good bacteria through its mother's breastmilk. If you don't have a good gut flora to begin with (and people with IBS or IBD do not), or your baby was delivered by cesarean section, then how can you pass on good bacteria to your baby? This is why it is absolutely crucial for every mother reading this book to take high dose oral probiotics prior to conception, during pregnancy and breastfeeding, and also to supplement your baby directly. Please see the *Probiotic Supplementation* section in Chapter Two for detailed probiotic dosage instructions for both you and your baby.

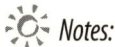 Notes:

Jini's Tried And Tested Supplements

Following are the supplements I have used during both my pregnancies (and during breastfeeding) and found to cause no adverse effects (and lots of benefits!) However, this is my experience only (and that of about ten others I've heard from) so use at your own risk/discretion. There's no 'published' information available on the safety of George's Aloe Vera Juice, Astragalus, or L-Glutamine during pregnancy. The other supplements are all published as being safe for pregnant women:

- George's 'Always Active' Aloe Vera Juice – but only this brand, do not substitute another! I know numerous pregnant women who've used George's successfully

- Natren brand Probiotics – Healthy Trinity capsules, or Megadophilus powder, Bifido Factor powder, Digesta-Lac powder and Life Start powder. Again, only use this brand, other brands of probiotics may deliver little benefit, and some will aggravate your condition. Continue taking Natren probiotics throughout breastfeeding as well, so your baby gets beneficial flora in his/her gut. See Chapter Two for detailed probiotic dosage guidelines for both mother and baby. Georges' Aloe Vera and Natren Probiotics both really help if you're experiencing heartburn (among their other benefits – see Chapter Two for more details).

- L-Glutamine – I've taken up to 1000 mg per day on an empty stomach (stops diarrhea) and up to 3000 mg per day when mixed in a protein shake (doesn't stop diarrhea when mixed with other foods but still highly beneficial for healing the mucosal lining).

- Full spectrum of vitamins and minerals, including trace minerals. I took Nature's Way Prenatal (capsules) while pregnant and breastfeeding.

- Up to 6000 mg of vitamin C per day in mineral ascorbate form only (do not use ascorbic acid) eg. calcium ascorbate, magnesium ascorbate. A product called Emergen-C is a really tasty naturally flavored drink packet with 1000 mg of Vitamin C per packet (in mineral ascorbate form) that you just mix with water.

- Up to 30 drops per day (in divided doses) of Herb Pharm's liquid tincture Astragalus when your immune system feels run down, or is battling a cold or illness (do not take if you already have a fever as it induces added sweating)

- 1 – 3 Absorb Plus elemental shakes per day (automatically contains 1000 mg L-Glutamine per shake) with 1 tbsp. of flax or Udo's oil per shake (great for fetal brain development), 30 mg CoEnzyme Q10, and 30 mg Pycnogenol or Grape Seed Extract added. I would also add my 2 prenatal multi-vitamin capsules (see above) and whip it all together in the blender, then pour over ice. A great way to get important nutrients for me and baby and about 500 calories per shake.

Flu/Cold Supplements

You can also take all these supplements (above) while breastfeeding and if your baby gets a cold, the Astragalus and vitamin C will get rid of it very quickly – but again, don't use Astragalus if your baby has a fever. If your baby is vomiting, has diarrhea or a bacterial infection, definitely take the Natren probiotics for the duration of the illness (also give *B. infantis* – Life Start – directly to your baby) and then for three months following. If there's a stomach flu bug going around your community, or a family member gets sick, then breastfeeding Mum should take all three Natren probiotics (ideally in powder form) 2 – 3 times per day to prevent Mum and Baby from contracting the illness. If you do get sick with an infection that causes vomiting or diarrhea, then sip the Natren probiotics (1 tsp. of each – Megadophilus, Bifido Factor, Digesta-Lac – mixed in room-temperature filtered water) in powder form every half hour until the vomiting or diarrhea subsides. Don't worry if you have to sip it very slowly and you still keep vomiting, just keep going with it, and the good bacteria will eventually take hold. Then take them three times per day for the next two weeks. Also *always* follow antibiotic use with probiotic supplementation, both for your baby and you. See Chapter Two for detailed instructions on probiotic supplementation.

Essential Supplements

So, here are the supplements I believe every mother should take during pregnancy (and ideally for three months prior to conception), for the duration of breastfeeding, and then for at least three months following weaning (to replenish your stores and health):

▶ Nature's Way Prenatal Multivitamin

▶ Udo's Oil (or flax oil) – at least 1 tbsp. per day

▶ Fish Oil – as directed on bottle, or to tolerance

▶ Absorb Plus or protein shake – at least once per day, or as needed

▶ Natren probiotics in powder form (Megadophilus, Bifido Factor, Life Start, Digesta-Lac) or capsules (if you prefer and have no diarrhea or heartburn).

> Pregnancy and lactation (breastfeeding) should be the most disciplined, healthy diet and lifestyle time of your life

- Follow the *Healing Diet* that suits your symptoms, or at *least* follow the *Maintenance Diet* strictly

Other supplements that would also be beneficial:

- Coenzyme Q10
- Pycnogenol or Grape Seed Extract
- Vitamin C in mineral ascorbate form
- Additional Multi-Mineral supplement

There have been many long-term studies done showing that the health of your baby in-utero will pre-determine your child's health until the late teenage years.[3] So please don't make the mistake of assuming that you can eat whatever you want whilst pregnant. Pregnancy and lactation (breastfeeding) should be the most disciplined, healthy diet and lifestyle time of your life. It is absolutely crucial that you strictly follow the guidelines in the *Maintenance Diet* and take the supplements recommended above to give your baby the best chance at good health, optimal brain functioning, and avoiding allergies and obesity. See Chapter Two for descriptions of why the supplements above are beneficial. If you experience nausea during the first trimester, you may not be able to take some of the supplements listed above. If this is the case, don't worry about it. Just try to drink the Absorb Plus shakes whenever you can, to keep your nutrient levels up and then begin supplementing whenever you can tolerate it.

An added bonus of ingesting the Udo's Oil and/or fish oil, is that you will probably not lose any hair following the birth of your baby. Doctors tell women this is inevitable, and is the result of hormonal changes. But I have had numerous friends take Udo's Oil daily after childbirth and none of them (including me) lost any hair. Another mother I know whose hair had already thinned considerably, began taking the Udo's Oil and her hair began thickening within a month.

> Your body is already in a weakened, compromised state and most likely coping with additional drug residues (or ongoing drug toxins), so it's imperative that you supplement with additional nutrients and healing substances during this very important time in your and baby's life.

If you experience rectal fissures either during or after giving birth (a common occurrence for even normal women), then you can use FissureHeal suppositories to heal them quite quickly. See the relevant sections in Chapter Two for healing both rectal fissures and/or hemorrhoids. Legally, Imix Naturals (the company that makes FissureHeal) has to warn against their use during pregnancy, because of the Comfrey contained in the product. Personally, I don't believe the Comfrey in FissureHeal will pose a problem during pregnancy, since it's in very small amounts, and as it is not ingested, it does not pass through your digestive system.

Natural Progesterone Cream

If you find yourself very sad, depressed, angry, irritable, or perhaps with a significant loss of short-term memory or other cognitive abilities (e.g., losing track of what you were saying in mid-sentence, going into a room or shop and being completely unable to remember why you needed to go there, etc.), then you may be suffering a hormonal imbalance. Many postpartum mothers find these problems resolve very quickly after supplementing with natural progesterone cream.

Progesterone is produced in massive amounts during pregnancy and then drops to virtually nothing following childbirth. Many theorize that this sudden drop is what triggers clinical postpartum depression in some women. These same symptoms, mentioned above, can also be caused by sleep deprivation. But even if they are, natural progesterone cream may still make a big difference. I used it after the birth of both my children, during the whole time I breastfed, and for several months following – and it changed my life. Without it I was extremely irritable, lost my temper at absurd things (often directed at my poor husband!), and couldn't think or remember properly. From day two of supplementing with natural progesterone cream, I was back to my normal self. Needless to say, my husband was amazed at the difference. I tested going off it a few times to see if it really was solely responsible for the improvements in my mind/emotions and every time I did, my husband asked me, "Did you use your progesterone cream today?" The change was that obvious!

Notes:

LISTEN TO YOUR GUT

Pick up Dr. John Lee and Dr. Jesse Hanley's book *What Your Doctor May Not Tell You About Premenopause* for excellent information on natural progesterone cream and hormonal balancing. If you're having trouble conceiving, then definitely pick up this book – they have helped thousands of women conceive who had tried everything else with no success. The important thing to remember about natural progesterone cream supplementation is that you must use a product that is completely natural. Synthetic progesterone will not have the same effect and is damaging to your body. Natural progesterone has been extensively tested and it is safe to use during pregnancy (for people with deficiencies, or to prevent miscarriage) and/or during breastfeeding. The type and concentration of natural progesterone is important and Dr. Lee has found that some brands work much better than others. He recommends several suitable brands in his book. I used one of the brands he recommended called Pro-Gest by Emerita and it's widely available.

Start with ¼ teaspoon of natural progesterone cream and rub it into your skin on either the soles of your feet, neck and face, inner arms and wrists, or the palms of your hands (where blood vessels are near the surface for quick absorption). Try to rotate application sites for maximum effectiveness, and don't use any other kind of cream or lotion on the areas you're applying it to. You may find that you don't need ¼ teaspoon and can get the same results from only ⅛ of a teaspoon (as I did). I also found that the soles of my feet were the best absorption site, so I alternated applying the cream once per day to either the soles of my feet, or my inner arms, wrists and neck. Keep the cream in the fridge to retain maximum potency.

If natural progesterone cream is going to work for you, you'll see a difference in two to three days. It works very quickly. If you don't see any improvement in postpartum symptoms, within three days, then your progesterone levels are probably fine and that's not the problem. If you have any emotional or cognitive irregularities following childbirth, I certainly recommend you give it a try.

☼ If you find yourself very sad, depressed, angry, irritable, or perhaps with a significant loss of short-term memory or other cognitive abilities, then you may be suffering a hormonal imbalance. Many postpartum mothers find these problems resolve very quickly after supplementing with natural progesterone cream.

BREASTFEEDING

Breastfeeding is absolutely crucial to the health of your baby. Even the American Medical Association has revised its recommendations based on scientific data, and now advises women to breastfeed for at least one year. Breastmilk contains hundreds of different components (from nutrients to immune system factors) and scientists have still not even isolated all the different components present. Breastmilk is also a dynamic, responsive feeding system, where your baby's body communicates with your body, and the composition of your breastmilk changes according to baby's needs! For example, if baby's brain is going through a growth or development phase, your breastmilk will automatically contain extra nutrients like essential fatty acids that support brain development. There is really no way formula feeding can even come close to breastfeeding in supporting your infant's growth and development. Breastfeeding also reduces allergies, improves immune system function, and reduces obesity (at all stages of life).

The emotional and soul-level benefits of breastfeeding are a whole other issue. I could go on and on about this topic alone, but suffice it to say that once you've experienced the level of communion, intimacy and bonding that occurs with breastfeeding, you wouldn't give it up for anything. Here's an excerpt from an article in *Mothering* magazine that I like for both its realism and beauty:

> "I nursed my son from the tender beginnings of skin-on-skin bonding just moments after his slippery entrance into this world until a few months after his second birthday, when he gracefully weaned himself from my breast. But many, many times it took so much concentration and self-discipline to sit there, just sit there, doing nothing, being still, feeding my baby, and waiting for him to finish. I'd fly through the full range of emotions – love, joy, gratitude, serenity, irritation, anger fear, impatience, selfishness, guilt, hopelessness, despair – all sometimes within a single nursing session. I'd fantasize that my body could get up and cook, clean, go to the bathroom, while my nipple stayed there in the chair nursing the baby. I would stare

> Even the American Medical Association has revised its recommendations based on scientific data, and now advises women to breastfeed for at least one year.

out the window at people passing by our San Francisco apartment, envious of the fantastic adventures they were living while I was stuck in my chair, ruled by his tiny mouth. While I nursed, I'd return calls, look through mail, and try to keep up with all the details of my life.

After about six months of this, I gave up and gave in. With each day that passed, I saw myself more and more as a mother, as a nursing mother, as a woman devoted to her child and to the importance of breastfeeding. I became an advocate for breastfeeding, trying to encourage it among all my friends and acquaintances. I awoke to the miracle of my milk and this intimate dance of nursing my child. A calmness began to quiet my restless energy, pulling me into the present moment. As Myla Kabat-Zinn says in her book, *Everyday Blessings: The Inner Work of Mindful Parenting*, "As I felt my milk let down, a wonderful haziness descended on me, and everything else became less important. I let go of the things I had planned to do, and instead let myself be pulled into the present moment, into being totally with my baby. It was a deeply meditative time for both of us."

One sunny afternoon we were nursing in our "big blue chair" (as we like to call our comfortable rocker), and I realized that I'd never before devoted myself to something so entirely. Of course I've devoted myself to my husband, to my family, to friends, to my writing, to mothering, and even to God and other spiritual endeavors at various points in my life. But in that moment, I realized, that as a breastfeeding mother, I'd completely given myself to this act of nursing in a way that I never had before. Nothing was more important than nursing my son. Nothing was put before it. There was no procrastination as with exercise, no excuses as with trying to stop eating sugar, no laziness as with housecleaning and other chores. Nursing had to be done, and I did it, over and over again, multiple times a day, for more than 800 days in a row. It was the closest thing to a spiritual practice that I'd ever experienced." [4]

Breastfeeding An Adopted Baby

If you're adopting a baby, you may be surprised to hear that you can still breastfeed. You simply put your adopted baby to your breast as many times per day and night as you can and eventually your breasts will produce milk. It is not usually enough milk to exclusively breastfeed your baby, so many adoptive mothers supplement with formula through a tube taped to the breast – so the baby still sucks on the mother's nipple and has the experience and intimacy of breastfeeding. *Mothering* magazine (www.mothering.com) has great articles about adoptive mothers breastfeeding, exactly how to do it, and further resources available in some of their back issues, so contact them for more information.

Difficulties Breastfeeding

I knew a woman who had been sexually abused and so couldn't bear to breastfeed her baby (at the time I met her, her child was already three years old). But, for the sake of her baby's health, she pumped breastmilk into bottles (which she hated as well) and exclusively fed her baby breastmilk for six months. What a gift to her child! In spite of her difficulties, she managed to do her best and give her baby that vital foundation of health. I admire her tremendously.

If you have been abused (physically or mentally) and find even the thought of breastfeeding repulsive or horrifying, then please see an EFT (Emotional Freedom Technique) therapist prior to birth, or conception, to heal yourself (see Chapter Six). You can completely heal this trauma/wounding from your body and psyche, and the healing will pervade and improve all areas of your life. Don't let your abuser continue to rob you of the riches of life.
You *can* be completely healed, and you will then be able to breastfeed your baby with joy and comfort.

If you're having difficulty breastfeeding for other reasons; insufficient milk supply, breast infection, extremely painful/wounded nipples, etc., I encourage you to not give up. La Leche League is an international organization dedicated to the promotion and encouragement of breastfeeding and they have many, many resources available to you.

> Breastmilk is also a dynamic, responsive feeding system, where your baby's body communicates with your body, and the composition of your breastmilk changes according to baby's needs.

 Notes:

You can go to a local meeting (they have chapters worldwide), and/or you can search their database of useful articles, questions & answers and varied resources available on their website: www.lalecheleague.org. Please do not give up. Breastfeeding is so crucial for your baby's physical and emotional health. Whatever your difficulty, there is a solution, you just need to find it. For example, anemia can cause insufficient milk supply, and this can be remedied through iron supplementation. Often, just supplementing with Mother's Milk tea (from Traditional Medicinals, available in most health stores) is enough to boost milk production. Definitely try EFT therapy as physical problems (in both baby and you) usually have emotional roots. If you've already given up on breastfeeding, it's not too late to start again! Remember that if adoptive mothers – who've never even been pregnant – can produce milk, then so can you. Just start putting your baby to your breast to suck for as long as it wants, as often as it wants. *Mothering* magazine (www.mothering.com) is another good resource for breastfeeding.

A Colicky Baby

The mainstream opinion on colic is that doctors still aren't sure what causes it. However, if you've ever had a serious abdominal pain attack due to trapped gas, stool, or spasming intestines – when you see a colicky baby, you'll know exactly why that baby is screaming! My son Oscar developed colic and I could see from the position and movement of his body, and the rigidity of his abdomen, that he was suffering the same kind of pain I had once suffered. I thought to myself, "Well, if the Bowel Queen can't figure out how to heal this, I don't know who can!"

As a result of my experimentation on Oscar, I worked out a very effective technique that combined *Colonic Massage* (see Chapter Six) with a number of other movements designed to release the abdomen and stimulate the relaxed passage of stool and gas. Within two weeks, Oscar's colic was completely resolved. Whenever I performed the technique on him, he would fart and poop on demand. I found this so funny that I called the routine 'Fart Aerobics'. Then of course I began teaching the technique to other mothers of newborns. Even if their baby didn't have colic, the routine still helped the baby to get their brand new intestines working properly – leading to less crying and improved sleep (for both mom and baby!). Like everything else in my life, demand led to a new product, and when my daughter Zara was born, we used her to shoot a video that I titled *BABY FART AEROBICS: And Other Natural Treatments For Colicky Babies*. I had to wait until Zara was born because I needed a newborn to demonstrate the technique on – newborns have to be handled in specific ways because they don't have head or limb control. I also included burping and positioning techniques to reduce the amount of upper gastrointestinal gas, and showed mothers a number of other techniques to make their babies more comfortable and help them sleep better.

Feedback to the DVD has been great from both midwives and mums, and I've even had mothers of three or four children, who said they learned something new from it. One mother (who was the buyer for a national children's book and video distribution agency) said it was the best video she's seen in fifteen years in the business, and she wished she'd had it when her kids were born! You can view a clip of the video and read more about what's in it at: *www.ColicInfant.com*.

Okay, and while I'm on the subject, I have to get in a plug for my *Sleeptime Stories* series of CDs for children aged 2 – 8 years. These CDs are recordings of stories I've used with my own children at bedtime, or any other time I want to calm them down, or keep them occupied. Each of the CDs features one story followed by half an hour of soothing music. The stories teach children concepts like deep breathing (meditative breathing) when faced with a puzzle or challenge – in order to get in touch with their body or creative self.

It's amazing how quickly kids pick up and utilize concepts like this. A few weeks after listening to the CDs, the kids and I arrived home after a busy day out and we were faced with a dilemma: Zara had fallen asleep in the car and really needed to sleep (if you move her, she wakes up), but Oscar wanted to go inside and do something. I was thinking out loud, trying to come up with a solution when Oscar piped up, "Mum, we should do some

> If you've ever had a serious abdominal pain attack due to trapped gas, stool, or spasming intestines – when you see a colicky baby, you'll know exactly why that baby is screaming!

deep breathing and wait for the answer to come." Just like he'd heard the characters say in the *Murray the Shark CDs*!

Anyway, these CDs are great for helping your kids go to sleep, or to calm them down before dinner, or keep them occupied on long car rides, etc. and one child I heard from used them whilst having her cavities filled! You can listen to a clip of the stories and the music at: www.MurrayTheShark.com.

FORMULA FEEDING

If you absolutely cannot breastfeed your baby, or if you have to supplement with formula feeding then there are things you can add to commercial formulas to increase their low nutrient value. But again, please go to a La Leche League meeting and/or search their website (*www.lalecheleague.org*), as there is so much help available for breastfeeding difficulties of all kinds.

If you're formula feeding a newborn, you'll need to add a number of crucial nutrients to facilitate proper brain development and help safeguard his/her gut. The best and most comprehensive instructions for infant formula supplementation can be found at *www.mercola.com* (search under "Infant Formula Fortification Protocol"). There's no point in me giving you additional instructions here, as Dr. Joseph Mercola has really covered it all (and gives a few different options) in this article on his website.

If you're exclusively formula feeding, contact Natren Inc. (*www.natren.com*, 1-800-992-3323) for guidelines on adding their probiotic (Life Start – *B. infantis*) to baby's formula bottles.

If you're using formula to supplement your breastfeeding, you should still read the article at *mercola.com* as the information is vital. Depending on the amount you're still breastfeeding, you'll either need to fortify your formula feedings as per Dr. Mercola's instructions, or you can use *Jini's Formula Supplement Protocol* below. My protocol assumes that you are taking the supplements recommended above (in *Essential Supplements*) – if you are not, then you need to follow Dr. Mercola's protocol instead. My protocol is also not to be used for newborns (0-4 months) and is nowhere near as good as Dr. Mercola's protocol. However, if you simply can't manage to implement Dr. Mercola's protocol, then this protocol is still far better than just plain formula.

Jini's Formula Supplement Protocol (5 months – 2 years)

- 8 – 9 ounces raw, organic goat's milk (or raw, organic cow's milk if raw, organic goat's milk not available)*
- 1 scoop of formula (or use amount as directed on label)
- ⅛ tsp. Life Start (*B. infantis*) probiotic until baby starts eating solids, then alternate/rotate with: ⅛ tsp. Life Start, ⅛ tsp. Megadophilus, ⅛ tsp. Bifido Factor (optional)
- ½ tsp. Udo's oil
- ½ Moducare capsule (plant sterols/fats) – boosts immunity after weaning. If breastfeeding three times per day or more, then you don't need to add Moducare.

Place formula, probiotics, Udo's oil, and Moducare in baby's bottle. Add 1 ounce of milk and mix with a spoon, crushing all lumps, until a smooth paste is formed. Then add the rest of the milk whilst stirring well. Put the lid on the bottle, block the nipple hole with your finger, and shake vigorously. It's okay to heat the milk to normal infant feeding temperature. Remember never to heat infant milk or formula in the microwave.

*If you can't get raw (unpasteurized, non-homogenized) goat's or cow's milk (see www.realmilk.com for suppliers) then just use your regular formula with water or rice milk. Do not ever use pasteurized cow's milk or soy milk.

Also give baby 1 – 2 Cod Liver Oil capsules per day (puncture capsule and squeeze contents into baby's mouth – do not add to bottle.)

> Never heat infant milk, formula, or breastmilk in the microwave. It denatures the ingredients and is harmful to your baby.

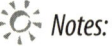 Notes:

COPING WITH A FLARE-UP WHILST PREGNANT

If you experience a flare-up of symptoms whilst pregnant or breastfeeding, you can use the supplements and diets in this healing program, along with Absorb Plus or protein shakes to provide adequate nutrition. Providing yourself and baby with enough nutrients to ensure proper development is vital, therefore I highly recommend you consume Absorb Plus shakes, or blend your own protein shakes (adding the extra supplements necessary), to provide you with nutrients that you know are actually being absorbed and utilized. Remember that during a flare, your digestive and absorptive capabilities can greatly deteriorate. So even if you're eating enough food, or you're overweight, your baby (and you) may still not be getting adequate nutrients. This is why I recommend the Absorb Plus shakes (*www.absorbplus.com*) – since they're completely pre-digested, they are absorbed very quickly into the bloodstream and the quality of nutrients is extremely high. As I mentioned before, I drank Absorb Plus shakes, off and on, throughout both my pregnancies and during breastfeeding both my children.

The IBD Remission Diet

If you experience a severe flare-up during pregnancy or breastfeeding, then the IBD Remission Diet (*www.caramal.com*), along with probiotics, may be the best solution for you to maintain your weight and nutrition, whilst avoiding drugs. A reader (with colitis that was later diagnosed as Crohn's) once contacted me in her second month of pregnancy. Anna was experiencing a severe flare with copious bleeding and diarrhea, and she was unable to eat much or absorb much nutrition from her food (the gastrointestinal transit time was too fast). Her doctor wanted strongly to put her on Prednisone and was afraid she'd lose the baby if she didn't go on it. Anna had been on the IBD Remission Diet before (and was very happy with the results that time), so she asked me if I thought she should go on the Diet again, rather than take Prednisone. After questioning her closely about her condition, symptoms, etc. I recommended that she go on the IBD Remission Diet with two modifications. First, I wanted her to amend the supplementation recommended in the Diet to comply with the list given above of safe supplements for pregnant women. Secondly, I advised her to try juicing vegetables and drinking them. By juicing and drinking fresh vegetables, the Diet was no longer elemental, but it would still be far easier for her body to extract nutrients from juices then from solid food. If she could tolerate the fresh vegetable juices, then that would be ideal because the baby would receive adequate phytonutrients as well. I felt the vegetable juices together with the Absorb Plus shakes, Udo's oil, and supplements should provide a fairly well-balanced diet with an adequate range of nutrients for a developing fetus. So, Anna tried the vegetable juices and found she could indeed tolerate them, and she stayed on the IBD Remission Diet along with the juices for about seven weeks until she was past her flare. The rest of her pregnancy went smoothly, her baby scored highly on the Apgar test at birth, and he was continuing to thrive at two years of age, when I last talked with Anna.

So far, Anna is the only person I've heard from who has attempted this variation of the IBD Remission Diet whilst pregnant. I have heard from numerous other readers who've used the Absorb Plus shakes along with the recommended supplements above during pregnancy and breastfeeding, but not exclusively. Initially, Anna was worried about whether the Diet and juicing would provide adequate nutrients. My view is that you have to balance it out against the alternative: What do you think will do more damage to your baby, Prednisone or missing a few nutrients for a while? When I think of what the average North American woman eats during pregnancy, I'm sure their babies are not getting adequate nutrition either!

If it happens that you need to go on the IBD Remission Diet during your pregnancy (or breastfeeding), then please post your story in as much detail as possible to my blog at: *www.ListenToYourGut.com* so that we can share information and other pregnant women can benefit from your experience.

> Remember that during a flare, your digestive and absorptive capabilities can greatly deteriorate. So even if you're eating enough food, or you're overweight, your baby (and you) may still not be getting adequate nutrients.

THE PHYSICAL & EMOTIONAL STRESS OF PARENTING

Conception, pregnancy, breastfeeding and parenting provide special challenges for people with IBD or IBS, for several reasons. Firstly, IBS and IBD are conditions that are triggered by emotional and physical stress. Parenting an infant and toddler is probably the most stressful thing you will ever do in your life. You may think I'm exaggerating, but I'm not. I have traveled and worked around the globe, I've moved countries seven times, I've owned my own business(es) since I was 19, been in car accidents, boat accidents, survived a hurricane (in a 20 foot wooden boat), fought my way out of a date rape, etc., etc. I have been through a lot of stressful experiences in my life, but nothing compares to the stress of parenting.

This is because the early years (newborn – age 2 or 3) often involve excruciating sleep deprivation. Ongoing sleep-deprivation results in immune system suppression, hormonal/endocrine malfunction, physical and mental exhaustion, loss of memory and other cognitive abilities, and many lesser effects. For a strong, healthy person these ramifications make life difficult. For people whose health is already compromised, ongoing sleep deprivation, combined with breastfeeding and daily chores, is devastating.

Emotional Stress

Next, is the emotional and mental stress of coping with an infant and toddler. Sure there is ongoing stress at all stages of parenting, but for someone with compromised health, the early years are definitely the worst. The parents I've seen who cope best with childcare are the people who are naturally high-energy and love running around all day. If you're this type of person by nature and you have the requisite energy, you'll have a much easier time of it. However, if you're more of an introspective, quiet person, who needs a fair amount of space and time alone – well, parenting is just going to wipe you out!

The emotional stress of wanting to provide the best possible care – for all levels of a developing human being – but being continually restricted by your physical health, can be wearing. It is also very difficult for a free and

---

☼ IBS and IBD are conditions that are triggered by emotional and physical stress. Parenting an infant and toddler is probably the most stressful thing you will ever do in your life.

unrestricted adult to suddenly become restricted in every way imaginable by this incredibly precious being who needs you (literally) all the time. Adjusting to this loss of freedom – and you almost need to develop new personality traits to cope effectively with your new reality – takes a fair bit of time and is very emotionally stressful.

Financial Stress

Then you have to weigh up the additional financial stress. If you're in poor health and your brain is not functioning well (due to sleep deprivation), you're probably not going to make as much money as you usually would. Then, not only do you have the added costs of the physical needs of your child, but you will also likely have added costs for additional childcare and home help. Unless you have outstanding family support – in the form of either monetary or physical support – the added financial pressure is going to be quite stressful.

Physical Stress

Another source of physical stress during the early years, is the difficulty of eating enough food to keep both you and your baby healthy. Why is it your infant always needs attention when you sit down to eat? If you're breastfeeding you not only have to eat (and absorb!) enough calories for yourself every day, but also for your baby. And God help you if you get a baby with a metabolism like my son Oscar's! I had to eat four meals per day, plus healthy snacks, just to maintain my weight. He fed (full feeds, both breasts) every hour or two, during the night, for the first six weeks. Then for the next seven months, he fed every two to three hours. Boy, was I glad I had formulated Absorb Plus and could drink that in place of a regular meal! Also, many people with IBD or IBS are not able to eat or digest properly when stressed. My kids are two and five right now, and yesterday I had to get up (all for good reasons) seven times just during breakfast. During supper tonight I was up three times (for varying lengths of time) and because my throat constricts during times of stress, it took me almost two hours to eat my meal. Sometimes it's just so stressful trying to eat that I give up and just have an Absorb Plus shake instead.

> For people whose health is already compromised, ongoing sleep deprivation, combined with breastfeeding and daily chores, is devastating.

Then there are the difficulties with food preparation itself. Most normal parents rely substantially on take-out and fast food during the first two years of their child's life. This is because they are simply too exhausted to shop, plan meals, and prepare meals from scratch. Unfortunately, you will not have that option because you physically cannot eat processed food with toxic additives. So, in spite of your exhaustion and ill health, you'll still have to cook your meals from scratch every day. Today I have made four meals (actually three – my husband cooked one) because my kids have large appetites. If I tried to eat fast food pizza or hamburgers on a regular basis because I'm too tired to cook, I'd be ill in no time. Plus, knowing what I do about health and diet, I could never feed such low quality food to my kids every day anyway! So you're stuck. You'll have to cook nutritious, unprocessed meals from scratch, for both you and your kids, and that takes a fair amount of time and energy.

You can reduce the load somewhat by buying frozen prepared meals at your organic grocer – but there's not a huge selection and this can get very expensive. If you have the funds, there are a growing number of personal chef services, who will deliver meals to you every week according to your dietary guidelines. Another option is to enlist the help of family and friends. If you have family members who can cook large meals (according to your tolerance/guidelines) and drop off the extra food to you, that can work well. If you're very organized you may be able to set up a 'cooking cooperative' with two or three other mothers/fathers where you each take turns cooking and make extra that the other families pick up close to dinnertime. But again, you'll have to find like-minded, health-conscious people who are willing to use quality ingredients and account for intolerances.

It is also a very good idea to get into the habit of cooking in volume, when you do cook, and cooking foods that can be frozen. When I make soup, stew, or lasagne, for example, I make a huge amount and then freeze the extra in single serving portions. It's not that much extra work to make triple (or quintuple!) the amount of food, but it does take planning.

Attachment Parenting

So, here you have your physical health, which is substantially (if not primarily) triggered by stress, and you are entering into (or have already entered into) the most stressful period of your life! If you leave your baby/child to cry themselves to sleep during the night, then you will probably avoid a good deal of the sleep deprivation and its subsequent stressors. For myself, I would never do that to my children. The last thing I want to teach my kids is that they can cry and cry, and mummy never comes. I don't want to abandon my children emotionally to that kind of body/mind/spirit trauma and I don't want to teach them that they are alone in this world. If I nurture my children with compassion, then they will grow to be nurturing, compassionate people. We have to be the change we want to see in the world, and that begins in utero and continues for the rest of your child's life. If you're going against the flow of western civilization by wanting to provide deep levels of attachment, intimacy and security for your child, then *Mothering* magazine is a fantastic resource and source of encouragement. It's available in many organic grocery stores, or online at: *www.mothering.com*. Kindred (an Australian magazine) is another excellent resource with lots of online articles: *www.KindredCommunity.com*. You've already read in earlier chapters of this book about the physical consequences I've suffered as a result of exhaustion and extended sleep deprivation. But I tell you, I revel in who my children are (their kindness, compassion, nurturing, intimacy, strength, charisma, fantastic health, joy in living, etc.) every day, and I don't regret a single sacrifice.

However, I sure wish someone had prepared me for the reality of childcare (as much as you can prepare someone who doesn't actually have children!) by outlining all the myriad stressors I would need to plan for – as I have done for you above. I'm also going to give you my advice as to what you need to have in place (or implement now) to minimize the deleterious effects of these stressors, as much as possible. Obviously, different people are going to have different levels of implementation for these suggestions due to their own belief system, support network and financial reality, but I'm going to give you my ideal and you can go from there.

> If I nurture my children with compassion, then they will grow to be nurturing, compassionate people. We have to be the change we want to see in the world, and that begins in utero and continues for the rest of your child's life.

Setting Up Your Home Help

When you are still pregnant, line up at least three months of daily help following the birth of your baby (six months would be ideal). This may seem like a lot to you, but remember that your needs are much greater than that of normal, healthy people and you need to take extra care of yourself to avoid a flare-up of symptoms. If you can have help at night too, that would be ideal. About three months prior to the birth of my second child, Zara, I said to my mum, "I need help for three months following the baby's birth, do you want to be that help, or should I hire someone? I'm fine either way, but I need to know now so I have enough time to interview and choose someone if you don't want to do it." My mother chose to come and stay with us for three months and she also took Zara at night, bringing her into my room to feed and changing her diaper when necessary. This took a huge load off me and greatly reduced the excruciating postnatal sleep deprivation. It also helped that Zara's metabolism is much slower than Oscar's, and she only needed to feed every three hours during the night. I also hired a cook/housekeeper to come in three afternoons per week during the whole time my mum was there. If someone's helping you do nights, you can't expect that person (even if they're perfectly healthy) to have the energy to do all the cooking and cleaning during the day as well.

So, make sure the help you set up for those first three months encompasses someone to at least do cooking, laundry, and clean the bathrooms and kitchen (these are the minimum essentials). You will also need to instruct your help in how to do their tasks (schedule this for 2 – 3 weeks before your due date), because it will be too stressful and exhausting to do this after you've given birth. Your help can consist of any combination of husband/partner, family members and paid help that may work for you. Don't expect yourself to be able to do anything other than recover from childbirth, nurse your baby, eat your meals, get out for a gentle walk each day, and spend quality time with your other children for the first three months. If you have other children, you'll need help arranged to look after a lot of their physical needs as well, so you can keep your energy for looking after their emotional and mental needs.

> Remember that your needs are much greater than that of normal, healthy people, and you need to take extra care of yourself to avoid a flare-up of symptoms.

After that initial three month period, arrange for regular home help to assist with cooking, cleaning and occasional childcare until your baby is two years old. No, I am not kidding, and I am not being excessive. Even just three hours per day, 4 – 5 days a week will change your life. Also, get your husband/partner or other family member/friend to do your grocery shopping (grocery shopping with young children can be a very stressful event). Remember, if you want to preserve your health and avoid a flare-up (where everyone loses, including your baby, husband/partner, and family), you're going to need a lot of help. You will not be able to parent your child properly if you are in the hospital, or unable to breastfeed. If you feel too guilty to get this amount of help, then use EFT (see Chapter Six) to get yourself over the guilt. You are not a normal, healthy person and you need a lot more help than most people/mothers around you. Accept this and you will have a chance at being able to care for and nurture your baby properly. Remember that if your health goes, you will not be able to feed or nurture your child properly – so what's the point? Feel guilty, go into debt to pay for it, ignore the sniping of others and do whatever it takes to get the help you need to keep yourself healthy.

It's also better to plan for more help than you think you'll need – because, if you haven't had children before, it's unlikely you'll be able to anticipate the amount of help you're going to need (all new parents are absolutely gobsmacked by how difficult and exhausting it is). If it turns out you don't need as much help as you arranged, then it's very easy to scale back. The last thing you need to be doing with a newborn is interviewing and training new home help because you don't have enough – that would be very stressful!

My friend Sarah in Hong Kong, who is perfectly robust and healthy, recently had her fourth child. Both she and her husband work for finance companies and hold demanding, well-paid positions. They have no family members in the city – they're all in Europe. So she has two nannies and a full-time maid during the day. With the birth of her fourth child, she hired a night nanny as well – to do what my mother did for me. This is a woman who has planned well for her extra needs, and this is probably one

> You need to have a support structure in place so that you have daily assistance with cooking, cleaning and childcare – otherwise, the overwhelming physical and emotional stress will degrade your health and then everyone loses. What use is having money in the bank, or being able to say 'we're debt-free!' when you're in the hospital and can't breastfeed your own child?

of the reasons she remains strong and healthy! So if you think what I'm advocating is excessive or unrealistic, just remember her story. If you feel guilty about arranging help, remember the fact that Sarah has never had a serious illness in her life, and she was still smart enough to arrange enough help to ensure her good health and vitality would continue.

But I Can't Afford It!

Over and over again I've had other mothers comment on my housekeeper and say, "That would be really nice, but we can't afford it." People routinely go into debt so they can build a bigger house, or renovate, buy a car, or go on a vacation. Compared to these things, isn't giving your child a foundation of health and security that will last their whole life, a much worthier reason to go into debt? Don't let financial excuses stop you from providing health, compassion, nurturing and security for your children and yourself. Nothing in life is more important than this. By choosing to have a child, I believe it is my responsibility to give that child the best emotional, physical and spiritual foundation I can. This is hard for even normal parents to do. It will be doubly hard for you because your health is compromised right from the start and you have a susceptibility that normal, healthy people do not. If you don't have family who are willing to step in and help out, then you will have to pay for help – and you may even need to have some combination of family and hired help.

Because of the extra demands of my health, I simply do not have the stamina and tolerance for stress that normal people do. It's like once you've had a bad knee injury, that knee is never going to be able to do the things that a healthy, non-injured knee can. You will always have to make special allowances for your knee. It's the same with your gut. Even though you may be perfectly healthy and strong when you get pregnant, your gut/health will not have the same tolerance level as that of someone who's never had a problem with their digestive system. So you need to be prepared. You need to have a support structure in place so that you have daily assistance with cooking, cleaning and childcare – otherwise, the overwhelming physical and emotional stress will degrade your health and then everyone loses.

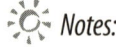 Notes:

What use is having money in the bank, or being able to say 'we're debt-free!' when you're in the hospital and can't breastfeed your own child? What use is money in the bank, when your vulnerable, young children or babies are in daycare 12 hours a day – having their core self formed by people who don't even love them? I read an article once where the author wrote something like, 'What does it say about us, when the richest country in the world cannot afford to raise its own children?'

Another option is to ask for financial help from family members – if they cannot, or don't want to, physically come over and help out. Don't let your guilt or pride stop you from asking for money to safeguard your health and raise healthy, secure children. Present your case to your parents or other family member – let them know that you have extra needs and you can't carry the workload of a normal, healthy person. You're not asking for money to enjoy a life of leisure, you're asking for money to keep you alive and help you take care of your most precious little ones. Don't worry (for those of you feeling guilty), even with all the help I've outlined above, you will still be exhausted every day. But hopefully, you won't be ill. And you'll be able to provide for your children's physical, emotional and soul-level needs, without winding up in the hospital.

Now, if you have the sense of self-worth and functionality necessary to move beyond survival (i.e. being exhausted every day, but not ill), then this is obviously ideal. However, since I'm only just beginning to approach that point myself, I don't feel qualified to write or give advice about it! But if you're already there, and you can set your life up to have actual 'ease' during these early childcare years (and why not!), then know that I'm admiring you and cheering you on with all my heart.

Hopefully, this chapter (along with the rest of this program) has given you enough tools and encouragement to have a healthy, drug-free pregnancy. I have already received many thanks from readers who were told, or believed, they'd never be healthy enough to bear children, but with the tools in this program, they have. As I mentioned earlier, please feel free to share your stories, struggles, triumphs at my website: *www.ListenToYourGut.com*.

> It's also better to plan for more help than you think you'll need – because, if you haven't had children before, it's unlikely you'll be able to anticipate the amount of help you're going to need.

Now go to the *Healing Journey Workbook* and complete the section for Chapter Nine, if applicable.

10

How To Use The Listen To Your Gut CD

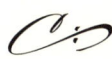

"Human beings living in modern industrialized societies are not so different from caged rabbits. Our environments have decreased the natural self-healing abilities that our wild brothers have retained.

The potential may still be there, however, and we need that special something extra to release it. We need the healing relationship – the loving touch, the positive expectancy, the sense of self-worth, even a bit of magic.

The healing relationship communicates high expectations for ourselves, our bodies, minds, and spirits, and motivates us to respect ourselves."

Dr. Jerry Solfvin, PhD

Now that you've finished reading the *Listen To Your Gut* manual, it's time to apply all this wonderful healing information to your own life. *The Listen To Your Gut CD* contains the various tools you'll need to implement this knowledge and produce healing in your own body. To get you started and excited about your Healing Journey, following is an outline of all the program tools that are available on the *Listen To Your Gut CD* – including how and when to use and implement each of the tools.

LISTEN TO YOUR GUT CD MENU

A. Healing Journey Workbook

B. Treatment Summaries
1. Jini's Optimum Treatment Plan
2. Jini's General Treatment Plan
3. Jini's Quick & Easy Treatment Plan

C. Health Assessment & Tracking Tools
1. Candida Symptom Test
2. Candida Saliva Test
3. Digestive System Test
4. Endocrine System Test
5. Nervous System Test
6. Symptom Tracking Chart No. 1
7. Symptom Tracking Chart No. 2
8. Food Diary
9. Food Reintroduction Chart
10. Maintenance Diet – Quick Reference Guide
11. Minimize Gas & Bloating Diet – Quick Reference Guide
12. Reduce Diarrhea Diet – Quick Reference Guide
13. Stop Intestinal Bleeding Diet – Quick Reference Guide

HEALING JOURNEY WORKBOOK

The *Healing Journey Workbook* takes you through the manual, one chapter at a time. It enables you to take the huge amount of information presented in the manual, and apply it directly to your situation. I suggest you print off the workbook and put it in a binder. Then, if you need extra room to answer certain questions, you can just insert an extra blank page where needed. You may also find it useful to get some colored sticky tabs to mark pages or sections that you need to come back to at a later date. Some sections (Chapter Four, for example) will take a long time to complete, so it's useful to have tabs to mark the questions you need to come back to. In six months, or one year's time, you may want to print out the workbook again and fill it in a second time, since your symptom profile, environment and treatment priorities will likely have shifted.

It's time to apply all this wonderful healing information to your own life.

TREATMENT SUMMARIES

The Treatment Summaries folder contains three separate action plans that give you a step-by-step treatment plan for what you need to do to heal yourself. Some plans are more thorough and comprehensive than others. You can choose which plan to follow depending on your current motivation, energy, and time available.

1. *Jini's Optimum Treatment Plan* – This is the best plan to ensure whole body healing. It guides you through creating your unique, customized, Optimum Treatment Plan based on your answers in the *Healing Journey Workbook*. This is the best treatment plan of the three offered, since it is the most thorough plan, and completely customized to your specific needs. *Jini's Optimum Treatment Plan* presents you with the highest chance of success in implementing the healing protocols in this program. However, you need to have completed the *Healing Journey Workbook* in order to fill out this plan.

2. *Jini's General Treatment Plan* – If you haven't had time, or don't want to, complete the *Healing Journey Workbook*, then this plan contains a

summary of generalized treatments for each illness (IBS, diverticulosis, colitis, Crohn's). Using a General Treatment Plan is not as good as compiling your own, individualized Optimum Treatment Plan, but it is the next best thing. Don't forget to read through the Quick & Easy plan as well, to get additional ideas.

3. ***Jini's Quick & Easy Treatment Plan*** – This plan is a list of quick-action points, for those of you who don't have the time or energy to follow either the Optimum Treatment, or General Treatment plans. Even if you just implement the first item on this list, you'll see an improvement in your health. Once you see an improvement, maybe you'll then have the energy or motivation to implement one of the more comprehensive treatment plans.

> *Jini's Optimum Treatment Plan is the best treatment plan of the three offered, since it is the most thorough plan, and completely customized to your specific needs.*

HEALTH ASSESSMENT & TRACKING TOOLS

The Health Assessment & Tracking Tools folder contains numerous different self-assessment tests that you can take to assess various aspects of your health. You'll be directed to take some of these tests at certain points throughout the *Healing Journey Workbook* to help you identify and compile your symptom lists. You may also find these tests useful to pinpoint other organs or systems in your body that need healing, but are beyond the scope of this book (e.g. nervous system, endocrine system, etc.). You can then address these health concerns with your naturopathic or holistic medical doctor. Again, you can perform these tests periodically (every three or six months) to help you track your progress and pinpoint areas that still need addressing.

This folder also contains two Symptom Tracking Charts that you can use to track your symptom progress and also evaluate which areas of your body still need healing. You'll be directed to use these Charts throughout the various Treatment Summaries.

Also in this folder are numerous tools to assist you in tracking and implementing the dietary guidelines from Chapter Three. They include a

Food Diary, Food Reintroduction Chart, and Quick Reference Guides for each of *The Healing Diets.* Use these tools as directed in Chapter Three of both the manual and the *Healing Journey Workbook.*

Here are the various self-assessment tests, symptom tracking charts, and diet charts included:

1. Candida Symptom Test
2. Candida Saliva Test
3. Digestive System Test
4. Endocrine System Test
5. Nervous System Test
6. Symptom Tracking Chart No. 1
7. Symptom Tracking Chart No. 2
8. Food Diary
9. Food Reintroduction Chart
10. Maintenance Diet – Quick Reference Guide
11. Minimize Gas & Bloating Diet – Quick Reference Guide
12. Reduce Diarrhea Diet – Quick Reference Guide
13. Stop Intestinal Bleeding Diet – Quick Reference Guide

So What Do I Do Now?

Start by filling out the *Healing Journey Workbook.* If you've already done that, then go straight to *Jini's Optimum Treatment Plan* (in the *Treatment Summaries* folder).

If you are not able to complete the *Healing Journey Workbook*, or you need an interim plan to use whilst you're working your way through the Workbook, then go to *Jini's General Treatment Plan* (in the *Treatment Summaries* folder).

If, for whatever reason, you're not able to implement any kind of comprehensive treatment plan, then go to *Jini's Quick & Easy Treatment*

Plan (in the *Treatment Summaries* folder), and just start with point #1 from the Quick-Action list.

Your Healing Journey Begins

My intent with this program has not been to overwhelm you, but rather to give you the tools and knowledge you need to take control of your life and health and begin the process of healing yourself. The timeline for that healing is going to depend upon the severity of your condition, length of time the dis-ease or imbalance has been present in your body, environmental and relational factors blocking you from health, and the commitment with which you choose to pursue your healing.

Also, as I've stated numerous times throughout this book, long-term healing involves healing all the aspects of your self – mental, emotional, spiritual and physical. This program should provide you with the template for your physical healing, and hopefully has also been a springboard to motivate you and make you aware of the other levels of yourself that also need healing.

As I mentioned at the beginning of this program, choose the area that's easiest for you to change/work on and start there. If all you do as a result of this book is point #1 from *Jini's Top Ten Quick-Action Points* – then great! You'll be better off than before and that's all that matters. Any change that we make for the better, is better than no change at all. So be kind and gentle with yourself, be patient. Give yourself the time and space that you need to implement change and heal yourself. Above all, love and accept yourself, seek out the joy in life and allow it to flow through you once again.

> Be kind and gentle with yourself, be patient. Give yourself the time and space that you need to implement change and heal yourself.

Footnotes

Chapter One

1. "Gut Feelings: The Surprising Link Between Mood and Digestion" by Chris Woolston, *Consumer Health Interactive*, 2001

2. "The Neurobiology of Stress and Emotions" by Emeran A. Mayer, M.D., *UCLA Mind Body Collaborative Research Center*, UCLA School of Medicine, California

3. *Spontaneous Healing: How to Discover and Embrace Your Body's Natural Ability to Maintain and Heal Itself* by Dr. Andrew Weil, Ballantine Publishing Group, 1995, pp. 235-236

4. *Mutant Message Down Under* by Marlo Morgan, HarperCollins Publishers, 1994, pg. 96

5. *Love Your Disease – It's Keeping You Healthy* by John Harrison, MD, Angus & Robertson, An imprint of HarperCollins Publishers, 1994, pg. 250

Chapter Two

1. *The Ultimate Nutrient Glutamine* by Judy Shabert MD, RD and Nancy Erhlich, ISBN 0-89529-588-1, pg. 21

2. *The Ultimate Nutrient Glutamine* by Judy Shabert MD, RD and Nancy Erhlich, ISBN 0-89529-588-1, pg. 37

3. "The Treatment of Poliomyelitis and Other Virus Diseases with Vitamin C" F. Klenner, *Journal of Southern Medicine and Surgery*, Vol. 111, 1949, pp. 209-214

4. "Effect of an enteric-coated fish-oil preparation on relapses in Crohn's disease" Belluzzi A, Brignola C, Campieri M, et al. *N Engl J Med*. 1996;334:1557–1560

5. *Optimal Wellness* by Ralph Golan, MD, Ballantine Books, pg. 157

6. "Uninvited Guests: The Impact of Small Intestinal Bacterial Overgrowth on Nutritional Status" by Oren Zaidel, M.D., Henry C. Lin, M.D., *Practical Gastroenterology*, July 2003

7. *Prescription for Nutritional Healing* by Phyllis Balch and James Balch, MD, Avery, 2000, pg. 71

8. "Medical Journalist Report of Innovative Biologics" by Morton Walker, DPM *Townsend Letter for Doctors & Patients*, #214, May 2001)

9. Excerpted from Chapter Three of *The Fungus Link* by Doug Kaufmann and Dave Holland, MD.
Available at: www.knowthecause.com

10. "Mechanisms of Action of Carvacrol on the Food-Borne Pathogen Bacillus cereus" by A. Ultee, E.P.W. Kets, E.J. Smid, *Applied and Environmental Microbiology*, Oct. 1999

11. "Promoting Gut Health with Probiotics" by Sara Horowitz, PhD, *Alternative & Complementary Therapies*, October 2003, pg.221

12. "Promoting Gut Health with Probiotics" by Sara Horowitz, PhD, *Alternative & Complementary Therapies*, October 2003, pg.223

13. "Promoting Gut Health with Probiotics" by Sara Horowitz, PhD, *Alternative & Complementary Therapies*, October 2003, pg.221

14. "Promoting Gut Health with Probiotics" by Sara Horowitz, PhD, *Alternative & Complementary Therapies*, October 2003, pg.223

15. *Probiotics: Nature's Internal Healers* by Natasha Trenev, Avery Publishing Group, 1998, pg. 164

16. "Crohn's: An Infectious Disease?" by Kelly Karper, PhD, RPh, *Drug Topics*, Nov. 3, 2003; 147:52

17. "Crohn's: An Infectious Disease?" by Kelly Karper, PhD, RPh, *Drug Topics*, Nov. 3, 2003; 147:52

18. "Invited Review: The Scientific Basis of Lactobacillus acidophilus NCFM Functionality as a Probiotic" by M.E. Sanders and T. R. Klaenhammer, *J. Dairy Science* 84:319-331, 2001

19. "Colonization of congenitally immunodeficient mice with probiotic bacteria" by R.T. Wagner, L. Robert, J. Farmer and E. Balish, *Infect. Immun.* 65:345-3351,1997

20. "Microbiologic Characteristics of Lactobacillus Products Used for Colonization of the Vagina" by V.L. Hughes and S. Miller, *Obstetrics and Gynecology* 75 (1990): 244

21. "Detection and activity of lactacin B, a bacteriocin produced by *Lactobacillus acidophilus*" by S.F. Barefoot and T. R. Kaaenhammer, *Appl. Environ. Microbiol.* 45:1808-1815, 1983

22. "Inflammatory Bowel Disease: Etiology and Pathogenesis" by Claudio Fiocchi, *Gastroenterology* 1998, Vol.115, pg. 185

23. "Lactobacillus and bifidobacterium in irritable bowel syndrome: Symptom responses and relationship to cytokine profiles" by Liam O'Mahony et al. *Gastroenterology* March 2005;128:541-551,783-785

24. *Fast Food Nation* by Eric Schlosser, Perennial 2002, pgs. 195, 196, 197

25. "Inflammatory Bowel Disease: Etiology and Pathogenesis" by Claudio Fiocchi, MD, *Gastroenterology* 1998, Vol.115, pg. 193

Chapter Three

1. "Acute fructose administration improves oral glucose tolerance in adults with type 2 diabetes" Moore MC, Mann SL, Davis SN, et al *Diabetes Care* 2001;24(11):1882-87

2. "Soy Formula Exposes Infants to High Hormone Levels" *The Lancet* July 5, 1997 350(9070) 23-27

3. "The USDA trypsin inhibitor study. I. Background, objectives and procedural details" Rackis, Joseph J. et al., *Qualification of Plant Foods in Human Nutrition*, vol. 35, 1985

4. "Homogenized Dairy, the Dependable Cardiotoxin" by Rodney Julian, *Well Being Journal*, Vol.12, Sept/Oct.2003

5. Dr. Bhupinder Sandhu *DDW Annual Meeting*: Abstracts 103976, 107178. May 19 & 21, 2002

6. Dr. Robert Canani *DDW Annual Meeting*: Abstracts 103976, 107178. May 19 & 21, 2002

7. "Diet in the Management of Crohn's Disease" by Workman EM, Jones AJ, Hunter JG., *Human Nutr.*1984:38A:469-473

Chapter Four

1. *Green Pharmacy: The History and Evolution of Western Herbal Medicine* by Barbara Griggs, Healing Arts Press, Rochester, 1991
2. *Alternative Medicine: The Definitive Guide* by The Burton Goldberg Group, Future Medicine Publishing Inc., 1994, pg. 169
3. *Alternative Medicine: The Definitive Guide* by The Burton Goldberg Group, Future Medicine Publishing Inc., 1994, pg. 168
4. "Inflammatory Bowel Disease: Etiology and Pathogenesis" by Claudio Fiocchi, *Gastroenterology* 1998, Vol.115, pg. 182
5. "Cigarette Smoking and IBD" by Guy L'Esperance MD, *IBD Round Table*, Quebec, 1994
6. "Physics and biology of mobile telephony" by Hyland G., *The Lancet* - Vol. 356, Issue 9244, 25 November 2000, pp. 1833-1836)
7. "Mobile phones and the illusory pursuit of safety" by Dendy PP *The Lancet* - Vol 356, Issue 9244, 25 November 2000, pp. 1782-1783 and "Physics and biology of mobile telephony" by Hyland G., *The Lancet* - Vol. 356, Issue 9244, 25 November 2000, pp. 1833-1836)
8. Professor Lawrie Challis, Chairman of the Mobile Telecommunications and Health Research Programme, UK
9. Dr. Stuart Porter, Department of Electronics at the University of York, UK
10. "Filtering Out Interference Signals with Cable Ferrites" By Jim May, *Compliance Engineering* magazine, Nov./Dec. 2002
11. Environmental Working Group, *EWG Report* May 2003
12. Environmental Working Group, *EWG Report* May 2003
13. Dr. Dan Harper, MD, The Hamilton Clinic, Montana, USA

14. "Comparative Study about the Influence on Man by Food Prepared Conventionally and in the Microwave-Oven" by Blanc, B. H., Hertel, H. U., 1992

15. *Journal of the Science of Food and Agriculture*, 83:1511-1516, online 2003

16. "The Truth About Immunization" by Dr. Robert Mendelsohn, MD, *The People's Doctor – A Medical Newsletter for Consumers*, Vol. 2, No. 4, Evanston, Illinois

17. *Vaccinations 100 Years of Orthodox Research* by Viera Scheibner, PhD, Co-Creative Designs, 1993

18. *Australian Journal of Medical Technology*, B. Allen, Vol.4, Nov.1973, pp. 26-27

19. *Universal Immunization: Medical Miracle or Masterful Mirage?* by Dr. Raymond Obomsawin
    Available at: *www.whale.to*

20. "Live Virus Vaccines and Genetic Mutation" by Buttram, H., *Health Consciousness*, April 1990, pp. 44-45

21. "Vitamin C in the Prophylaxis and Therapy of Infectious Diseases" McCormick, W.J., *Archives of Pediatrics*, Vol.68, No.1, January 1951

22. US House of Representatives, *Hearing on HR* 10541, pg. 113

23. *British Medical Journal*, Stewart, G.T., Jan.31,1976

24. "Viral Vaccines Vital or Vulnerable" Dettman, G and Kalokerinos, A., *Australasian Nurses Journal*, August 1980

25. *Universal Immunization: Medical Miracle or Masterful Mirage?* by Dr. Raymond Obomsawin, pg. 12
    Available at: *www.whale.to*

26. "The National Childhood Encephalopathy Study", Alderslade, R. et al, *Whooping Cough: Reports from the Committee on Safety of Medicines and the Joint Committee on Vaccination and Immunization*, Department of Health and Social Security, Her Majesty's Stationery Office, London 1981, pp. 79-154

27. Editor of Postgraduate Medicine, summarizing the following article: "Allergic Reactions Associated with Viral Vaccines" by Zimmerman B. and Stone A., *Progress in Medical Virology*, Vol.82, No.5, October 1987, pp. 225-232

28. "The Truth About Immunization" by Dr. Robert Mendelsohn, MD, *The People's Doctor – A Medical Newsletter for Consumers*, Vol. 2, No. 4, Evanston, Illinois

29. *Immunization: The Reality Behind the Myth* by Walene James, Greenwood Publishing Group, 1995

30. "Viral Vaccines Vital or Vulnerable" Dettman, G and Kalokerinos, A., *Australasian Nurses Journal*, August 1980, pg. 27

31. "Autistic Spectrum Disorders, Changes in the California Caseload: 1999-2002" *California Department of Developmental Services*, May 7, 2003

32. "Mortality and Morbidity from Invasive Bacterial Infections During a Clinical Trial of Acellular Pertussis Vaccines in Sweden" Storsaeter, J., et al, *Pediatrics Infectious Disease Journal*, Vol.78, 1988, pp. 637-645

33. *The Medical Time Bomb of Immunization Against Disease* by Dr. Robert Mendelsohn, MD, pg. 52.
Available at: *www.whale.to/vaccines/mendelsohn.html*

34. "Bringing Vaccines Into Perspective" Buttram, H.E. and Hoffman, J.C., *Mothering*, Vol.34, 1985, pg. 42

35. *Immunization: The Reality behind the Myth* by Walene James, Greenwood Publishing Group, 1995, pg. 15

36. "The Case Against Immunization" Markowitz, R., *Journal of the American Institute of Homeopathy*, Washington, DC, 1983

37. *Immunization: The Reality behind the Myth* by Walene James, Greenwood Publishing Group, 1995, pg. 15

38. *Universal Vaccination: Medical Miracle or Masterful Mirage?* by R. Obomsawin, pg. 56.
Available at: *www.whale.to/*

39. Barbara Fisher in a talk before the International Chiropractic Pediatricians Association, Boston, MA, March 19, 1993

Chapter Five

1. *Hands of Life: Use Your Body's Own Energy Medicine for Healing, Recovery, and Transformation* by Julie Motz, Bantam, 1998
2. *Green Pharmacy: The History and Evolution of Western Herbal Medicine* by Barbara Griggs, Healing Arts Press, Rochester, 1991
3. *How To Raise a Healthy Child…In Spite of Your Doctor* by Robert Mendelsohn, MD, Ballantine Books, 1984
4. *How To Raise a Healthy Child…In Spite of Your Doctor* by Robert Mendelsohn, MD, Ballantine Books, 1984
5. *Tales From the Medicine Trail: Tracking Down the Health Secrets of Shamans, Herbalists, Mystics, Yogis, and Other Healers* by Christopher Kilham, Rodale Press, 2000
6. "Recurrent Crohn's disease in transplanted bowel" Sustento-Reodica N, Ruiz P, Rogers A, Viciana AL, Conn HO, Tzakis AG, *The Lancet* – Vol. 349, Issue 9053, 1997, pp. 688-691
7. "Short bowel syndrome: a nutritional and medical approach" by K.N. Jeejeebhoy. Reprinted from, *CMAJ* 14 May 2002; 166(10), Page(s) 1297-1302 by permission of the publisher. © 2002 CMA Media Inc.
8. *When The Body Says No: The Hidden Cost of Stress* by Gabor Mate - MD, Vintage Canada, 2004
9. Data presented by Pfizer at *Digestive Disease Week* 2003

Chapter Six

1. *Family Therapy Networker*, Nov./Dec.1997
2. *Utne Reader*, March-April 1998, pg. 79

Chapter Seven

1. *Molecules of Emotion: The Science Behind Mind-Body Medicine* by Candace Pert, PhD, Scribner, 1999

2. *Healing and the Mind* by Bill Moyers, Main Street Books, 1995
3. *You Can Heal Your Life* by Louise L. Hay, Hay House, 1999 and *Heal Your Body A-Z* by Louise L. Hay, Hay House Lifestyles, 2001

Chapter Eight
No footnotes.

Chapter Nine
1. *How To Raise a Healthy Child...In Spite of Your Doctor* by Robert Mendelsohn, MD, Ballantine Books, 1984
2. "Bifidobacterial species differentially affect expression of cell surface markers and cytokines of dendritic cells harvested from cord blood" by Young SL. et al., Clinical and Diagnostic Laboratory Immunology. 2004;11(4):686-90.
3. "Fetal programming and adult health" by Godfrey K.M., Barker D.J., *Public Health Nutrition*, April 2001, vol. 4, no. Special Issue 2B, pp. 611-624(14)
   and
   Integrating the early nutritional influences into a life course approach" by Diana Kuh, *MRC National Survey of Health and Development*, Royal Free and University College Medical School, London UK
4. "Breathing in, I am nursing my baby: breastfeeding as a spiritual practice" by Leslie Davis, *Mothering* Sept/Oct. 2003

Chapter Ten
No footnotes.

Appendix A
Recommended Reading

Love Your Disease – It's Keeping You Healthy
By John Harrison, MD
(Angus & Robertson, an imprint of HarperCollins Publishers, 1994)

When The Body Says No: The Hidden Cost of Stress
By Gabor Maté, MD
(Vintage Canada, 2004)

Mutant Message Down Under
By Marlo Morgan
(HarperCollins Publishers, 1994)

Instant Healing
By Serge Kahili King, PhD
(Renaissance Books, 2000)

Nutrition and Physical Degeneration
By Weston A. Price, DDS
(Keats Pub, 2003)

How To Live Between Office Visits: A Guide to Life, Love and Health
By Bernie S. Siegel, MD
(HarperCollins, New York, 1993)

Energy Medicine
By Donna Eden
(Jeremy P. Tarcher/Putnam, New York, 1998)

How To Raise a Healthy Child…In Spite of Your Doctor
By Robert Mendelsohn, MD
(Ballantine Books, 1984)

Spontaneous Healing: How to Discover and Embrace Your Body's Natural Ability to Maintain and Heal Itself
By Andrew Weil, MD
(Ballantine Publishing Group, 1995)

RECOMMENDED READING | APPENDIX A

Vibrational Medicine: New Choices for Healing Ourselves
By Richard Gerber, MD
(Bear & Company, 1998)

Molecules of Emotion: The Science Behind Mind-Body Medicine
By Candace Pert, PhD
(Scribner, 1999)

Hands of Life: Use Your Body's Own Energy Medicine for Healing, Recovery, and Transformation
By Julie Motz
(Bantam, 1998)

Autobiography of a Yogi
By Paramahansa Yogananda
(Self-Realization Fellowship, 1993)

Wellness Workbook: How to Achieve Enduring Health and Vitality
By John W. Travis, MD and Regina Sara Ryan
(Celestial Arts; 3rd edition, 2004)

Passion To Heal
By Echo Bodine
(Nataraj Publishing, California, 1993)

Braving The Void: Journeys Into Healing
By Michael Greenwood, MD
(Paradox Publishers, Victoria)

Full Catastrophe Living: Using the Wisdom of Your Body and Mind to Face Stress, Pain, and Illness
By Jon Kabat-Zinn
(Delta, New York, 1990)

Transformation Through Birth
By Claudia Panuthos
(Bergin & Garvey Publishers, 1984)

The Experience of Childbirth
By Sheila Kitzinger
(Penguin Books, 1987)

Eating For IBS – 175 Delicious, Nutritious, Low-Fat, Low-Residue Recipes to Stabilize The Touchiest Tummy
By Heather Van Vorous
(Marlowe & Company, New York, 2000)

Nourishing Traditions: The Cookbook that Challenges Politically Correct Nutrition and the Diet Dictocrats
By Sally Fallon with Mary G. Enig, PhD
(New Trends Publishing, 1999)

Food and Healing
By Annemarie Colbin
(Ballantine Books, 1996)

A Consumer's Dictionary of Food Additives
By Ruth Winter, MS
(Three Rivers Press, New York, 1999)

Appendix B
Practitioner Resources

Contact these organizations for referrals to practitioners or suppliers in your area, or for more information. Many of them also offer free catalogues and newsletters.

Acupressure

Acupressure Institute
1533 Shattuck Avenue, Berkeley, California 94709
Tel: 510.845.1059
www.healthy.net/acupressure

Acupuncture

American Association of Oriental Medicine
PO Box 162340, Sacramento, CA 95816
Toll free: 866.455.7999
Fax: 916.443.4766
www.aaaomonline.org

Bio-Kinesiology

International College of Applied Kinesiology
6405 Metcalf Avenue, Suite 503, Shawnee Mission, KS 66202
Tel: 913.384.5336
www.icakusa.com

Biological Dentistry

The International Academy of Oral Medicine & Toxicology
www.iaomt.org

Environmental Dental Association
10160 Aviary Drive, San Diego, CA 92131
Toll free: 800.388.8124

Consumers for Dental Choice
www.toxicteeth.org

Certified Organic Meat & Produce

Contact these organizations for a list of suppliers, supermarkets and mail-order companies that carry organic meat and produce:

Organic Trade Association
PO Box 547, Greenfield, MA 01302
Tel: 1.413.774.7511
Fax: 1.413.774.6432
www.ota.com

The Organic Center for Education and Promotion
www.organic-center.org

A Campaign for Real Milk
www.realmilk.com

Craniosacral Therapy

Upledger Institute
11211 Prosperity Farms Road, Palm Beach Gardens, Florida 33410
Tel: 561.622.4334
Toll free: 1.800.233.5880
Fax: 561.622.4771
www.upledger.com

Holistic Medicine

American College for Advancement in Medicine
23121 Verdugo Drive, Suite 204, Laguna Hills, California 92653
Tel: 949.583.7666
www.acam.org

American Holistic Medical Association
6728 Old McLean Village Drive, McLean, VA 22101
Tel: 703.556.9728
www.ahmaholistic.com

Homeopathy

National Center for Homeopathy
801 North Fairfax Street, Suite 306, Alexandria, Virginia 22314
Tel: 703.548.7790
www.homeopathic.org

North American Society of Homeopaths
PO Box 450039, Sunrise, FL 33345.0039
Tel: 206.720.7000
Fax: 208.248.1942
www.homeopathy.org

Massage Therapy

Massage Online
www.massageonline.net

American Massage Therapy Association
www.amtamassage.org

International Massage Association
www.imagroup.com

Mind/Body Medicine

The Center for Mind/Body Medicine
5225 Connecticut Ave., NW, Suite 414, Washington, DC 20015
Tel: 202.966.7338
Fax: 202.966.2589
www.cmbm.org

Naturopathy

The American Association of Naturopathic Physicians
3201 New Mexico Avenue, NW Suite 350, Washington, DC 20016
Toll free: 1.866.538.2267
Tel: 202.895.1392
Fax: 202.274.1992
www.naturopathic.org

American Naturopathic Medical Association
www.anma.com

Canadian College of Naturopathic Medicine
1255 Sheppard Ave. E., Toronto, ON M2K 1E2 Canada
Toll free: 1.866.241.2266
www.ccnm.edu

Osteopathy

American Academy of Osteopathy
3500 De Pauw Boulevard, Suite 1080, Indianapolis, Indiana 46268
Tel: 317.879.1881
www.academyofosteopathy.org

Appendix C
Products & Suppliers

Following is the contact information for brands or products that have been recommended in this book. If your local health store doesn't carry the product you want, give them the contact information so they can order it in for you.

Remember, you can order almost every product on this list from my online health store, we're open 24 hours a day, 7 days a week, and we ship worldwide:

LTYG Holistic Health Shoppe

www.LTYGshoppe.com
Toll free: 1.888.866.7745
Tel: +1.360.977.5357

Even if you don't want to use the LTYG Holistic Health Shoppe, feel free to view the listings for products that have been chosen and approved by me – so as to not aggravate your sensitive system – then you'll know exactly which brands to get at your local health store.

Aloe Vera Juice

George's Always Active Aloe Vera Juice
Warren Laboratories
1656 IH 35 S, Abbot, TX 76621
Toll free: 1.800.232.2563
Tel: 254.580.9944
www.warrenlabsaloe.com

Bentonite Clay

Great Plains Bentonite
Yerba Prima Inc.
740 Jefferson Avenue, Ashland, OR 97520
Toll free: 1.800.488.4339
Tel: 541.488.2443
www.yerba.com

Cold Pressed Oils

Udo's Choice Ultimate Oil Blend
Flora Manufacturing & Distributing Ltd.
Burnaby, BC, V5J 5B9
Toll free: 1.800.446.2110
Tel: 360.354.2110
Fax: 360.354.5355
www.florahealth.com

Omegaflo – Omega Nutrition
1695 Franklin Street
Vancouver, BC V5L 1P5
Toll free: 1.800.661.3529
Tel: 604.253.4677
Fax: 604.253.4228
www.omeganutrition.com

Spectrum Organic Products, Inc.
5341 Old Redwood Hwy., Suite 400
Petaluma, CA 94954
www.spectrumorganics.com

Deglycyrrhizinated Licorice (Dgl)

Chewable DGL
Enzymatic Therapy
Green Bay, WI
Toll free: 1.800.783.2286
www.enzy.com

Elemental Diet Supplements

Absorb Plus
Imix Naturals Inc.
1124 Fir Avenue #176, Blaine, WA 98230
Toll free: 1.800.460.8606
Tel: 360.647.3238
www.absorbplus.com

Alpha ENF / PMX
Environmed Research Inc.
PO Box 2660, Sechelt, BC, V0N 3A0
Tel: 604.885.9007
www.nutramed.com

Fish Oil

Omega-3 Fish Oils
Nordic Naturals, Inc.
94 Hangar Way, Watsonville, CA 95076
Toll free: 1.800.662.2544
Tel: 831.724.6200
Fax: 831.724.6600
www.nordicnaturals.com

Carlson Cod Liver Oil
J.R. Carlson Laboratories Inc.
15 College Drive, Arlington Heights, IL 60004.1985
Toll free: 1.888.234.5656
Tel: 847.255.1600
www.carlsonlabs.com

Herbal Teas

Green Tea with Kombucha and Chinese Herbs
The Yogi Tea Company
2545 Prairie Road, Eugene, Oregon 97402
Tel: 1.800.964.4832
www.yogitea.com

Huckleberry Tea
Flora Manufacturing & Distributing Ltd.
Burnaby, BC, Canada, V5J 5B9
Toll free: 1.800.446.2110
Tel: 360.354.2110
Fax: 360.354.5355
www.florahealth.com

Immune System

Astragalus
Herb Pharm
P.O. Box 116, Williams, OR 97544
Toll free: 1.800.348.4372
www.herb-pharm.com

Echinacea
Eclectic Institute
36350 SE Industrial Way, Sandy OR 97055
Toll free: 1.800.332.4372
www.eclecticherb.com

Grifron Maitake
Maitake Products
New Jersey, NY
www.maitake.com

Intestinal Healing

MucosaHeal
Imix Naturals Inc.
1124 Fir Avenue #176, Blaine, WA 98230
Toll free: 1.800.460.8606
Tel: 360.647.3238
www.mucosaheal.com

Robert's Formula
Gaia Herbs
108 Island Ford Rd., Brevard, NC 28712
Toll free: 1.800.831.7780
Tel: 828.884.4242
www.gaiaherbs.com

N-Acetyl Glucosamine (NAG)
Jarrow Formulas
1824 S. Robertson Blvd, Los Angeles, CA 90035
Toll free: 1.800.726.0886
Tel: 310.204.6936
Fax: 310.204.2520
www.jarrow.com

Iron Supplements

Ferrasorb
Thorne Research Inc.
www.thorne.com
*They only sell to doctors.

AUXIMA Fera
Sandoz Nutrition S.A.
Gran Via de les Corts Catalanes, 764, 08013 Barcelona, Spain
Distributed by: Inno-Vite Inc.
www.inno-vite.com

Floradix Formula
Salus-Haus, Bruckmuhl, Bavaria, Germany
Distributed by: Flora Manufacturing & Distributing Ltd.
Burnaby, BC, Canada, V5J 5B9
Toll free: 1.800.446.2110
Fax: 360.354.5355
Tel: 360.354.2110
www.florahealth.com

Probiotics

Megadophilus, Bifido Factor, Digesta Lac, Life Start Powders Healthy Trinity Capsules
Natren Inc.
3105 Willow Lane, Westlake Village, CA 91361
Toll free: 1.800.992.3323
Tel: 805.371.4737
www.natren.com

Progesterone Cream (Natural)

Pro-Gest Emerita
621 SW Alder Street, Suite 900, Portland, OR 97205
Toll free: 1.800.648.8211
Tel: 503.226.1010
www.emerita.com

Suppositories

FissureHeal
Imix Naturals Inc.
1124 Fir Avenue #176, Blaine, WA 98230
Toll free: 1.800.460.8606
Tel: 360.647.3238
www.fissureheal.com

Vitamins & Minerals

Prenatal Multivitamin
Nature's Way
10 Mountain Springs Parkway, Springville, UT 84663
Tel: 801.489.1500
Fax: 801.489.1700
www.naturesway.com

Multivitamin Iron-Free
Nature's Way
10 Mountain Springs Parkway, Springville, UT 84663
Tel: 801.489.1500
Fax: 801.489.1700
www.naturesway.com

Multi-Mineral Complex
Nature's Way
10 Mountain Springs Parkway, Springville, UT 84663
Tel: 801.489.1500
Fax: 801.489.1700
www.naturesway.com

Adult's Chewable Multi-Vitamin/Mineral

Natural Pineapple Flavor
Nature's Plus
Division of Natural Organics Inc.
548 Broadhollow Road, Melville, NY, 11747
www.naturesplus.com

TriVita Vital Four

Sublingual B12 complex
Health Basics
Toll free: 1.866.553.5507
Tel: 604.951.2583
Email: healthbasics@telus.net

*This is a MLM product, so only available from this phone number (I'm not a member, I don't receive commissions). I've included it since it's the best B12 I've ever tried. It's a fantastic blend that includes B12, Folate, Vit.B6, Biotin, Inositol, Taurine, Dimethylglycine, Lysine, CoQ10, Cysteine, Methionine, and Choline.

Weight Gain Supplements

Absorb Plus

Imix Naturals Inc.
1124 Fir Avenue #176, Blaine, WA 98230
Toll free: 1.800.460.8606
Tel: 360.647.3238
www.absorbplus.com

Wild Oregano Oil

Oil of Oregano

Joy of the Mountains
Box 1058, Lumby, BC, V0E 2G0
Tel: 1.866.547.0268
www.joyofthemountains.com

Oreganol

North American Herb & Spice
PO Box 4885, Buffalo Grove, IL 60089

Appendix D

Research & References

Chapter Two

Here are the details for the study referenced in the excerpt from *The Fungus Link* by Doug Kaufman and Dave Holland, MD:

Hesman, T. "WU Researchers have developed controversial Crohn's treatment". *St. Louis Post-Dispatch*. Nov 8, 2002. You can read the whole article at: http://aisweb.wustl.edu/alumni/atwu.nsf/crohns

Chapter Five

If you've had intestinal surgery, or have Short Bowel Syndrome, then please see this article for information on nutrients that your gastrointestinal tract may not be able to absorb properly:

"Short bowel syndrome: a nutritional and medical approach" by K. N. Jeejeebhoy, *Canadian Medical Association Journal*, Vol. 166 No. 10, 2002

Following are a list of references substantiating my statement that colonoscopes (and other endoscopes) are often not properly sterilized:

1. "Unsterile Devices Prompt Warnings; Use of dirty endoscopes in colon and throat exams can pass along infections, activists say" by John M. Glionna. *The Los Angeles Times*, Los Angeles, Calif.: Feb 13, 2003. pg. B.1
   Excerpts from the article:
   "The nation's leading manufacturer of endoscopes has known for a decade that some scopes contain cavities inaccessible to cleaning by hand but has failed to fix the oversight, said David Lewis, a University of Georgia research microbiologist who has conducted research for the federal Environmental Protection Agency on the issue of dirty endoscopes. There is wide consensus that it is difficult to sterilize the devices, which can cost $28,000 each, without using temperatures so high that the scopes themselves become damaged. The scopes have numerous cavities that are difficult to clean, even by hand, critics say. Even the government can't agree on how long is needed to clean the devices. The FDA says endoscopes should be disinfected for 45 minutes to kill tuberculosis bacteria, but the Centers for Disease Control believes the job can be done in 20 minutes, Lewis says. He and other microbiologists advocate sterile disposable parts for endoscopes as well as the use of a condom-like sheath for each new patient. But they say manufacturers and health-care providers have resisted such solutions because of added costs." You can read the entire newspaper article at: http://www.sheller.com/NewsDetails.asp?NewsID=22

2. This next article highlights the ongoing debate over how exactly to effectively sterilize endoscopes (include bronchoscopes, sigmoidoscopes, colonoscopes, gastroscopes, etc.). The sterilant most widely used for scopes which are damaged by high heat (and most are) is Gluteraldehyde. See the next article to see why Gluteraldehyde is NOT a good sterilant for the patient receiving a colonoscopy.
"Endoscope decontamination: Where do we go from here?" by Babb J.R., Bradley C.R., *J Hosp Infect* 1995;Vol 30, Iss Suppl.:543-551

3. In this article we find that Gluteraldehyde on colonoscopes (the residue left after sterilization), can result in toxic colitis – symptoms within 48 hours of the colonoscopy included cramps and abdominal pain, tenesmus (painful, urgent straining to defecate), rectal bleeding and in some cases, hemorrhaging. Also, if you've been diagnosed with ischemic colitis, you may in fact have Gluteraldehyde-induced toxic colitis!
"Glutaraldehyde colitis: radiologic findings" by Birnbaum B.A., Gordon R.B., Jacobs J.E., *Radiology* 1995;195:131-134

4. Also important to note, is that Gluteraldehyde (the most commonly used disinfectant for endoscopes) is not very effective against mycobacterium (remember that *Mycobacterium Avium* Paratuberculosis has been detected in 92-100% of Crohn's patients – incidence varies between studies). The normal amount of time a hospital immerses a colonoscope in Gluteraldehyde is 10-20 minutes. This article shows that even after 45 minutes, mycobacterium still remained in four out of five scopes:
"Mycobacteria and glutaraldehyde: Is high-level disinfection of endoscopes possible?" by Urayama S., Kozarek R.A., Sumida S., et al, *Gastrointest Endoscop* 1996;Vol 43, Iss 5:451-45

5. Here we have another article assessing endoscope sterilization procedures – in this case gas sterilization, and the conclusion is again: unable to properly/reliably sterilize: "The inability of all sterilizers, including the 12/88, to kill organisms in narrow lumens reliably when serum and salt were present raises concern about the current practice of gas sterilization of flexible endoscopes."
"Comparison of ion plasma, vaporized hydrogen peroxide, and 100% ethylene oxide sterilizers to the 12/88 ethylene oxide gas sterilizer" by Alfa M.J., Degagne P., et al, *Infect Control Hosp Epidemiol* 1996; Vol 17, Iss 2:92-100

6. This article points out that even if a hospital does have an effective sterilization or disinfection method in place – the endoscope will NOT be sterile if it has not been thoroughly cleaned BEFORE sterilization/disinfection takes place. And this is where the frequent occurrence of human error, lack of time, lack of staff, etc. comes into play:
"High-level disinfection or "sterilization" of endoscopes?" by Muscarella L.F., *Infect Control Hosp Epidemiol* 1996;Vol 17, Iss 3:183-187

7. This article highlights the fact (in a TWO YEAR study) that whether manual or automated sterilization procedures were used, colonoscopes were more often contaminated than gastroscopes or bronchoscopes:
"Evaluation of bacteriological contamination of gastrointestinal and pulmonary endoscopes after cleaning and disinfection procedures" by Duc D.L., Sing J.S.C., Mallaret M.R., et al, *Med Mal Infec* 1996;Vol 26, Iss 2:99-104

8. This study shows that following standard colonoscope sterilization procedures, 62.3% of the outside surfaces were still contaminated and 40.3% of the channels were still contaminated with infectious bacteria. Instituting further sterilization procedures reduced the bacterial contamination but did not eliminate it – i.e. the colonoscopes still were not sterile:
"Quality improvement in gastrointestinal endoscopy: Microbiologic surveillance of disinfection" by Merighi A., Contato E., et al, *Gastrointest Endoscop* 1996; Vol 43, Iss 5:457-462

Chapter Six
Hypnosis Research Summaries

The following are a selection of study summaries, excerpted from *www.ibshypnosis.com*, compiled by Dr. Olafur S. Palsson, Psy.D. Dr. Palsson is a licensed clinical psychologist. He is Associate Professor of Medicine in the Division of Gastroenterology and Hepatology in the School of Medicine at the University of North Carolina at Chapel Hill.

Controlled trial of hypnotherapy in the treatment of severe refractory irritable-bowel syndrome

This study was placebo-controlled and results showed a dramatic difference in symptoms between the hypnosis group and the placebo group. Thirty patients with severe symptoms unresponsive to any other treatment were randomly chosen to receive (a) seven sessions of hypnotherapy (15 patients) or (b) seven sessions of psychotherapy with placebo pills (15 patients).

The psychotherapy group showed a small but significant improvement in abdominal pain and distension, and in general well-being, but no improvement in bowel activity pattern. The hypnotherapy patients showed a *dramatic* improvement of *all* central symptoms. Equally significant, the hypnotherapy group showed no relapses during the 3-month follow-up period.
(Whorwell PJ, Prior A, Faragher EB. "Controlled trial of hypnotherapy in the treatment of severe refractory irritable-bowel syndrome"
The Lancet, 1984, 2: 1232-4.)

Hypnotherapy in severe irritable bowel syndrome: further experience.
In this report, 35 patients were added to the 15 treated with hypnotherapy in the 1984 Lancet study (above). For the whole 50 patient group, the success rate was 95% for classic IBS cases, but substantially less for IBS patients with an atypical symptom picture, or significant psychological problems. The report also observed that patients over age 50 seemed to have a lower rate of success from this treatment.
(Whorwell PJ, Prior A, Colgan SM. "Hypnotherapy in severe irritable bowel syndrome: further experience" *Gut*, 1987 Apr, 28:4, 423-5.)

Individual and group hypnotherapy in treatment of refractory irritable bowel syndrome.
This study used only four sessions of hypnosis per subject and the success rate was lower than in other studies. This shows that a larger number of hypnotherapy sessions is required to achieve positive, lasting results. Twenty out of the 33 patients with refractory irritable bowel syndrome treated with four sessions of hypnotherapy in this study improved. Improvement was maintained at a 3-month treatment. Interestingly, these researchers found that hypnosis treatment for IBS in groups of up to 8 patients seems as effective as individual therapy.
(Harvey RF, Hinton RA, Gunary RM, Barry RE. "Individual and group hypnotherapy in treatment of refractory irritable bowel syndrome." *The Lancet*, 1989 Feb, 1:8635, 424-5.)

Symptomatology, quality of life and economic features of irritable bowel syndrome – the effect of hypnotherapy.
This study compared 25 IBS patients (with severe symptoms) treated with hypnosis, to 25 patients with similar symptom severity, treated with other methods.

The study demonstrated that in addition to significant improvement in all central IBS symptoms, hypnotherapy recipients had fewer visits to doctors, lost less time from work than the control group and rated their quality of life more improved. Those patients who had been unable to work prior to treatment resumed employment in the hypnotherapy group but not in the control group. The study quantifies the substantial economic benefits and improvement in health-related quality of life which result from hypnotherapy for IBS, on top of clinical symptom improvement.

(Houghton LA, Heyman DJ, Whorwell PJ. "Symptomatology, quality of life and economic features of irritable bowel syndrome – the effect of hypnotherapy" *Aliment Pharmacol Ther,* 1996 Feb, 10:1, 91-5.)

Gut focused hypnotherapy normalises rectal hypersensitivity in patients with irritable bowel syndrome (IBS).
Twenty-three patients each received 12 sessions of hypnotherapy.
Significant improvement was seen in the severity and frequency of abdominal pain, bloating and satisfaction with bowel habit. A subset of the treated patients who were found to be unusually pain-sensitive in their intestines prior to treatment (as evidenced by balloon inflation tests) showed normalization of pain sensitivity, and this change correlated with their pain improvement following treatment. Such pain threshold change was not seen for the treated group as a whole.

(Houghton LA, Larder S, Lee R, Gonsalcorale WM, Whelan V, Randles J, Cooper P, Cruikshanks P, Miller V, Whorwell PJ. "Gut focused hypnotherapy normalises rectal hypersensitivity in patients with irritable bowel syndrome (IBS)" *Gastroenterology* 1999; 116: A1009.)

Chapter Eight

Here are some relevant articles regarding the dangers of bacterial soil organisms:

Kniehl E, Becker A, Forster DH. "Pseudo-outbreak of toxigenic Bacillus cereus isolated from stools of three patients with diarrhoea after oral administration of a probiotic medication" *Journal of Hospital infection,* 2003;55(1):33-8.

Matsumoto S, Suenaga H, Naito K, Sawazaki M, Hiramatsu T, Agata N. "Management of suspected nosocomial infection: an audit of 19 hospitalized patients with septicemia caused by Bacillus species" *Jpn J Infect Dis.* 2000 Oct;53(5):196-202.

Mikkola R, Kolari M, Andersson MA, Helin J, Salkinoja-Salonen MS. "Toxic lactonic lipopeptide from food poisoning isolates of Bacillus licheniformis" *Eur J Biochem.* 2000 Jul;267(13):4068-74.

Oggioni MR, Pozzi G, Valensin PE, Galieni P, Bigazzi C. "Recurrent Septicemia in an Immunocompromised Patient Due to Probiotic Strains of Bacillus subtilis" *J. Clin. Microbiol.* 1998 36: 325-326.

Pease P. "Identification of bacteria from blood and joint fluids of human subjects as Bacillus licheniformis" *Ann Rheum Dis.* 1974 33: 67-69.

Richard V, Van der Auwera P, Snoeck R, Daneau D, Meunier F. "Nosocomial bacteremia caused by Bacillus species" *Eur J Clin Microbiol Infect Dis.* 1988 Dec;7(6):783-5.

Rowan NJ, Deans K, Anderson JG, Gemmell CG, Hunter IS, and Chaithong T. "Putative Virulence Factor Expression by Clinical and Food Isolates of Bacillus spp. after Growth in Reconstituted Infant Milk Formulae" *Appl. Envir. Microbiol.* 2001 67: 3873-3881.

Rowan NJ, Caldow G, Gemmell CG, Hunter IS. "Production of Diarrheal Enterotoxins and Other Potential Virulence Factors by Veterinary Isolates of Bacillus Species Associated with Nongastrointestinal Infection." *Appl. Envir. Microbiol.* 2003 69: 2372-2376.

Sagripanti JL, Bonifacino A. "Bacterial Spores Survive Treatment with Commercial Sterilants and Disinfectants" *Appl Environ Microbiol.* 1999;65(9):4255

Spinosa MR, Wallet F. et al. "The Trouble in Tracing Opportunistic Pathogens: Cholangitis due to Bacillus in a French Hospital Caused by a Strain Related to an Italian Probiotic?" *Microbial Ecology in Health and Disease.* 2000;12(2):99-101.

Tuazon CU, Murray HW, Levy C, Solny MN, Curtin JA, Sheagren JN. "Serious infections from Bacillus sp." *JAMA.* 1979 Mar 16;241(11):1137-40.

Wainwright M. "Extreme pleomorphism and the bacterial life cycle: a forgotten controversy" *Perspectives in Biology and Medicine.* 1997;40:407-14.

Young RF, Yoshimori RN, Murray DL, Chou PJ. "Postoperative neurosurgical infections due to bacillus species" *Surg Neurol.* 1982 Oct;18(4):271-3.

Agerholm JS, Jensen NE, Giese SB, Jensen HE. "A preliminary study on the pathogenicity of Bacillus licheniformis bacteria in immunodepressed mice" *APMIS.* 1997 Jan;105(1):48-54.

Banerjee C, Bustamante CI, Wharton R, Talley E, Wade JC. "Bacillus infections in patients with cancer" *Arch Intern Med* 1988 Aug;148(8):1769-74

Bisset KA, Bartlett R. "The isolation and characters of L-forms and reversions of Bacillus licheniformis var. Endoparasiticus (Benedek) associated with the erythrocytes of clinically normal persons" *J. Med. Microbiol.* 1978 11: 335-349.

Blue SR, Singh VR, Saubolle MA. "Bacillus licheniformis bacteremia: five cases associated with indwelling central venous catheters." *Clin Infect Dis.* 1995 Mar;20(3):629-33.

European Commission, Health & Consumer Protection Directorate-General. "Opinion on the use of certain micro-organisms as additives in feedingstuffs" Expressed 26 September 1997, updated 25 April 2003.

Hoa NT, Baccigalupi L, et al, "Characterization of Bacillus Species Used for Oral Bacteriotherapy and Bacterioprophylaxis of Gastrointestinal Disorders" *Appl Environ Microbiol.* 2000;66(12):5241-5247

Hoa TT, Duc LH, Isticato R, Baccigalupi L, Ricca E, Van PH, Cutting SM. "Fate and dissemination of Bacillus subtilis spores in a murine model" *Appl Environ Microbiol* 2001 Sep;67(9):3819-23

Logan NA. Bacillus species of medical and veterinary importance. *J Med Microbiol.* 1988 Mar;25(3):157-65.

Index

A

Absorption
    intestinal 121, 123, 186
    skin 254, 268, 274
Acid reflux 87, 338, 340
    treatment summary 90
Acidic foods 212, 222
Acidolin 156
Acidophilin 156
Acidophilus 87, 161, 162
Acne 399
Acupressure 188, 331, 341
Acupuncture 188, 331, 341
Adrenal gland 188, 295, 302, 309
Affirmations 362
AIDS 30
Ajna chakra 349
Albumin 237
Alcohol 212
Alkalizing agents 189, 203
Allergies/intolerance
    environmental 260
    food 217, 241, 381
    testing 242, 383
Allopathic medicine 291
Almond milk 207
Aloe vera
    freeze-dried 391
    gel 103
    juice 60, 103, 385
    suppository 132
Aloin 53, 103
Amaranth 203, 204
Amino acids 70, 206, 238
Ammonium perfluorooctanoate
    (C-8) 266, 270
Anal
    fissures 132
    sore 225
    sphincter 315, 345, 369
Anemia 58
    exercising 359
    treatment summary 64
Antibiotic 27, 99, 140, 175, 387
Antibodies 277, 282, 383
Antifungal 140, 145, 152
Anti-inflammatory 144, 322
Antimicrobial 99, 140, 145
Antioxidants 187, 276
Antiviral 140, 145, 152
Anti-yeast 140, 145, 152
Apo-prednisone 305
Applied kinesiology 332
Artificial
    colors/flavors 211
    sweeteners 213
Asacol 302, 305
Ascorbic acid 54, 66
Ashwaganda 392
Aspartame 213, 255

Astragalus 94, 97, 406
Attachment parenting 423
Auto-immune 277, 283
Autonomic nervous system 347
Ayurvedic medicine 378, 392
Azathioprine 304
AZT 30
Azulfidine 306

B

Bacillus cereus 145, 386
Bacteria (see also "Probiotics")
    lose tolerance in inflammation 170
    small intestine bacterial
        overgrowth (SIBO) 134
    supplementation 155
Bacterial soil organisms 54, 386
Bakeware 272
Barium enema 318
Basal body temperature 400
Bedding 266
Bentonite clay 74, 384
Beta-glucan 95
Betaine HCL 54, 87, 244
BHA/BHT 255
Bifidobacterium bifidum (B. bifidum)
    see "Probiotics"
Bifidobacterium infantis (B. infantis)
    170 (see also "Probiotics")
Bioflavonoids 92

Bio-kinesiology 332
Biological terrain analysis (BTA) 189
Birth control 399
Birthing 339, 376
Bisphenol A 273
Bleeding
    danger signals 100
    hemorrhoids 91, 100
    large intestine 99, 108, 114
    pregnancy 418
    small intestine 99, 113
    stop bleeding 99, 108, 113, 114, 230, 235
Bloating 84, 220, 354
    treatment summary 86
Blood
    cleansing 62
    transfusion 63
    type diet 380
Blueberries 54
Bodybuilding 125
Bowel rest 122, 235
Brain-gut axis 17, 347
Breast cancer 206
Breastfeeding 397, 411
    adopted baby 413
    difficulties 413
    supplements 407
Budesonide 306
Butyrate 156

C

Cabbage family vegetables 204, 214
Caesarean birth 339
Caffeine 90, 212
Calcium 186
Calendula 111
Calories 124
Canasa 305
Candida albicans 146, 147, 156, 203, 384
    treatment 148, 203, 221
Capsule endoscopy 322
Carbohydrates 203
    complex vs. simple 215
Carbonated drinks 213
Carcinogenic 190, 203, 255, 273, 318
Carrageenan 211, 219
Carvacrol 145, 150
Casein 124
Catechins 391
Cause of IBD & IBS 24, 27, 257, 312
CD-ROM 430
Cell phone 262
    ferrite bead 264
Certified organic food 196
    healthier rats 198
Cervical cancer 206
Chakras 349, 357
Cherries 54
Chi 357
Children with IBD/IBS 37
    diet changes 216
    dosage instructions 56
    steroids 295
Chinese medicine 379
Chlorine 269
Chlorophyll 62
Chocolate 90
Cholesterol 156
Cigarette smoking 260
Ciprofloxacin (Cipro) 304

Citrus foods/juices 54, 212
Coccyx 339
Coenzyme Q10 95, 104
Coffee 90, 212
Cold-pressed oils 219
Colic 68, 339, 414
Colitis
    infectious disease 159
    probiotic trials 157, 158
    treatment summary – see CD-ROM
Colon cancer 190, 203, 318
Colon cleansing (colonics) 385
Colonic massage 352
Colonoscope 323
Colonoscopy 313, 318
    dangers 318, 323
    questions to ask 322
    treatment following 178, 318, 355
Colostomy 312
    pouchitis 71
    surgery (j-pouch) 312
Comfrey 108
    controversy 111
    salve 109, 133
Compassion 423
Conception 402
Condom 399
Constipation 65, 353
    treatment summary 67
Cookware 272
Corticosteroids 187
Cortisol 309
Cous-cous 203, 204
Cramping 67, 356, 373
    treatment summary 68

Craniosacral therapy
  babies/children 339
  esophageal valve 88
  physical 335
  somato-emotional 336
  strictures 136
Crohn's
  infectious disease 159
  probiotic trials 157, 158
  treatment summary – see CD-ROM
Cruciferous vegetables 204, 205, 214

D

Dairy
  intolerance 124, 211
  mycobacterium avium paratuberculosis (MAP) 159
  products 211, 220
Debt 426
Deglycyrrhizinated licorice extract (DGL) 112
  lozenges 88, 130
Deltasone 305
Detoxification 75, 239, 383
DHEA 310
Dialoguing with your body 350
Diapers 401
Diarrhea 69, 356, 384
  diet treatment 225
  herbal treatment 69, 407
  treatment summary 76
Die-off effect 149, 171
Diet
  blood type 380
  elemental 122, 235
  Gottschall 381
  healing 209
  IBD remission 236, 238, 418
  raw food 205
  specific carbohydrate (SC) 381
  vegetarian 204
Digestive enzymes 85, 204
  inhibitors 206
Dioxin 401
Disposable enema 108
Diva cup 401
Diverticulae 353
Diverticulitis
  treatment summary – see CD-ROM
Domestic help 424
Doshas 378
Dreams 317
Drugs
  attitude towards 293
  pregnancy 402, 418
  side-effects 187, 301, 304
  symptom suppression 295
  weaning/tapering 217, 306
Dry curd 70

E

Echinacea 94
Elaine Gottschall 216, 381, 383
Electrolytes 100
Elemental diet 122, 235
  induce remission 236, 238
  pregnancy 418
Emotional
  healing 17, 19, 336, 341, 360
  stress/trauma 27, 289, 336, 420
Emotional Freedom Technique (EFT) 341, 362, 413
Endocrine system 309, 399
Enema kits 108
Energy healing 292, 313, 336
Entocort 306
Environmental toxins 27, 256, 258, 259, 265, 270
Epsom salts 79
Erythema nodosum 117, 297
Esophageal valve 89
Essential fatty acids 104, 411
Estrogen 206, 273, 309
Etiology of IBD & IBS 24, 27, 257, 312
Euphrasia eye drops 118
Evening primrose oil 105
Exercise 357
  to gain weight 125
  to lose weight 128
Eye inflammation 118

F

Family dynamic 37
Fast food 422
Fear 324, 374
Fecal occult blood test 322
Ferrite bead 265
Ferrum phosphoricum 63
Filtered water 203
Finances 300, 343, 421, 426
Fish
  farmed vs. wild 207
  medium-oily 224
  non-oily 234
  oil 105
  protein 392

Fissures 132
Fistulas 77
    client story 388
    syringing wild oregano oil 78
    treatment 77
    treatment summary 83
Flagyl 305, 388
Flare/flare-up 34, 36, 210, 243, 298, 320, 388
    pregnancy 418
Flatulence 84, 86, 220, 354
Flax seed oil 105, 123
Flu 406
Fluoride 268
Folic acid 186
Food
    allergies/intolerance 217, 241
    combining 215
    diary 245
    poisoning 145, 184
    reintroduction chart 251
    sensitivity testing 241
    toxins 261
Foot and mouth disease 146
Formula feeding 390, 416
    supplementation 416
Free radicals 59, 186
Fructooligosaccharides (FOS) 54
Fructose 201
Fungus 143, 144, 146, 387

G

Garlic 140, 141
Gas 84, 220, 354
    treatment summary 86
Gastro-esophageal reflux disease
    (GERD) 87, 338, 340
    treatment summary 90
Gastroscopy 318, 323
Glucosaminoglycans 107
Glycemic response/load 202
Glycogen 202
Goat milk 207, 220
Gottschall diet 381
Grains 203
Grape seed extract 104, 191
Grapefruit seed extract 141
Green tea 391

H

Hair loss/thinning 408
Hay fever 118
Healing
    crisis 34, 36, 308
    journey 23, 32, 44
    layers/spirals 34, 36
Healing implant enema 108
Healing journey workbook 40, 431
Health assessment tools 42, 432
Heartburn 87, 338, 340
    treatment summary 90
Helicobacter pylori 156
Hemoglobin 101, 275, 359, 387
Hemorrhaging 101, 108, 114, 237
    danger signals 100
    pregnancy 418
    stop 108, 114, 230, 235
Hemorrhoids 91, 353
    treatment summary 94
Hemp
    protein 124, 204, 207
    seed oil 105, 224

Herbal medicine 49, 296
Herbal tinctures 97-98
Herbal supplements 49, 296
    aggravating/avoid 52, 54
    children's dosages 56
    good companies 50
    how to introduce 55
    introduction order 191
    pregnancy/breastfeeding 404
    testing 55, 393
Herpes 128, 146
Herxheimer reaction 149
Hesperidin 92
High blood pressure 200
High fibre foods 205, 214
High fructose corn syrup 202
Higher self 32, 33
Hirtum 150
HIV 30
Holistic health shoppe 50, 193
Home help 424
Homeopathic
    iron 63
    remedies 393
Homeostatic mechanism 36, 377
Honey 201
Hormones
    animals 197
    balance 309, 399
    food 206, 273
    plastics 273
Horse chestnut 92
Huckleberry tea
Hydrogenated oils 213, 219
Hypnotherapy 346
Hypothyroid 311

INDEX

I

IBD
    pathogenosis (cause) 24, 27, 257, 312
    remisssion diet 236, 238, 418
IBS (see "Irritable bowel syndrome")
Ileocecal valve 335
    bacterial infection 183
    craniosacral treatment 335
Immune system
    boosting, strengthening 94, 98, 335
    stimulation results in remission 143
    suppression 20, 157, 319
Immunosciences laboratory 144
Immunosuppresive drugs 236, 283, 309, 312
    pregnancy 402, 418
    side effects 304
Imodium 220
Implant enema 108
Imuran 304, 309
Infant formula 390
    supplement protocol 416
Infection 77, 144, 147
Inflammation 99, 147
    eye 118
    joint 117, 120
    lose tolerance to bacteria 170
Infliximab 304
Insulin 202
Intestinal
    bleeding 99, 113, 114, 230, 235
    infection 77, 144, 147
    mucosa 48, 137, 157, 383
    obstruction 134
    rupture/perforation 101, 134, 313
    transplant 312
Intrauterine Device (IUD) 399
Intravenous
    iron 63
    needle insertion 64
Intuition 350, 382
Inulin 54
Iron
    absorption 61
    infusion 63
Iron-rich foods 61
Irritable bowel syndrome (IBS)
    acidophilus trial 158
    B. infantis trial 170
    hypnosis 347
    infectious etiology 159
    stress 347, 349
    treatment summary – see CD-ROM

J

Jini's EFA salad dressing 106
Jini's formula supplement protocol 417
Jini's healing implant enema 108
Jini's probiotic retention enema 138
Jini's wild oregano oil protocol 152
Joint pain & swelling 117, 297
    treatment summary 120
J-pouch 312
Juice
    fast 384
    fruit 223
    vegetable 205

K

Kamut 203, 204
Kegel excercises 369
Kinesiology 332
Kombucha 390

L

Label 31
Lactation 397, 411
    adopted baby 413
    difficulties 413
    supplements 407
Lactic acid 156
Lactobacillus acidophilus (L. acidophilus) 87, 161, 162
(see also "Probiotics")
Lactobacillus bulgaricus (L. bulgaricus) – see "Probiotics"
Lactose intolerance 124
Large intestine
    bleeding 99, 114
    inflammation 99, 116
    ulceration 99, 116
Laxative 65
Leukerin 305
Leukocytes 275
Levaquin 388
L-glutamine 70
Licorice 112
    lozenges 88, 130
Liquid diet 122, 235
    pregnancy 418

Listen to your gut CD-ROM 430
Liver 111, 188
    problems 92, 390
    tonic 92
Lotronex 170

M
6-MP 305
Magnesium 54, 66, 186
    deficiency 186, 327
Maitake mushroom 95, 97
Malabsorption 121, 123, 186, 419
Malnutrition 120, 419
Mantra 349
Maple syrup 201
Margarine 213
Marijuana 213
Marshmallow root 108, 112
Martial arts 375
Massage therapy 334
Meal planning/preparation 422
Medical labeling 29
Meditation 348, 361, 373
Menstruation 400, 401
    products 401
Mercaleukin 305
Mercaptopurine 305
Mercury
    amalgam fillings 267
    in fish 208
Mesalamine 305
Methyl-sulfonyl-methane (MSM) 53, 54, 391
Metronidazole 305
Microwave 275

Milk
    intolerance 124, 211
    mycobacterium avium paratuberculosis (MAP) 159
    products 211, 220
Millet 203
Minerals 186, 189, 190, 316
Miscarriage 418
Mobile phone 262
    ferrite bead 264
Monosodium glutamate (MSG) 211
Morning sickness 403
Mouth ulcers 128, 337
    treatment summary 131
Mucosal lining 48, 112, 137, 157, 383
Mucus 112, 241, 381, 384
Muscle-testing 333
Musco-skeletal 358
Mycobacterium avium paratuberculosis (MAP) 148, 159
    infection 147
    milk 159
    testing 144, 148
    treatment 160
Mycoplasma 142, 148
    testing 144
Mycotoxins 144

N
N-acetyl glucosamine (NAG) 107, 112
Natural progesterone cream 310, 400, 409
Naturopathic physician 49, 326
Nausea 403
Nervous system 18

Neurogastroenterology 18, 360
Neuropeptides 362
Neurotoxins 211
Neurotransmitters 17
Novo-prednisone 305

O
Obstruction 134, 353, 372
Olive leaf extract 80, 141-143
Olive oil 150
Omega-3, omega-6, omega-9 104, 207
Orasone 305
Oregano oil 80, 140, 142, 145
    fistulas 77
    Jini's wild oregano oil protocol 152
    mouth ulcers 129
    pregnant or breastfeeding 151, 403
    usage 153
Organic food 196
    healthier rats 198
Organochlorines 273
Orthotics 339
Ovulation 400
Oxidative injury 187

P
Pain management 373
Panchakarma 378
Parasites 28, 148
Parenting 343, 396, 420, 423
Pathogen 24, 28, 48, 84
    die-off effect 149, 171
Pathogenesis 27, 257, 312
Pentasa 305

INDEX

Peppermint 54, 90, 189
Perforated intestine 101, 134, 313, 373
Perianal 311, 345
Peristaltic mechanism 371
Pesticides 197, 199, 256
pH level 189
Phytic acid 206
Phyto-estrogen 206
Pill (birth control) 399
Pine bark extract 104
Pituitary gland 309
Plant sterols/sterolins 389, 417
Plastic 273
Potassium 186
Pouchitis 71
Prana/pranic 336
Prebiotics 54, 168
Pre-digested food 235, 237
Prednisone 295, 297, 309, 388, 402, 418
   alternative 143, 158, 236
   children 295
   life threatening 296
   side effects 295, 305
Pregnancy 237, 402
   flare-up 418
   supplementation 404
Premenopause 410
Prescription drugs
   attitude towards 293
   pregnancy 402, 418
   side-effects 187, 301, 304
   symptom suppression 295
   weaning/tapering 217, 306
Primordial sound meditation 349

Probiotics 155-185
   benefits 156
   centrifugal extraction 167
   contraindications 170, 175, 399
   die-off effect (Herxheimer reaction) 171
   different species packaged together 164
   dosage guidelines 172-185
      antibiotics 178
      babies 180
      barium enema 178, 318
      cautious approach 175
      colonoscopy 178, 318
      fast approach 177
      moderate approach 176
      ongoing 184
   filter extraction 167
   freeze-drying 166, 167
   pregnancy 404
   retention enema 138, 158, 171, 181
   selection criteria 164-168
   species/strains 160
Processed food/preservatives 211
Progesterone 309, 400, 409
Projectile vomiting 339
Prostate gland 310
Protein
   allergy 124
   hemp 124, 204, 207
   shakes 123, 238
   soy 206
   whey 124
Proteoglycans 107
Protostat 305
Psychic 344

Psychoneuroimmunology 360, 362
Psychotherapy 331, 342
Psyllium seed powder 66, 74
Pulse diagnosis 378
Purinethol 305
Pycnogenol 104, 191

Q

Qigong 336
Quercetin 93
Quinoa 203, 204

R

Rapadura sugar 201
Raw
   fish 208
   food 205
   milk 207, 211
Rectal
   abscess 78, 388
   stricture 136
Rectal fissures 132
   treatment summary 133
Recurrence rates 16, 312
Refined sugar 201
Reiki 336
Reishi mushrooms 95
Remicade 304, 309
Remission 158
   diet 236, 238
   via immune stimulation 143
   via probiotics 158
Resection 312
Rice milk 207
Rolfing 20
Roughage 205, 214

Rowasa 305
Rupture 101, 134, 313
Rutin 92

S

Saccharomyces boulardii 163
Salad dressing 106
Salazopyrin 306
Saliva method/testing 400
Salmon 207
Salmonella 156
Salofalk 305
Sashimi 208
Scoliosis 334, 340
Selenium 186, 187
Senna 66
Shigella 156
Shock 100
Short bowel syndrome 74, 316
Sigmoidoscopy 318
    disposable 323
Simple carbohydrates 215
Sleep
    deprivation 22, 146, 299, 420
    environment 266
Slippery elm bark 108, 112
Small intestine
    bacterial overgrowth (SIBO) 134
    bleeding 99, 113, 230
    inflammation 99, 116
    ulceration 99, 116
Soda pop 213
Sodium benzoate 103
Solar plexus 90
Somato-emotional release 330, 336

Sore bum remedy 225
Soy
    products 206
    sauce 224
Spasming 67, 237, 373, 368, 372
    treatment summary 68
Specific carbohydrate (SC) diet 381
Spelt 203
Spermicide 399
Sphincter 315, 345, 369
Spiritual healing 36, 313
Spring water 203
Squatting position 65, 352
Stainless steel 272, 273
Staphylococcus 156
Steaming vegetables 200
Steroids 187
    alternative 143, 158, 236
    children 295
    life threatening 296
    side effects 295, 305
Sterols/sterolins 389, 417
Stevia 201, 203
Stomach
    bleeding 99, 113
    inflammation 99, 116
    ulceration 99, 116
Stress 20, 23, 33, 319, 349, 360, 420
Strictures 134
    rectal 136, 314
    throat 314
    treatment summary 139
Sublingual 315
    vitamin B12 61, 187
Sugar 201

Sulphasalazine 188, 306
Supplements 49, 296
    aggravating/avoid 52, 54
    children's dosages 56
    good companies 50
    how to introduce 55
    introduction order 191
    pregnancy/breastfeeding 404
    testing 55, 393
Support network 36, 424
Suppository 51, 132
Surgery 311, 340, 355
    recurrence rates 16, 312
Sushi 224
Symptom
    as message 298
    recurrence 210, 217, 308
    suppression 295
    tracking charts 432

T

Tai chi 357, 373
Tailbone 339
Taste buds 351
Tea tree oil 79
Teflon 270
Tegarosod 170, 306
Tempeh 206
Testosterone 309
Theophylline 391
Thought patterns 363
Thymol 145, 150
Thyroid 206, 309
Tofu 206
Tomatoes 212, 380

Total parenteral nutrition (TPN) 242
Touch for health 332
Toxins
   drug 297, 308
   environmental 27, 256, 258, 259, 265
   food 261
   kitchen 270
   release 34, 36, 308
Traditional chinese medicine 379
Transcendental meditation 349
Transdermal 268, 315
Trans-fatty acids 213, 219
Treatment summaries 42, 431
Trichozole 305
Tuna 209
Turbinado sugar 201

U

Ulceration 99, 116
Ulcerative colitis
   infectious disease 159
   treatment summary – see CD-ROM
Ultrasound 340
Uterine cancer 206

V

Vaccination 27, 276
   adverse reactions 281
   immune support 286
   long-term effects 282
   political/economic aspect 285
   side effects 280
Vaginal fistula 81
Vegetarianism 204

Vinegar 222
Visualizations 364
Vitamin
   A 186, 191
   absorption 316
   B 191
   B12 61, 187
   C 61, 66, 96
   chewable 190
   D 186
   E 105, 186, 190
   E oil 109
   K 187
   reduce colon cancer risk 190
   transdermal spray 190
Vomiting 339, 384, 407

W

Weight
   gain 120, 239
   loss 128, 240
   training 125, 357
Wheat 242, 380
Wheatgrass 62
Whey protein 124
White light 367, 375
White rice 233
Wild oregano oil 80, 140, 142, 145
   fistulas 77
   Jini's wild oregano oil protocol 152
   mouth ulcers 129
   pregnant or breastfeeding 151, 403
   usage 153
Workbook (healing journey) 40, 431

X

Xenoestrogens 273
Xylitol 214

Y

Yeast 242
   infection 146, 147, 148, 384
Yoga 334, 357, 358, 373
Young's Formula 57

Z

Zinc 186
Zelnorm 170, 306
Zoloft 303

About The Author

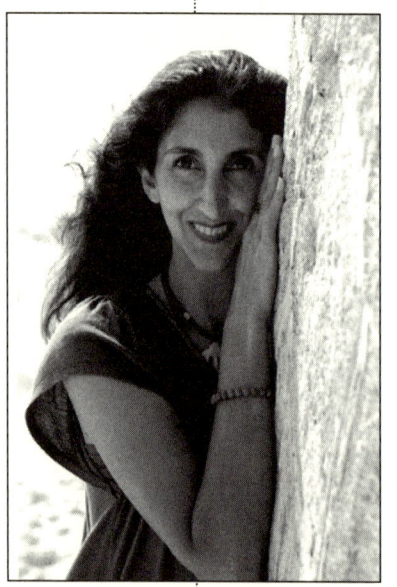

Jini Patel Thompson was diagnosed with widespread Crohn's Disease in 1986. For the next three years she adhered to medical treatment protocols until it became clear they were not helping her. She spent the next seven years researching and experimenting with alternative healing methods and therapies as she lived and worked in Canada, Japan and England. Jini has since remained drug and surgery-free for over 20 years. She continues to manage her symptoms and heal flare-ups using the natural methods described in her books *Listen To Your Gut* and *The IBD Remission Diet*. Jini has also produced a DVD titled *BABY FART AEROBICS: And Other Natural Treatments for Colicky Babies* and a line of children's stories on CD called *Murray the Shark Sleeptime Stories* (all available at *www.ListenToYourGut.com*).

Jini Patel Thompson has a Bachelor's degree in English and Sociology from the University of Alberta (1989). She then worked as a journalist and magazine editor in Tokyo, Japan for two years, followed by three years in the music business in London, U.K. She set up a telecommunications company in Vancouver, BC, sold it five years later and started a publishing company. Jini's health articles have been published in numerous magazines and newspapers throughout North America, Europe and Australia and she has appeared on radio and TV shows in the U.S., as an expert on natural management/healing for digestive diseases. Jini currently runs her own publishing and consulting business and travels often throughout North America, Asia and Europe. She lives with her husband and three children in White Rock, BC, Canada.